The Ultimate Guide for Horses in Need

CARE, TRAINING, AND REHABILITATION FOR RESCUES, ADOPTIONS, AND HORSES IN TRANSITION

STACIE G. BOSWELL,
DVM, DACVS

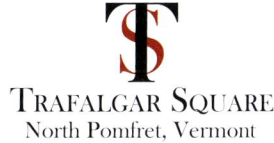

Trafalgar Square
North Pomfret, Vermont

First published in 2020 by
Trafalgar Square Books
North Pomfret, Vermont 05053

Copyright © 2020 Stacie G. Boswell

All rights reserved. No part of this book may be reproduced, by any means, without written permission of the publisher, except by a reviewer quoting brief excerpts for a review in a magazine, newspaper, or website.

Disclaimer of Liability
The author and publisher shall have neither liability nor responsibility to any person or entity with respect to any loss or damage caused or alleged to be caused directly or indirectly by the information contained in this book. While the book is as accurate as the author can make it, there may be errors, omissions, and inaccuracies.

This book describes medical care and treatment of horses that have been neglected or abused. Naturally, these horses may behave unpredictably. Additionally, they may have ongoing medical needs. Although meant as an educational guide, it is always best to consult a professional for training and medical care, especially if your horse is worsening rather than improving.

The names of horses and people in this book have been changed to protect privacy.

Trafalgar Square Books encourages the use of approved safety helmets in all equestrian sports and activities.

Library of Congress Cataloging-in-Publication Data
Names: Boswell, Stacie G., author.
Title: The ultimate guide for horses in need : care, training, and rehabilitation for rescues, purchases, and adoptions / Stacie G. Boswell, DVM, DACVS.
Description: North Pomfret, Vermont : Trafalgar Square Books, 2020. | Includes bibliographical references and index. | Summary: "Dr. Stacie Boswell's goal is to restore health and comfort to every horse in transition, and to help him learn how to function as the horse he is expected to be-from the Thoroughbred off the track to the grade pony from the field down the road. She has compiled hundreds of case studies highlighting the areas of concern in the horse "in need," and in these pages details proactive methods of handling common medical problems and health issues, from nutrition and dentistry to deworming and hoofcare to traumatic injury and emergency rescue scenarios. Dr. Boswell then explains the ways that, as a new horse is rehabilitated physically, specific training techniques can help him adapt to the positive changes in his care and environment"-- Provided by publisher.
Identifiers: LCCN 2020000722 (print) | LCCN 2020000723 (ebook) | ISBN 9781570769627 (paperback) | ISBN 9781646010257 (epub)
Subjects: LCSH: Horses.
Classification: LCC SF285 .B69 2020 (print) | LCC SF285 (ebook) | DDC 636.1--dc23
LC record available at https://lccn.loc.gov/2020000722

All photographs courtesy of Stacie Boswell except Cover photo (Jake Mosher) 1.1, 1.2, 2.4, 16.3 (Jennifer Williams, PhD, Bluebonnet Equine Humane Society, College Station, Texas); 2.10 (Walkin' N Circles Rescue, Stanley, New Mexico); 3.2, 5.1 diagrams (Brianna Rigdon), 3.18 (Sue Barton, founder of Remus Horse Sanctuary, Essex, United Kingdom); 4.1 B, 7.11 C (Am Kuglin); 4.6 A & B (Tasha Marie Anthony and family, Big Horn Ranch and Rescue, Busby, Montana); 5.22 A–F, 7.4, 7.15, 14.4 A–D, 14.5, 14.7 B (Crystal Sharp); 7.17 A & B, 16.1 (Lori Walton); 8.8 (Chief Doug Monaco); 8.9 A & B (Dr. Melissa T. Hines, University of Tennessee); 9.6 (Dr. Steve Adair, University of Tennessee); 10.2 (Dr. Bill Layton, Diagnostic Laboratory of the State of Montana); 12.1, 12.2, 14.2 A&B diagrams (Rachael Roberts), 12.3 (Val Siegel, Siegel Reining Horses, Wilsall, Montana); 12.5 A & B, 14.8, 14.9, 15.2 (Janice Cartwright, Montana Horse Sense); 13.6 A (Four Corners Saddlery, Bozeman, Montana); 14.4, 14.5, 14.7 (Halter Courtesy Steele Halters, Belgrade, Montana); 16.2 A & B (Emily Hutton); 17.1 (Julia Kennedy, 3H Humans, Horses, and Herds, Tijeras, New Mexico).

Book design by Lauryl Eddlemon
Cover design by RM Didier
Index by Andrea Jones (JonesLiteraryServices.com)
Typeface: Candara
Printed in Hong Kong

10 9 8 7 6 5 4 3 2 1

For suffering horses—that they
may find wellness and homes.

Contents

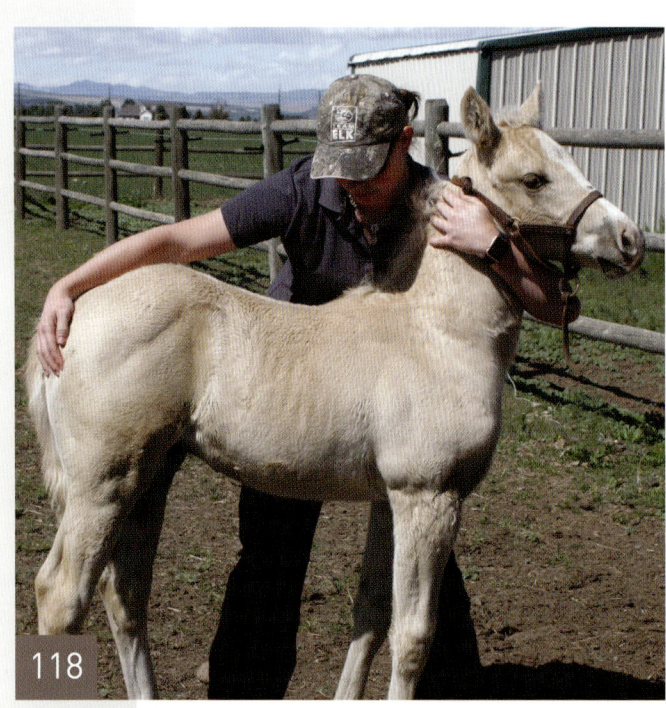
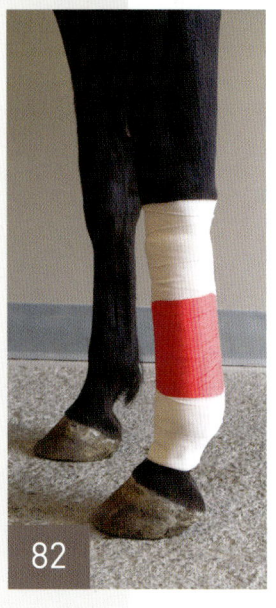
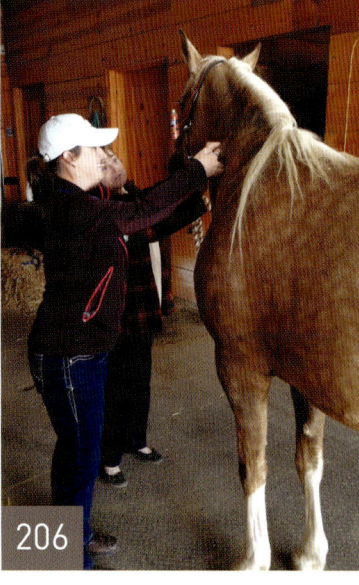

Note to the Reader	ix
Preface	xi

PART I: CARING FOR HORSES IN NEED — 1

Chapter 1: Where They Come From: Horses in Need — 2

The Unwanted or Neglected Horse	3
Economic Factors	4
Horse Population Changes	6
Confiscation or Assistance	7
How to Take Proper Care of Your Rescued Horse	8

Chapter 2: Bringing Him Home: Traveling and Intake of Your Rescue Horse — 10

Get Ready to Roll	10
Trailer Safety	10
Travel Stress of Horses	13
Federal Regulations for Transport	15
Other Regulations	15
Identification	16
Permanent Identification	16
Temporary Identification	19
Traceability	20
Ownership	20
Quarantine	21
Veterinary Examination	22
Laboratory Testing	23
Make Time to Bond	25

Chapter 3: Digestion: Nutrition, Dentistry, and Colic — 26

Nutrition — 26
Body Condition Scoring — 26
Starvation — 27
   Refeeding Syndrome — 27
   Safely Feeding the Starved Horse — 27
   Feeding Program — 30
Forages — 32
   Forage Selection — 32
   Forage Facts — 32
Other Feeds — 34
   Grains — 34
   Feeding Fats — 35
   Use of Probiotics — 35
Long-Term Weight Changes — 36
   Monitor His Weight — 36
Other Considerations for Refeeding Rescue Horses — 36
   Psychological Effects of Starvation — 38
   Extra Winter Care for the Emaciated Horse — 38
Dentistry — 38
Other Reasons for Weight Loss — 43
   Gastric Ulcers — 44
Colic — 44
   Signs of Colic — 44
   Types of Colic — 45
   Preventing Colic — 47
   Veterinary Evaluation and Treatment of Colic — 47
Understanding Is Critical for Success — 48

Chapter 4: Germs and Worms: Vaccination and Parasite Management — 49

Parasite Management and Deworming — 49
   Parasite Management — 49
   Toxicity and Environmental Concerns — 50
   Manure Management — 51
   Fecal Egg Count — 52
   Special Cases and Considerations — 53
   Deworming Needy Horses — 54
Ectoparasites and Skin Conditions — 54
   Other Skin Conditions — 55
Vaccines — 55
   Tetanus — 57
   Rabies — 58
   Mosquito-Borne Viruses That Affect the Nervous System — 58
   Respiratory Diseases — 59
   Respiratory Disease in Needy Equines — 60

Chapter 5: Keeping Them Moving and Sound: Hoof Care, Lameness, and Wounds — 61

Foot Anatomy — 61
Routine Hoof Care — 63
   Factors Affecting Hoof Structure and Growth — 64
Recognizing Lameness in Rescue Horses — 66
   Evaluating the Feet of a Rescue Horse — 67
   Monitoring Movement — 69
When to Shoe — 69
   When Wear Exceeds Growth, Shoes are Necessary — 71
   When the Horse Experiences Foot Pain, Shoes are Necessary — 71
   Shoeing Horses with Abnormalities — 72
Causes of Lameness — 73
   Injuries That Damage the Hoof — 73
   Hoof Abscesses — 74
   Laminitis — 75
   Chronic Generalized Arthritis — 76
Wounds — 79
   Wound Evaluation — 80
   Wound Treatment — 81
   Bandaging — 82

Extensive or Deep Wounds	83
Infected Wounds	84
The Reality of Lameness	84

Chapter 6: Birth Control: Managing Mares and Castrating Colts — 85

Castration of Males	85
Anesthesia	85
Routine Castration	87
Routine After-Care	87
Long-Term Expectations	88
Castration Complications	89
Cryptorchid Castration	90
The Proud-Cut Myth	91
Paraphimosis	93
Pregnancy Evaluation in Mares and Fillies	93
Pregnant Mare Nutrition	94
Vaccines for Pregnant Mares	96
Spaying Mares	97
A Goal of Preventing Pregnancies	97

Chapter 7: Little Lives: Rescuing Foals — 98

The Birthing Process	98
Predicting Foaling Time	98
Timing: Foaling Happens Quickly	100
Foal Positioning Problems	101
Red Bag	101
Normal After-Birth Sequence	102
Foal Examination	104
Temperature	104
Heart	104
Respiration	105
Examination of the Limbs	105
Normal Foal Behavior	110
The Orphan Foal	110
Feeding Orphan Foals	111
Orphan Socialization	115

Halter Training	116
When to Begin	116
Putting on the Halter	117
Learning to Lead	118
Picking Up Feet	120
Other Training	121
Aim for a Healthy, Solid Citizen	121

Chapter 8: Unable to Rise: The Down Horse — 122

Safety	122
Normal Sleeping Patterns	123
Reasons for a Horse to be Down	124
Identifying Underlying Problems	125
Treating Underlying Problems	126
How to Get the "Down" Horse Up	126
Identify and Remove Obstacles	127
Rolling a Horse	128
Sliding to Reposition	129
Get Him Up (Prepare and Assist)	129
Long-Term Treatment of Underlying Problems	130
Long-Term Down Horse	130
Bed Sores and Skin Injuries	132
Use of Slings	133
The Quality of Life Question	133

Chapter 9: Urgent Rescue: Working in Disasters — 134

Disaster Preparedness	134
Learn About Your Locale	134
Plan Ahead	134
Prepare for Transport	135
Identify Your Horse	136
Guidelines for Working in Natural Disasters and Accidents	138
Communication	138
Technical Large Animal Emergency Rescue	139

First Aid for Horses	**140**
Leg Wounds	140
Eyes	140
Wounds on the Body	141
Specific Disasters and Their	
Equine Health Consequences	**141**
Fire	142
Floods	142
High Winds	142
Heat Waves	142
Blizzards and Snow	142
Falling Through Ice or into a	
Swimming Pool	144
Be Prepared	**144**

Chapter 10: A Good Goodbye: Euthanasia — 145

Making the Decision	**145**
Compassionate Guidelines	**145**
Other Reasons for Euthanasia	146
Euthanasia Procedure	**147**
Most Common Procedure	148
Confirming Death	149
Aftercare	149
Cost	150
Take Home Message	**150**

PART II: TRAINING HORSES IN NEED — 151

Chapter 11: Understanding Unique Training Considerations — 152

Training Appropriate by Body	
Condition Scoring (BCS)	**152**
BCS 1 to 2	152
BCS 3	153
BCS 4	154
BCS 5 to 6	154
BCS 7 to 9	154

Chapter 12: How Horses Sense and Respond: Sensory Physiology, Training Concepts, and Thought Processes (Fear) — 155

Sensory Physiology	**155**
Equine Vision	155
Other Senses	158
Understanding His Senses	159
Training Principles	**159**
Positive Reinforcement	159
Intrinsic Reward and Bribery	159
Negative Reinforcement	161
Approach-and-Retreat	161
Punishment	161
The Fearful Horse and Rescue Training	**162**
The Fear Response	164
Recognizing Fear—What Your	
Horse Is Telling You	165
Physiology of Fear	166
Recognizing Relaxation—	
What Your Horse is Telling You	167
Changing Fear	168
Helping Others Improve	
Their Training Skills	**168**
Mutual Understanding	**168**

Chapter 13: Restoring Trust: Developing a Relationship — 169

Readiness Review	**169**
Social Integration	**169**
Develop a Foundation of Trust	**170**
Routine and Respect	170
Behavior and Weakness	171
Rebuild Muscle	171
Consistency and Fairness	172
Training Stress	**172**
Novelty and Anxiety	173
Overcoming Fear	**175**
Medically Addressing Fear	175

Mealtime Anxiety	177
Handling Feet and Legs with Trust	180
Picking Up the Feet of a Trained Adult	180
Training for Hoof Care	181
A Basic Foundation	183

Chapter 14: Fearless: Halter Training Adult Horses — 184

Readiness Review	184
Horse Personality	184
The Flight Zone	185
Enclosure Guidelines	186
Reduce Flight Zone	186
Round Pen	187
Initiate Touch	187
Haltering and Halter Types	188
Flat Halters	188
Rope Halters	189
Halter Fit	190
Applying the Halter	190
Halter Training	192
Tying	193
The Sick Horse	194
A Crucial Step	194

Chapter 15: Patient Training: Skills for Medical Care — 195

Readiness Review	195
Reviewing Approach-and-Retreat	195
Advanced Leading Skills—Tight Spaces and New Situations	196
Thinking About His Options	197
Advanced Leading Skills	199
Small Spaces	199
Physical Examination	203
Physical Touch	203
Evaluating Gums	203
Rectal Temperature	203
Nervous Nellies	204
Companionship for Reassurance	204
Oral Medications	204
Injection Training	205
Retraining Needle-Shy Horses	207
Desensitize Your Horse to Injections—Long-Term Training	207
Preparation for Intranasal Treatments	208
Building Toward Health with a Respectful Horse	208

Chapter 16: Getting Going: Groundwork — 209

Readiness Review	209
Safety First	209
Health Status of the Horse	210
Considerations of the Mental Status of the Horse	211
Longeing	212
Longeing Movements	213
Halting When Longeing	214
Increasing Speed	215
Tacking Up	217
Saddle Pad	217
Saddle	218
Beginning to Make a Difference	219

Chapter 17: Final Steps: Riding — 220

Readiness Review	220
Before Riding	220
Lameness Evaluation	222
To Bridle or Not to Bridle	222
Bridle Fit	224
Mounting	226
The Best Gift	230
End Notes	231
Acknowledgments	241
Index	243

Note to the Reader

The inception of this book came because there was a serious deficiency of information available to help people help horses in need that they either had acquired or worked with via a rescue organization. Some people say that "buying" a horse and "rescuing" a horse is not the same thing, but in my view, these acts are part of a broad continuum with a lot of gray zones and overlap.

There are now terrific, active organizations that emphasize adoption as a primary means of finding your next equine partner. This is a wonderful option, and supporting an official adoption center through volunteering, donating, fostering, or adopting ensures that your desire to help makes a positive impact.

In addition, hard-working groups are aspiring to intentionally define some terms relevant to rescuing horses, with the recognition that horses typically have more than one owner or career in their lifetime. Terms that have been defined may not always match the word usage I currently see from rescue groups or veterinary clients (and which I used in the writing of this book). Know that I recognize the evolving definitions as part of a large and important effort to increase awareness of horses in need, as well as increase the number of equine adoptions worldwide. The various explanations for describing a horse in need and what I, in the pages ahead, label a "rescue horse" or "rescue organization" are slightly different, but the intent and meaning concur.

As we join each other to support horses in need, we come from different areas of the horse industry, and we need to recognize our commonalities more than our differences. It's so important for the equine rescue and adoption community to work together. After all, we share a common goal of helping horses.

Preface

As a horse lover, my heart goes to my patients and their owners. As a veterinarian, I have worked in several states across the United States that made me aware of the universal, critical need for knowledge on the care and treatment of horses that come from neglectful or abusive situations. While watching rescuers navigate the muddy waters of providing for these horses, I have seen the need for a resource that will help caring and compassionate people take care of them.

Horses in need of rescue or rehabilitation come from auctions, off the range, from neighbors or family who are having financial trouble or pass away, and a variety of other sources. Many horses have a unique story, and sometimes the humans in the story have suffered, too. In fact, the incident that solidified my resolve to write this book was one where a beloved horse lost her life, and her people lost their well-being.

As I practice veterinary medicine, I see repeated issues, similar problems, and patterns in the needs of these horses. I can help each one as an individual, but I'm limited in where I go and how many I can assist. More horses can be helped with education and awareness, which I hope this book fulfills.

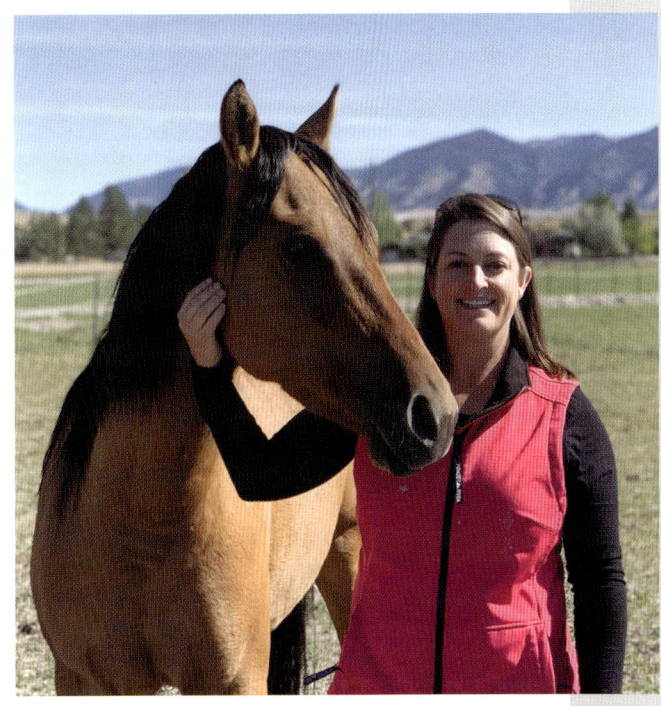

My passion for horses and my experiences as a veterinarian and horse owner motivated me to write this book. My beloved Paint mare Piñon is with me in this photo.

It takes you from the moment you acquire your horse, all the way through riding a horse that is restored to full health. Rescue horses have special needs, both physically and mentally, and there is no other fully formed set of guidelines available.

I was inspired to write because of the shift I have observed in the horse industry over the last 20 years. This change has been gradual and periodic, with peaks and plateaus in developments and advances. Over time, we have grown to appreciate and love horses in a new light. We don't depend on them like we once did, and yet, we are still undeniably drawn to their presence.

The mindset of modern humanity has changed to desire horses as companions. Horses still carry us willingly; when we ride, we entrust our physical body to the horse, and he also lifts our spirits. We value horses as sentient beings. With this change, society has begun to realize that horses should not be discarded and sent, as the saying goes, to the "glue factory." Unfortunately, their sheer size elicits an economic burden that sometimes forces their caretakers to make very hard choices. So, we must "rescue" them, from auctions, from the track, from homes that can't support them.

Until now, there have been no consolidated guidelines addressing both the medical and mental needs of horses transitioning from difficult situations to new homes. This book aims to guide us on the path of helping heal a horse—physically, emotionally, or both—restore him safely to full strength, and protect him through all his future days.

Stacie Boswell, DVM, DACVS

PART I

Caring for Horses in Need

CHAPTER 1

Where They Come From:
Horses in Need

Why rescue a horse? Anyone who has spent time in the world of horses has seen heart-wrenching cases of abuse or neglect, either in person or online. For me, it is impossible to forget the horses' sad faces or how thin they are—these animals that are desperate for food, water, and shelter.

Rescue is defined as "to free or deliver from confinement, violence, danger, or evil."[1] In this book, I define a "rescue" horse as one who has come to you from a situation where his physical or mental needs have not been met. My goal is to help you provide him with a home that will meet those needs, whether by volunteering at a horse rescue, buying a horse from an auction yard, finding an abandoned or stray horse, or otherwise obtaining a needy equine (fig. 1.1). You will be able to get this horse out of his current plight and do everything you can to help him. He will probably need a lot more than just food. When you take him home, you may find that he has a respiratory illness, an injury, or behavioral problems—he may have all of those things at one time. According to Tracy McGonigle, Executive Director of the Hooved Animal Humane Society in Woodstock, Illinois, the

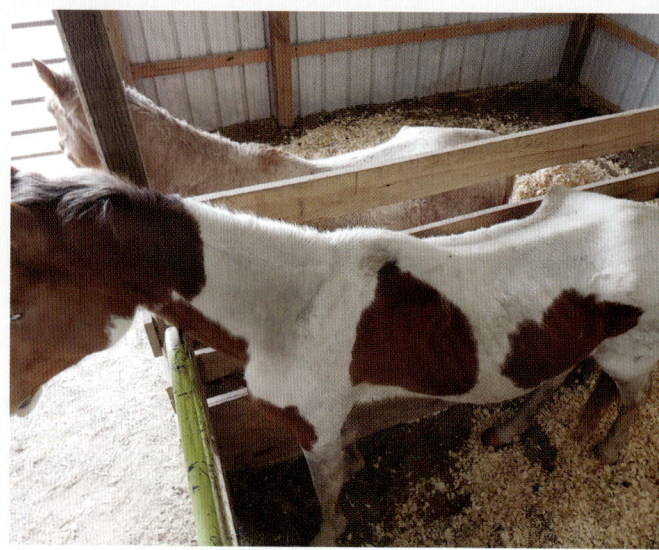

1.1 Recently rescued: two very thin horses, Wren (the roan at the top of the photo) and Boomerang (the pinto). Both had been badly neglected, but Boomerang was in worse condition. Wren bounced back pretty quickly, and it was discovered she was broke to ride. She went to a youth rider to be worked with for four months, and when they competed together in the Bluebonnet Rescue Horse Training Challenge, the mare was adopted at the event.

"number one ailment seen ... is malnourishment, followed by foot issues, then emotional issues."[2]

Taking in a rescue horse is different than buying a healthy, sound horse who has had excellent care throughout his life. However, you can be deeply rewarded by the experience and give him freedom, love, and comfort, making his world a better place.

Once you have your needy equine, you need to know where to start and what problems are most important to address first. I have laid this book out as a series of guidelines, starting with bringing a needy horse home. Guidelines and science are supported by real-world experiences and inspirational anecdotes. Your goal is to restore health and comfort and help him learn how to function as the horse he is expected to be.

Every horse, situation, and caretaker capability is unique, but as a veterinarian, I have observed broad commonalities among many rescue situations. Aside from universal horse health needs, I will discuss common medical problems. As your horse recovers physically, you will concurrently be training him. Emergency rescue, horses unable to rise, and euthanasia are also covered. It's important to acknowledge that it is possible that the full health of a rescue horse may never be restored.

THE UNWANTED OR NEGLECTED HORSE

When the "Five Freedoms" (see sidebar) are not met, a horse's situation needs improvement. These horses can come from any number of places. For example, an elderly person may pass away and the heirs may not want her horses, or a rescue group may work with law enforcement and look after horses after they have been confiscated. Social media and internet sites have rescue networks, including those for orphan foals. I have treated horses that wandered into somebody's semi-rural yard. Gathered Mustangs[4,5] and off-the-track Thoroughbreds are looking for homes and jobs. Some people buy horses at auction yards that are "known" for allowing kill-pen buyers to bid and buy stock.

The phrase "unwanted horse" means "...horses that are no longer wanted by their current owner because they are old, injured, sick, unmanageable, or fail to meet their owner's expectations."[6] The horse may or may not have an injury, lameness, or illness, or he could be the wrong color or gender.

The Five Freedoms[3]

1. Freedom from hunger and thirst
by ready access to fresh water and diet to maintain health and vigor.

2. Freedom from discomfort
by providing an appropriate environment including shelter and a comfortable resting area.

3. Freedom from pain, injury or disease
by prevention or rapid diagnosis and treatment.

4. Freedom to express normal behavior
by providing sufficient space, proper facilities and company of the animal's own kind.

5. Freedom from fear and distress
by ensuring conditions and treatment which avoid mental suffering.

His problem could be either immediately life-threatening or chronic and manageable. He may also have a behavioral problem that ranges from mild to severe. In the United States, it is estimated that 100,000 to 150,000 horses per year are unwanted.

Any horse can end up in a bad or neglected situation; through my career, I have noticed that a horse in a high-dollar, high-level performance barn can have similar bloodlines, capabilities, and temperament to a horse that ends up in a muddy paddock with minimal care. What makes the difference?

Luck.

Economic Factors

Many of us have a hard time understanding the root of this problem, since culturally we regard horses as magnificent, sentient beings. They capture our spirits and hearts, so the idea of neglecting them is horrifying.

Yet there have been, and probably will always be, people who are unable to provide appropriate food, shelter, or medical care to the animals that depend on them.[7] The well-being of these unlucky horses truly suffers. A survey taken in 2012 determined that half of horse owners in the United States had an annual income of less than $50,000.[8]

A Cautionary Tale

It was early January, the air was biting, and a week's worth of snow came up around my boot tops as I traipsed across the yard and knocked on the door. Rose and Dan, an elderly couple, were wearing coats and hats inside the house—it was almost as frigid inside as it was outside. The neighbors had been calling the authorities for weeks and reporting their horse Cookie's emaciated appearance. In most jurisdictions, a veterinarian must examine an animal before it is confiscated because of neglect, so I had been called to examine the horse in question.

We slowly walked together out to the barn. Dan explained, "We have to subsist only off our Social Security checks. I have bad knees and a bad heart, and my company's retirement fund was lost when the economy crashed."

"I'm sorry to hear that," I replied.

Dan continued, "We had a great place in east Texas, always had grass! We couldn't afford to maintain that property, so we downsized and moved out here to the desert."

Rose told me, "We used to have three horses, but we were able to sell the others before we moved. Cookie was my favorite, so we kept her." She went on to say that after the move, when they realized they wouldn't have Dan's retirement income, they had tried to sell Cookie. She had become thin and nobody wanted to buy her. Rose had also talked to some people at the local horse rescue group, but they didn't have room for any more horses and were underfunded. She had been told there was a waiting list, although the rescue had never called back. The couple had even tried to give her away. Only one person had come to inquire, and Rose had feared he would sell Cookie to slaughter, so she didn't let the man take her.

When the economy crashed in the late 2000s, people and horses were left starving and out in the cold.

Around the same time, the federal budget no longer provided funding to the U.S. Department of Agriculture (USDA) to maintain the three equine slaughter facilities in the country. Without the economic support of the horse industry that slaughter provided, many horses were adversely affected by this federal policy change. Problems worsened with the coincident economic recession.

Horse slaughter is a complex issue, but since it has been unavailable in the United States for over a decade, it is unlikely to return. I shudder to think of any of my own beloved horses consigned to a fate of slaughter. However, I also recognize that the horse market was suddenly flooded, and with no long-term solution to quell the population, the ultimate fate of many horses was prolonged suffering.

At this time, when a horse goes to slaughter, it is in another country. The trailer ride is long. There is no USDA oversight of foreign slaughter facilities to ensure humane handling. Try as we might to prevent this

Cookie was in the barn. She was a kind horse, with soft eyes and relaxed ears, but was emaciated. Rose and Cookie looked at each other with love and sadness. In the dusty aisle, there was a single bale of fresh hay, and a single bag of grain that had been purchased in anticipation of my arrival. The mare was eating. When we talked about how to help Cookie, I emphasized how sudden dietary changes could be dangerous to horses who were this thin. Dan told me that although Cookie lost weight each winter, she always picked back up and was fine during warmer months.

A few days later, I received another call from Rose. Cookie was down in the snow, and couldn't get up. When I arrived, it was obvious her body had shut down. Cookie had experienced a severe metabolic problem called refeeding syndrome. I gave her medications and fluids directly into her vein. We tried to help her up with support and encouragement, but it was a losing battle. We all cried as Cookie took her last breath.

Rose and Dan weren't able to pay the invoices to the veterinary practice. In a few months, we found out that they had filed bankruptcy and lost their home. Rose and Dan knew Cookie was thin, and cared deeply about her. They couldn't feed her because they had no money—they couldn't keep heat on in their home or feed themselves. They had honestly tried to the best of their ability and had lost their beloved friend. For me, this case was a wake-up call about the judgment that we sometimes feel without knowing the entire situation. Please help your neighbors. Please learn more about their struggle before assuming the worst of them. Cookie's situation happens hundreds or thousands of times over the world.

fact, an average 68,000 horses per year were exported from the United States to Canada or Mexico for slaughter from 2007 to 2017. This is between 1 and 2 percent of the total U.S. horse population, and may be as much as half of the unwanted horse population. The horses that are killed are mainly used for human consumption in Europe and other countries.[9, 10]

Horse Population Changes

The 2018 American Horse Council (AHC) Foundation Economic Impact of the US Horse Industry Report stated that between 2005 and 2017, the horse population declined by about two million (from 9.2 to 7.2 million horses).[11] Most breed registries in North America reported overall declines in new horse registries from about 2000 to 2015. For example, the Jockey Club is the second largest registry of horses in North America. The Jockey Club has had fewer and fewer foal registries since 1990—well before the most recent economic recession. In 1990, 44,143 foals were registered. After the recession, in both 2010 and 2011, there was more than a 12 percent decline, although this decline has stabilized in recent years. Fewer Thoroughbred foals than ever were born in 2018 (10,500). For perspective, consider that more than twice that number were born in 1990.[12]

The key feature when looking at foaling trends is to acknowledge that horses live a very long time. A horse born in 1990 could still be alive in 2019 at 29 years of age. Caring for a horse is a real long-term commitment. Financial circumstances of some horse owners through that period of time may well have changed so the problem of overpopulation could ricochet for years given that unwanted and aging horses already existed before the recession.

While the horse market "corrected" itself and breeders decreased the number of foals they raised during the last decade, many horses are still in need of rescue. Between 2008 and 2018, the University of Tennessee alone treated 114 horses for emaciation and neglect, of which 28 died despite aggressive medical therapy.[13]

During the worst part of the decline, there were dark days for horses, with reports of people turning their herds out in the forests of the central United States or in remote areas of the West. Nobody knows for sure how many horses this happened to or what became of them.

The Horse Industry Improves

Ownership transfers of adult horses can serve as an estimate of how many horses exchange hands, but not all registries track

Large North American Breed Registries

1. American Quarter Horse Association
2. Jockey Club of North America, which maintains records for Thoroughbred horses and races
3. American Paint Horse Association
4. U.S. Trotting Association, which maintains records for Standardbred horses and races
5. Tennessee Walking Horse Breeders and Exhibitors' Association
6. Arabian Horse Association

this information. Transfers decreased from 2005 to 2015. From 2016 to 2018, small increases have been recorded, showing that the horse industry is recovering.

We are now more than a decade beyond the start of the severe recession. Rescue groups are better organized and financial resources have stabilized. According to the AHC Horse Industry Report, the horse population was 7.2 million in 2016. You will find horses in all areas of the country, in cities and in rural areas. You will find working horses (used by mounted police, carriage drivers, ranchers, and backcountry tourists), racehorses, show horses, and beloved companions.

The AHC report counted 602 equine rescues or sanctuaries that handled 24,000 horses. These rescues added 438 jobs and a $42 million value to the U.S economy. Unfortunately, rescue groups handled only about 20 percent of unwanted horses.

The 2018 AHC survey documented that just over one percent of U.S. households own horses, and 16 percent of households participate in horse activities. Rescue is one activity that attracts horse enthusiasts who don't own horses. There is an untapped network of millions of people that could become rescue donors, volunteers, and adopters. The United Horse Coalition (UHC) is one group that intends to help rescuers, adopters, and economically challenged horse homes. The UHC educates prospective and current horse owners, advocates for good horse welfare, and assists with the cost of castration (gelding), microchipping, hay, veterinary care, and euthanasia.[14]

Some states register and inspect equine rescue groups. Many rescue groups have a working partnership with local law enforcement, which helps both groups serve their purpose more effectively. Rescue groups must stick to specific guidelines during the rehabilitation process. Following science-supported guidelines improves a horse's chance of recovery, and can help prove in court that a horse was neglected.

Confiscation or Assistance

When evaluating a horse's situation, consider if he is not cared for because of a short-term or a permanent problem (fig. 1.2). For example, a family that ordinarily allows their horses to graze on pasture can experience severe drought. A herd that normally accesses low-land winter pasture can experience a particularly snowy year, preventing access to forage.

For temporary problems, keeping a horse in the home he already has is best. Moving him out of the owner's hands often turns him into an unwanted horse and

---

Technology in Rescue

The recent internet and social media explosion has positively impacted horse rescue. Dozens of Facebook groups and Instagram accounts focus on rescue horses. Rescue organizations use email lists. Netposse.com focuses on recovering stolen horses. We have our smartphones with us, so we can check on that cute palomino (lot #115) and donate to her plight while we are in line at the grocery store.

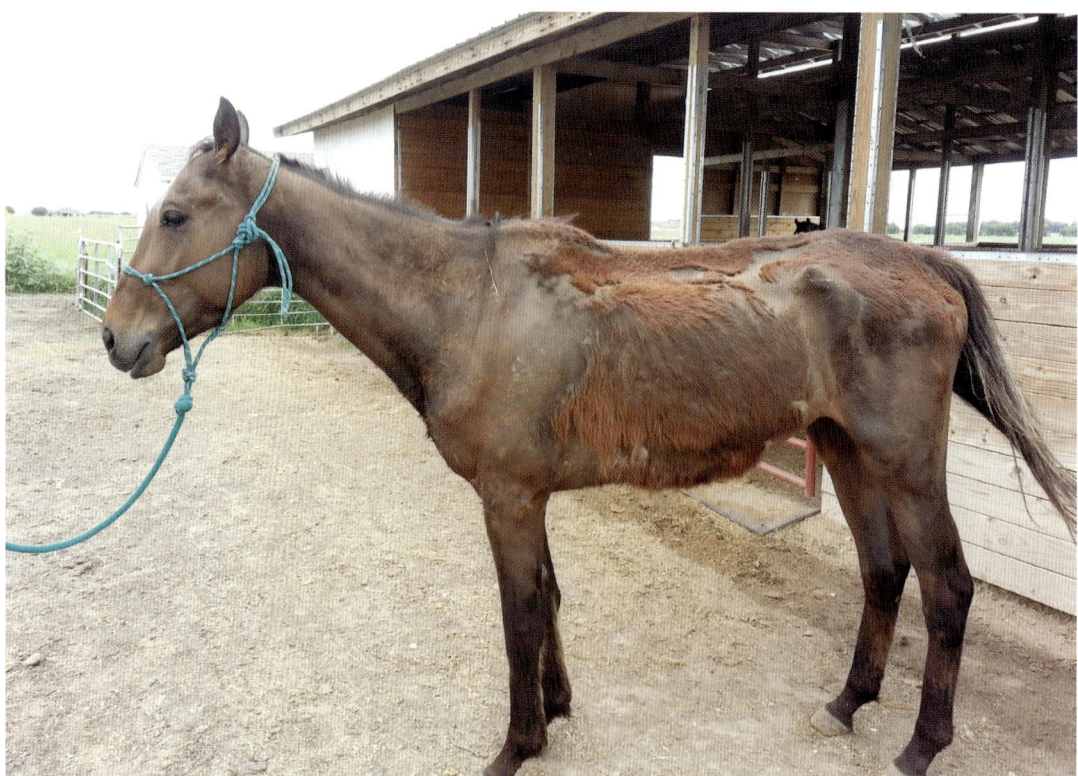

1.2 This horse was neglected. "Bingo" was around 12 years old and had a lip tattoo that didn't match any U.S. racing breeds, so his previous history is unknown. When he was rescued, he had a Body Condition Score of 1 (see p. 28). When this photo was taken he was shedding the long, coarse hair many malnourished horses grow. Once he gained weight and was healthy, it was discovered that he was lame and so he was adopted as a pet/companion. His adopter was able to give him several years peaceful retirement.

further burdens the system that is managing the horse overpopulation problem.

We can educate and assist people to improve the plight of their stock. Funding can be acquired from state or local government or non-profit assistance. Reaching out to help the humans as much as possible helps horses. We often don't know the whole story and sometimes people just need a boost.[15]

HOW TO TAKE PROPER CARE OF YOUR RESCUED HORSE

This book is going to help you take care of your horse. I have used organized scientific data as well as personal veterinary experience to compile the information it contains. It starts with the first day when your horse arrives at his new home with you, then progresses to address your horse's ongoing needs, both medical and mental.[16, 17]

This is no easy task. The daunting facts are that we cannot save every single horse in need. Money is a huge factor in restoring health. We may have to choose between the possibility of helping a horse with a very expensive problem or helping four or five other horses with less severe problems. It may take six months to a year to restore a starved and neglected horse to maximal health. There may be lingering health or behavioral consequences that last his lifetime.

Morally, we must help alleviate suffering. Horse people are strong people, and this is even truer for people who rescue horses. By working together to learn what each horse needs, we can better help horses who depend on us for their fate.[18, 19, 20]

Long-Term Consequences

This is one of several medical cases that inspired me to write this book. I treated a rescued horse, Chico, for colic. Chico was sleek and fit. His owner, Sheila, fed him high-quality alfalfa hay from a large feed trough as was common in the region. Feeding in the trough allows a horse to eat at ground level, as his body is designed to do, but prevents him from ingesting dirt. Chico was up to date on regular veterinary care, vaccines, and parasite control. They went on rides several times a week. Sheila loved Chico.

As part of the examination for colic, I palpated him per rectum to identify abnormalities. I could feel a hard impaction in his large colon—severe, high constipation. Worse yet, his colon was displaced from its normal location in the abdomen. The impaction felt like it had a gritty texture. There was an additional unusual finding: small black gravel and coarse sand in his feces. I was pulling out handfuls of sand rather than handfuls of normal fecal balls of digested forage. At Sheila's home, Chico lived in a high desert paddock of fine red dirt. He had been living there for the last seven years. Sheila and I were confused. Where had the black sand come from?

Sheila showed me photographs of where Chico had lived with his previous owner, and we realized that he had lived on black and gray sand. In the photograph, he was dirty and skinny. Some of the soil he had eaten while starving and neglected remained in his gut for seven years. As part of his episode of colic, his colon became displaced and the sand had been shifted around. There was no other plausible explanation.

Chico, sadly, continued to be in pain. His colic worsened, despite hospitalization, intravenous fluids, and other treatments to combat the sand problem and displaced colon. Sheila could not afford the cost of surgery, and Chico was not getting better. Finally, we made the sad, difficult decision to euthanize him.

Sheila's grief was bittersweet. "I guess that is the tough part of rescue. You never know what is going to happen. I'm going to miss Chico very much. We loved each other! I'm grateful I could make his years with me happy and carefree."

CHAPTER 2

Bringing Him Home:
Traveling and Intake of Your Rescue Horse

The point of helping a horse is to move him to a better situation, so nearly all rescued horses will need to travel in a trailer. In this chapter, I'll first describe salient points related specifically to travel and federal regulations related to shipping horses.

Once you get your new horse home, there is a lot to do. Identification of your horse and subsequent documentation of your ownership is the first step. When a new horse arrives, it is critical that he is housed in a quarantine area, both for his own protection as well as the horses in your already established herd. It's also important to have a veterinarian examine him to make a plan to treat the problems you already know about and, maybe, identify new issues. Your veterinarian's evaluation will include recommended lab tests. You—or your rescue group, if you belong to one—may also have a formal intake process that includes legal ownership forms, documentation of a horse's condition, and medical and behavioral assessments.

During this time, you are going to establish a trusting relationship. Your horse is going to be wholly dependent on you for all of his needs. Remember, he comes from a situation where other humans have failed

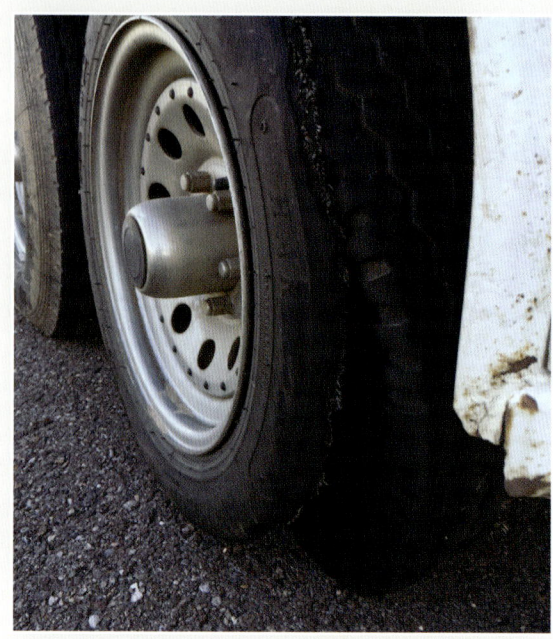

2.1 *Unexpected events, such as this tire blowout, can arise when traveling with horses, but maintenance will prevent many problems.*

him. Now is your chance to make a real change in his life.

GET READY TO ROLL

Trailer Safety
Mechanical problems can occur with both truck and trailer, but regular inspection and repair will prevent many of them. Loose or weak floorboards, a malfunctioning braking

system, or a tire blowout can cause a calamity (fig. 2.1). Therefore, keeping your trailer in good repair is paramount. Choose a trailer with a double axle. Make sure the truck and trailer coupler and ball are size-matched and engaged correctly, and the trailer is level when it is hooked up (figs. 2.2 and 2.3).

Using a pre-drive checklist (see sidebar) helps you avoid errors and malfunctions. In addition, each year you should have your trailer professionally inspected.

Driver Safety: Develop your confidence with the truck and trailer you will be driving. Practice, practice, practice with your rig empty. Make a contingency plan with another driver in case you are injured or become ill.

Pre-Drive Checklist

- Truck and trailer ball or coupling are size-matched and engaged correctly.
- Lights and brakes are plugged in and functioning.
- Trailer emergency braking system battery is charged and connected.
- Windows and doors are latched.
- Lug nuts on wheels are tightened to manufacturer specifications.
- Tires and spare have proper air pressure.
- Safety chains are hooked up.
- Manure from last trip has been cleaned out.

Professional Trailer Inspection

- Evaluate integrity of the floor.
- Check wheel bearings and packing.
- Check trailer brakes and emergency brake battery.
- Check hardware and latches.
- Examine hitch, including bolts.
- Ensure tires and spare are in good repair.
- Check lights and electrical system.

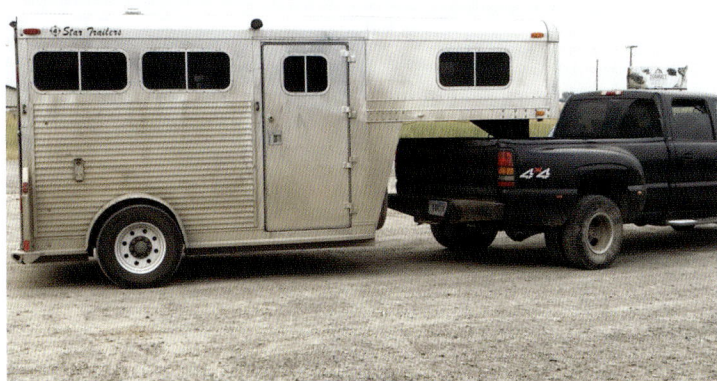

2.2 A single-axle trailer is not as safe for hauling horses as a double-axle trailer. Fortunately, this one is used for farrier supplies rather than live animals.

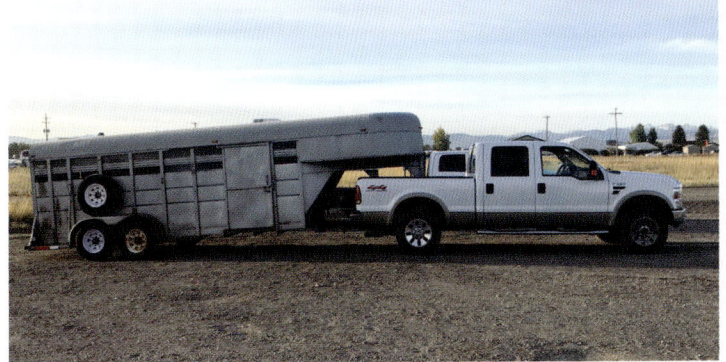

2.3 This trailer is not level to the ground and adjustments need to be made to the gooseneck coupler or a lift should be put on the trailer, which would raise the back end relative to the front end where it is coupled. Horses are safer and more comfortable when traveling in a level trailer.

Aside from bringing your horse home, it is important to be confident about trailering so you could take your horse to an equine hospital if necessary.

Use your headlights for improved visibility—you want other drivers to see you. Drive slower than usual, allowing for longer braking distances. A smooth, confident ride prevents your horse from slipping and falling. Imagine a cup of coffee sitting on your dash, and drive in such a way that it wouldn't spill.

Driving when drowsy is not worth the risk, so be well-rested and alert. Drivers should not have cell phones out while shipping horses. Pull over to use the phone or have a passenger assist with communication or maps.

Loading Your Horse: Safety is the number-one priority. You cannot afford an injury; you have a horse to care for! In the ideal world, your horse is halter-broke and trained to load fearlessly into the trailer.

In the rescue world, you may be backing your trailer up to the opening of a pen or

Watch Your Step

As a veterinarian, I observe people of all levels of experience load their horses in and out of trailers. One nice, older gentleman, Norman, brought his mare Barbie for a dental appointment. Unfortunately, Norman's timing was so poor that he was unable to communicate with her effectively—he did not release the pressure he applied to her halter and lead rope in a way that encouraged the horse to do what he was asking. Whatever Barbie was doing, Norman was pulling on her halter and lead, putting constant pressure on the mare. Even after sedation, we were unable to get her to go where we needed her to be.

Fortunately, Barbie was a nice mare with an otherwise pleasant demeanor, so I worked on her teeth outside.

To return home, Norman tried to get Barbie back in his trailer for over an hour. He pulled and pulled on her. If she was standing still, he was pulling on her; if she was moving her feet, he was still pulling on her. She looked at the floor of the trailer, and he pulled her head up. She swung her hindquarters from right to left then left to right. Guess what? Norman was still pulling. Barbie could do nothing to get relief from the pulling, so she did what must have been easiest for her: she stood firmly.

In the meantime, I had other patients waiting for me, so Norman had to work with Barbie alone. He became tired and took a break to go inside and pay his bill. He tied Barbie to the back corner of his open livestock trailer. While he was inside, I watched the mare through the clinic window. She sniffed and pawed the floor of the trailer a few times, and then loaded herself right in, swinging her hip around to accommodate her head position because she was still tied. Barbie knew what she was supposed to do, but she needed to have some relief from the pulling and some freedom to inspect her footing before stepping in.

chute then "chasing" a horse into it using his flight instinct. You still want to move him as deliberately as possible. Being in a hurry may cause him to panic, resulting in injury to human or horse. As you are pushing your horse to the trailer, allow him to inspect it and the footing before insisting he goes forward. If this is his first experience in a trailer, try not to scare him, as that will make subsequent trailer training more difficult.

Know Your Horse: You should be able to identify each horse in your care. In case of an emergency, it is important that horses have identification attached to their halter or a neck collar.

When shipping multiple horses, do your best to divide horses into compatible groups. Don't ship a foal or pony with adult horses as they could get crushed. More space per horse results in fewer injuries, so don't overcrowd them.[21, 22]

Travel Stress of Horses

A horse is stressed during travel because his main defense—flight—has been eliminated. Travel disrupts herd social structure. Stress of transportation weakens his immune system at the same time he is being exposed to new horses and the contagious diseases they may carry, increasing his risk for illness.[23]

Horses can experience adverse changes in muscle metabolism and dehydration. They can also lose up to 6 percent of body weight—only half of which is recovered in the following 24 hours. The longer a horse's journey, the higher the risk of respiratory problems, gastrointestinal problems, and death from any cause.[24, 25]

Stopping for breaks is important for you as the driver as well as for your horse's health.

Preventing Respiratory Illness While Traveling: Keep trailer vents open to maintain fresh, cool air and reduce respiratory problems. Without air flow, ammonia build-up from urine results in damage to the cells that line the respiratory tract, thus increasing the risk of pneumonia.

Don't put dusty shavings on the floor of the trailer, as inhalation of these small particles predisposes a horse to pneumonia. If you hang a hay bag, reduce dust by wetting it down, which also adds a small amount of water consumption.

Travel Time: A recent study concluded that equine respiratory tract inflammation is minimal to absent for most horses traveling less than two and a half hours,[26] though pneumonia is more likely with increased travel time. Contamination of the respiratory tree increases with time traveled as well as inability to clear the airway.[27] Your horse should be able to clear his airway by coughing, and to cough he must be able to put his head down to the level of his knees. Stop for a few minutes and allow your horses to rest, cough, and drink.

Reducing Stress—Rest Your Horse: Stopping the trailer for a break during a long journey will allow physiologic stress to normalize, and rest tired muscles. Whether or not you can offload the horse you are shipping, providing food and water during the rest time is ideal.

A follow-up study found that interrupting 24 hours of total transport time with a 12-hour rest period allowed white blood cell counts to recover.[28]

Other Ways to Reduce Stress: When you are picking up a single halter-broke horse, consider taking a well-seasoned buddy along for the ride as a companion.

If possible, allow your horse to face the direction in the trailer that he chooses. Horses often choose to stand at a diagonal, facing the rear of the trailer. This position seems to be less stressful (mentally and physically) for them. If the horse trailer has stalls, it is ideal when horses are able to see each other.[29]

For non-starved horses, making sure your horse has free-choice access to food and water prior to the journey and immediately upon arrival helps prevent muscle problems and may reduce stress-induced stomach ulcers. In cases of starvation, refer to chapter 3 (p. 27) before feeding.

Make sure hay nets or bags are not hung where a horse can get a leg or foot entangled. Nervous or unbroken horses may be fearful of nets or bags blowing in the wind, so putting the hay on the floor of the trailer may be the best option.

Halter and Tie Your Horse Properly: For horses who are halter trained, use a halter that fits correctly. Use either a breakaway halter or tie. I explicitly recommend not using a rope halter for shipping. Rope halters are thinner than nylon or leather halters, so they have more "feel," which helps achieve the desired response from a horse as the pressure that is applied is more concentrated. However, if a horse is riding in the trailer and balances himself by partially leaning on the halter, it is unfair to have the extra "bite" of the thin rope punishing him. Additionally, the halter-and-rope combination doesn't meet the breakaway requirement needed for trailer travel.

With few exceptions (for example, a horse that fights with his neighbor) your horse should be tied in such a way that he can get his head down below the point of his shoulder. This will allow him the physical space to cough and clear his airway.

How your horse is tied can affect his stress level and immunity. One study evaluated several factors that affect immunity and compared values from cross-tied horses versus those that had a small space in the trailer but traveled loose for a 24-hour period. Based on the results, the researchers concluded by recommending that shippers should allow "…horses during long-term transportation to travel loose in small compartments."[30]

Don't allow a horse to stick his head out of your trailer in any way while the vehicle is moving. This can result in injury to his head or eyes.

Dress Your Horse Properly: Because many people like to protect their horse as much as possible, use of such equipment is discussed here, though using this gear is not always recommended. Any items your horse will be wearing should be clean, in good repair, and the correct size. Also, the horse should be trained or desensitized to wearing the garments prior to the trip. When a horse is not accustomed to wearing leg wraps, he may become agitated and kick or stomp. This behavior can result in trailer damage, injury to himself, and injury to other horses. Studies have documented that head bumpers, leg wraps, and blankets or sheets are actually associated with an increased risk of injury. Wraps or boots may cause rubs or sores when they are ill-fitting.

When sitting in the sun, and especially when warm horses are added into it, the trailer quickly becomes 20 degrees warmer than the outdoor ambient temperature, and horses can rapidly overheat, sweat and become dehydrated. Dressing horses in shipping boots and blankets or sheets increases the risk of overheating. Horses in enclosed trailers generally don't need a blanket as they are more likely to sweat than to become cold, even in winter weather. Sweating leads to dehydration and loss of electrolytes, which can lead to colic. As the trailer moves, ventilation and airflow help to keep animals cool. Make sure all vents are open, especially during hot weather.

If you are hauling your horse in an open or livestock-type trailer where your horse will be exposed to wind, other considerations apply. Your horse should wear a fly mask to prevent particles from injuring his eyes or face. Low air temperatures combined with high wind velocity or precipitation may justify a blanket.

FEDERAL REGULATIONS FOR TRANSPORT

If you adopt a wild Mustang from the Bureau of Land Management (BLM), there are specific regulations for transport. A BLM employee will give your trailer final approval prior to loading your Mustang. These regulations are good guidelines for *any* situation where you are moving untrained horses. Therefore, I have paraphrased these regulations below:

- Animals will ride loose and must have enough space to turn around.
- No one-horse trailers.
- No pick-ups with stock racks.
- Trailer must have a rear swing gate (no trailers with only a drop ramp).
- Trailer must have a covered top, but allow ample head room.
- Standard covered stock trailers and horse trailers large enough to accommodate four or more horses are ideal.
- Two-horse trailers are only allowed when it is a stock type with no internal dividers.
- Internal dividers of slant-load trailers must be removed or securely folded back.[31, 32]

Other Regulations

The only laws that govern general or individual horse transport fall under anti-cruelty legislation in 33 states.[33] Federal regulations mainly govern horse transport for slaughter. The aim of the regulations is to ensure that horses are transported humanely. The original Horse Transportation Safety Act of 2001 had loopholes and problems, so it was revised during 2013/2014. It outlaws use of double-decker trailers,[34] ensures that horses that travel are able to stand and meet certain health requirements. Regulations also dictate that horses should have the opportunity to rest and have access to food and water before and after their journey. Enforcing these laws is difficult, and I recommend the reader be familiar with it so that individuals who do not follow the regulations can be recognized and potentially reported. I also recommend understanding that these are *mimimum* guidelines for humane transport and that you yourself do not function outside these guidelines with your own horses. Transport can be stressful and dangerous to horses, so we must do everything we can to ensure their safety and welfare.[35, 36]

Trailering rescue horses is necessary to get them to their new home, as well as for medical care. The driver should be confident, and the truck and trailer should be in good working order. Maintaining good hydration, preventing stress, and optimizing air quality is critical for preventing illness. Federal guidelines and regulations are the minimum standard for shipping horses and should be followed.

2.4 An example of a horse identification form from the Bluebonnet Equine Humane Society.

IDENTIFICATION

There are many ways to identify a horse, both temporarily and permanently.[37] It's important that every person handling a group of horses can distinguish individuals. If a large number of horses arrive as a group, it can be difficult to achieve this. Tracking who is who and being able to make notes about each individual is ideal for getting to know the new horses, and for providing medical care each one may need (fig. 2.4).

Permanent Identification

Natural Features: Using a horse's natural features is the most common way his identification is documented in legal paperwork. Basic information includes breed, color, sex, age, markings or scars, and hair whorl patterns. This information has the advantage of being permanent, but the disadvantage is that it requires paper to be useful.

Natural identification of a horse by his unique iris (eyeD™) or his chestnuts (callous-like tissue on the inside of the leg just above the knee or below the hock) is possible, but these methods have not gained widespread use.

Brands: Branding a horse is a permanent method of identification. A *freeze* brand results in white hair and a *hot* brand causes scarring that results in no hair growth (figs. 2.5 A & B). Many states require registration of the brand in a database—you can't just go out and put a marking on your horse. When you register the brand with the state, the species (cattle, horse, sheep) and location of the brand is specified (for example, right or left side of the animal, and on the hip, shoulder, jaw, or other body area).

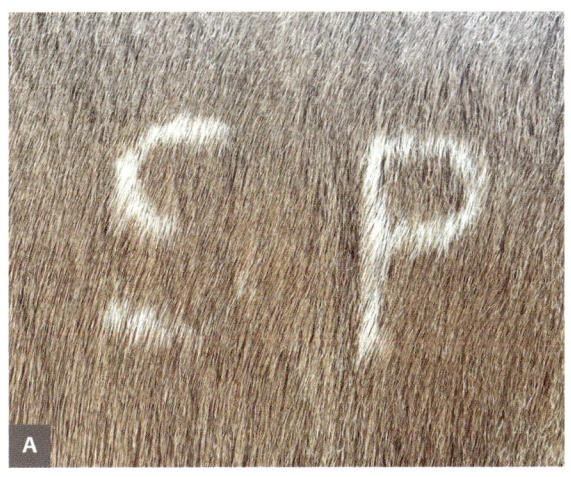
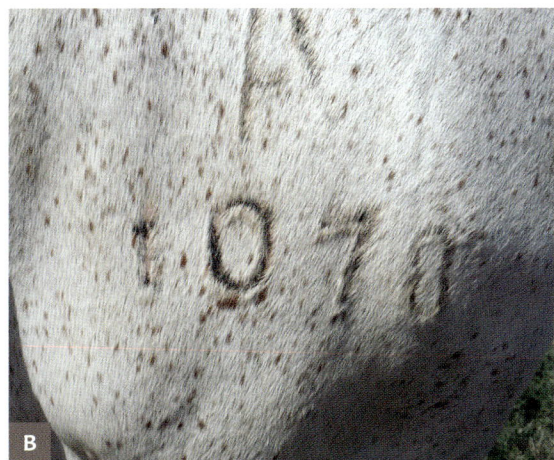

2.5 A & B A freeze brand (A) and a hot brand (B).

Brands are typically a combination of letters and simple symbols.

Another method of freeze branding, the *angle code* system, contains information about the horse (fig. 2.6). Each symbol represents a number, so information such as the year of birth or other numeric information can be permanently marked on the horse. Mustangs gathered by the BLM are marked on the left side of the neck, and information from the brand can be entered into the BLM database to trace the location and time when a Mustang was gathered. Other breeds (namely Arabians and Standardbreds) also use the system, but those horses are branded on the right. Any horse can be branded with this system to help identify the horse and thus, deter theft.

Lip Tattoos: Thoroughbred, Standardbred, Quarter Horse, and Arabian racehorses have a permanent *lip tattoo* (fig. 2.7). A racetrack official verifies identification before each race. Although these are permanent marks, they do not cause an external blemish. Like angle code freeze branding, there is information inherent in the marking. Each of the

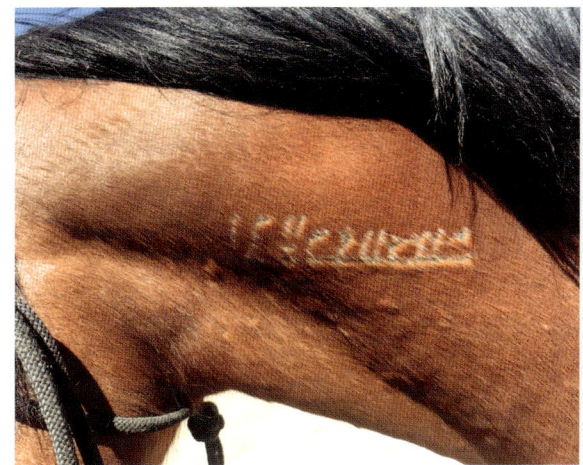

2.6 An angle-code freeze brand on a BLM-gathered Mustang.

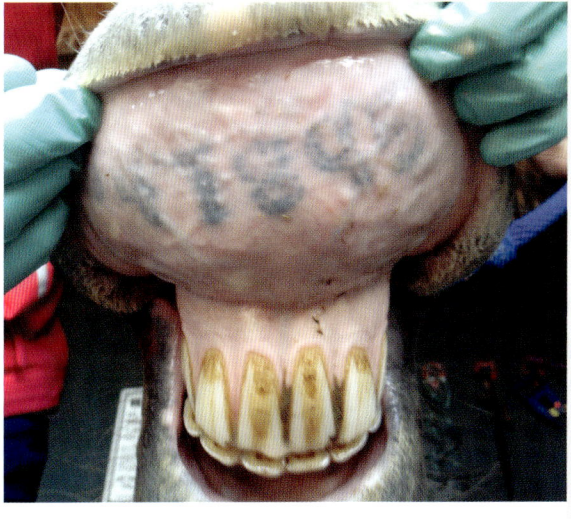

2.7 A lip tattoo on an older Thoroughbred. As occurs over time with most tattoos, this one is partially illegible.

Part I: Caring for Horses in Need—17

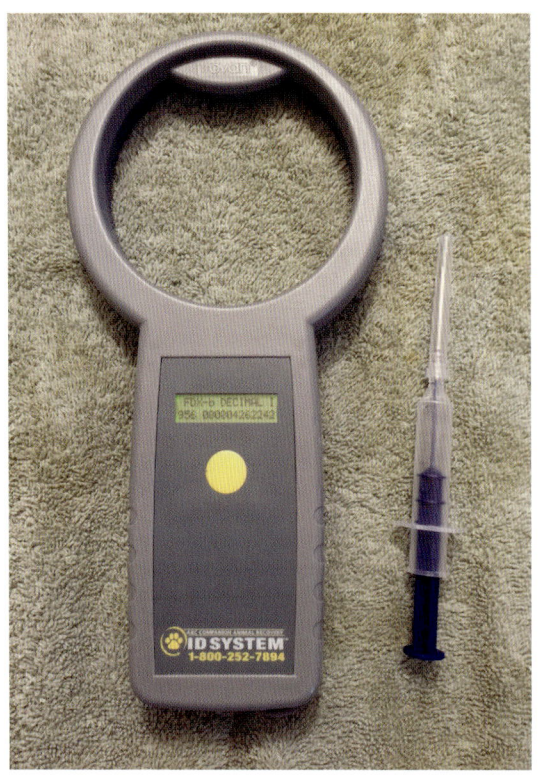

2.8 A microchip scanner and microchip in its syringe ready to be implanted.

racing industries uses a slightly different system, but the concept is similar. For Thoroughbreds, the tattoo begins with a letter that designates the year the horse was born. The letter D designates the year 2000, the letter E 2001, and so forth. After reaching the end of the alphabet, the Jockey Club begins again with the letter A. It is easy to tell the difference between a 26-year-old horse and a yearling when they have the same letter on the tattoo. Now, lip tattoos are being phased out in favor of microchips.

The American Quarter Horse Association (AQHA) requires a horse to be genotyped before registration and lip tattooing. Genetic markers in DNA are unique to each horse. After genetic testing determines the genotype, DNA markers of the horse are compared with the markers of the horse's sire and dam to verify his parentage.

Microchipping: A radio frequency identification microchip can be implanted in the nuchal ligament of a horse's neck as a method of permanent identification (fig. 2.8). The microchip should meet National Animal Identification System recommendations and is useful for reuniting horses separated from their owners as well as identifying horses at shows and races.

Advantages of microchipping are that it does not cause an exterior blemish, and the information is treated as legal permanent identification, much like the permanent vehicle identification number on your car. There are some disadvantages to microchipping, though. If you don't have a microchip reader, you cannot trace the horse. This means when your horses accidentally get out and your neighbor finds them, their identification and ownership may not be immediately

Never Look a Gift Horse in the Mouth

A horse was gifted to a client of mine and his children by a church parishioner and friend of theirs. Reddy was a sweet horse, and the people had determined her presumed age solely by looking at her left corner incisor. It was small and square, so both the new owners and the former owner thought she was a two-year-old. But, Reddy had a serious dental imbalance and the right incisor was nearly three inches long. This horse didn't have a lip tattoo, but after fully evaluating all of her dentition, looking at her body shape, and the gray hair around her eyes and face, I estimated her age to be between 25 and 30. A classic case of not looking a gift horse in the mouth!

obvious. Also, microchips are only as good as the data stored in association with them. There currently is not a centralized database for equine microchip information, so if you move and do not update contact information, it may not be possible to reunite your horse with you.

Some breed associations and show or racing authorities require microchips and maintain the information in their own databases. This is a list of a few examples:

- The Jockey Club of North America requires microchips for all registered Thoroughbreds born after 2017.

- The U.S. Hunter Jumper Association (USHJA) requires microchipping for horses competing in their sanctioned shows.

- The Fédération Equestrian Internationale (FEI), which is the governing body for international equestrian sporting events, also requires microchipping for identification and showing.

- Louisiana requires a microchip, lip tattoo, or other permanent identification to be documented on a horse's Coggins test (see p. 23).

Temporary Identification

Tags and Collars: Temporary name tags have become popular for horses traveling to trail rides or shows (figs. 2.9 A–C). These are easy to read, just like finding a lost dog with a collar. Name tags are inexpensive and safe.

While some people keep a tag on their horse's halter or bridle, I prefer the

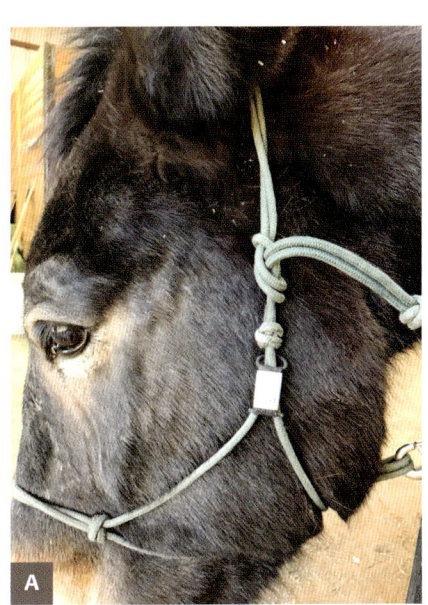
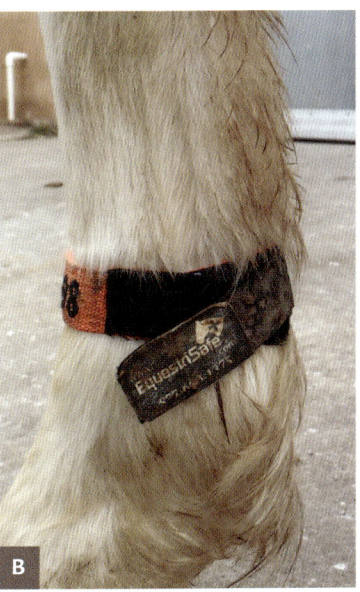
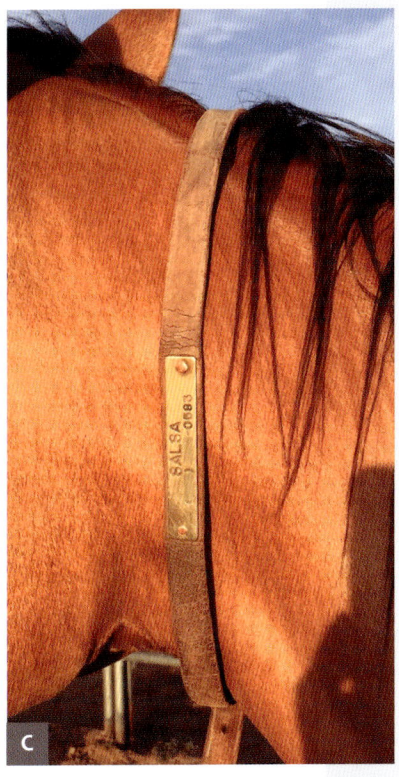

2.9 A–C Three examples of temporary tags and collars: The first tag is designed to be affixed to a rope halter (A). It is preferable for tags to be on the animal independent of halters or tack, like a fetlock band attached with Velcro (B). When using neck collars, a leather collar is safest because it can break in an emergency (C).

Part I: Caring for Horses in Need—19

identifier to remain attached to the horse all the time. This way, should the horse not be wearing tack, he can still be found. For example, a small tag can be braided into a horse's mane or tail, although they have to be re-braided regularly.

Velcro bands can be embroidered with contact information and placed around the horse's leg. Another way to attach identification to the horse is with a neck collar. These are commonly used in large herds that have multiple people working with many horses, such as university research herds. Neck collars are available in both plastic and leather. Leather has a breakaway function (it will break if your horse catches it on a fencepost), so it can be safely worn at all times. A nameplate can have a horse-identification number for the herd, or information such as your horse's name and your phone number. A rescue group with multiple new horses and multiple volunteers will find this form of identification useful.

Although temporary identifiers can be lost or separated from your horse, a huge advantage is that anyone who finds him can read the tag and use the attached information to reunite you.

Traceability

Because of the advantages and disadvantages of each form of identification, every horse should have a permanent, traceable form of identification as well as a visible temporary identifier at all times, no matter how long you have had or will have him. Depending on the situation, one form of identification may be better than the other. If you think about how much effort and care you are about to put into this horse, you will want to ensure he is traceable. It would be a tragedy to help a horse, re-home him, and then lose track of him. You care about your horses, so make sure you can follow up.

OWNERSHIP

Identifying a horse is not the same thing as providing proof of ownership. When you acquire a horse, documentation of your ownership is necessary. Transfer of ownership of neglected horses may be complicated by court proceedings or legal issues. Save any papers, such as a bill of sale, or communications from the previous owner. If the courts or authorities were involved in confiscation or ownership transfer, a "Chain of Custody" form should be maintained and copies kept. If the horse is registered, communicate with the breed association and make sure the ownership change is recorded.

In most of the United States, proof of ownership can be documented via a bill of sale or updated registration papers. If neither of these documents are available for an individual horse, the Coggins test paperwork and affidavits or records from equine professionals (farriers, trainers, or veterinarians) can help prove ownership.

In some Western states, a brand inspection is required. In these states, there are only two ways to legally prove ownership: 1) a horse is branded with a symbol officially registered to the horse owner in that state; 2) a brand inspector issues an official identification card or certificate from that state's livestock board. In this case, features such as markings, unregistered brands, scars, and tattoos are considered "distinguishing marks" and will be recorded by the brand inspector. States that require this include New Mexico, Montana, Colorado, Idaho,

Nevada, Utah, Wyoming, and portions of Oregon, South Dakota, and Washington.

QUARANTINE

Depending on the circumstances, you may not know much about your newly acquired horse. He may have an uncertain vaccine status. Travel exposes him to contagious diseases, especially if he commingled with others at a livestock auction or other holding area.

A new horse should be quarantined from your other horses for at least three weeks (fig. 2.10). Quarantine distance should be a minimum 40 feet, which is based on a horse's ability to sneeze or cough and spray droplets up to 15 feet, and accounts for additional wind dispersal. Another way respiratory diseases are spread is carriage by fomites—objects such as buckets, brushes, or clothing that have come into contact with infected horses.

Quarantine time period and distance recommendations are designed to prevent contagious respiratory diseases such as Equine Herpes Virus (*rhinopneumonitis*), influenza, and strangles (*Streptococcus equi ssp. equi*) from infecting the established herd. During the quarantine period, you should monitor the temperature of your new horse each day because a fever sometimes occurs before obvious disease. Spread of other contagious diseases that cause diarrhea (such as *Salmonella spp.*) are minimized by using proper quarantine procedures. Finally, quarantine protects your established herd from both external and internal parasites such as lice or strongyles.

During quarantine, you should implement biosecurity measures, including a sanitizing foot bath and protective barrier gear, such as gloves, disposable barrier coveralls or gown, and a hat or mask, especially if there are any signs of illness. A horse can sneeze or breathe into the caretaker's hair, and the virus particles can then be carried to other horses.

Another technique is to care for your established horses first, and then the new horse. Washing your hands between horses or groups is an easy and effective way to reduce the spread of infectious agents. You should attend to the healthy horses first, then any horses possibly exposed to illness or disease that are not yet showing signs. Take care of sick horses last.

A horse should be fully vaccinated and medically cleared before being moved from quarantine to general housing. A very thin

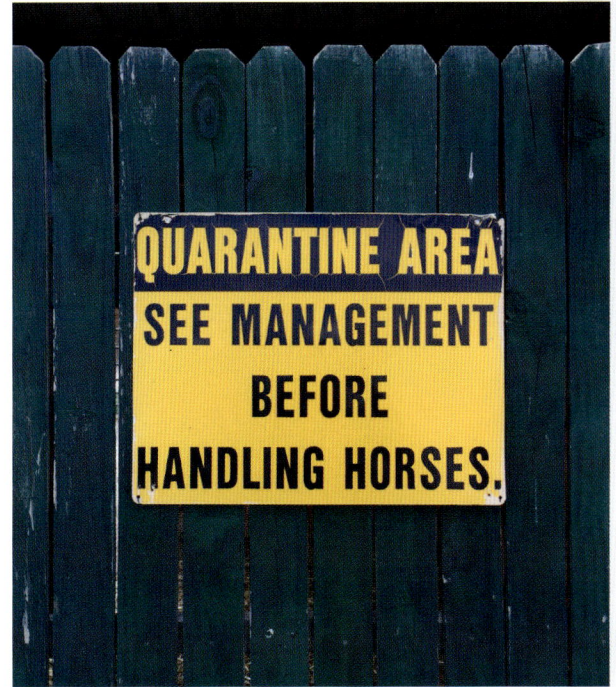

2.10 *Quarantining a rescue horse is important for reducing the chance of contagious diseases and parasites spreading.*

or sick horse may remain in quarantine for a longer period of time.

Quarantine should also account for a horse's mental well-being. Maintain previously established groups, if possible. For instance, if a group of yearlings arrive together, they should continue to live together. Spend time haltering, brushing, petting, and bonding with your new arrivals. Quarantine pens are typically small, so if you have an untrained, untouchable horse, this is a great time to befriend him and begin the halter-training process. When you consistently provide food and water to a horse who has been neglected, this is the first step to showing him that you are trustworthy.

A horse who lives alone may feel stressed out. This is not ideal as stress weakens the immune system. When you adopt a single new horse into your group, he may need a companion during the quarantine time. A fully vaccinated, mature gelding with a steady personality can be used as a quarantine companion. Remember, the "companion" horse cannot be returned to the established herd until the quarantine period is over. A mare is not ideal as she could be impregnated by a newly rescued colt that has not been gelded. A goat can also be used as a companion, without the risk of contracting an equine respiratory disease.

VETERINARY EXAMINATION

As soon as your new horse is home, call a veterinarian for a physical examination. Your veterinarian is a big part of your team—she will help you establish a medical record, legally documenting your horse's condition on arrival. She will also identify subtle or underlying problems, perform laboratory testing, and make a plan to restore your horse to full health. As the new owner, willingness and financial ability to provide medical care supports your legal ownership, should it ever be questioned. She may also have suggestions about effective quarantine for your particular farm or situation. Finally, establishing a relationship between your horse and your veterinarian is important because if he gets sick, she already knows him, his normal behavior, and vital signs.

As part of the examination, your horse's body condition score (BCS) will be recorded (see Body Condition Scoring, p. 28). For now, just know that this is a system of documenting how thin a horse is, and there are established legal precedents. If you are nursing a thin horse back to health, having your veterinarian document this specific parameter is useful, especially if there is a court case pending.

Although less accurate in older horses, your veterinarian will be able to estimate your horse's age. With this information, and taking into consideration your rescue horse's BCS, you and your veterinarian can formulate an appropriate health care and nutrition plan.

A physical examination evaluates all body systems. If you expect to ride your horse, it is important to know neurologic status and identify lameness. This may not be possible to precisely determine for a weak horse who has a decreased muscle mass. Thin horses should be reassessed after weight gain.

If the horse has traveled, especially over a long distance, evaluating the respiratory system for any early signs of disease is necessary. His skin and hair coat should be assessed for the presence of *ectoparasites* such as mites, lice, or ticks. You definitely don't want these bugs spreading through your herd. Early identification of diseases optimizes successful intervention.

Laboratory Testing

Laboratory testing for a newly acquired horse should always include a fecal evaluation and a Coggins test. Your veterinarian may recommend additional blood work. There is a lot of testing, but it helps to remember that your goal is to make life better for your horse.

Fecal Evaluation: A full fecal analysis looks for both sand and parasites (fig. 2.11). Undernourished horses are more likely to ingest sand, gravel, and other footing or bedding due to starvation. When sand is identified, an individualized treatment plan for getting rid of the sand will be developed. Psyllium husk (pelleted and sold under the brand name SandClear™, among others) is used to help clear the sand.

We will discuss deworming and parasites more thoroughly in chapter 4 (p. 49). For now, understand that the choice to deworm a rescue horse may depend on his parasite load and overall health status. Parasites might not be a problem, and you cannot tell for sure without a fecal. It may show that deworming is not yet necessary.

Also, if a horse is debilitated, deworming him before his strength returns could cause harm. A newly acquired rescue horse has many risk factors for colic: travel, a change in food, and a change in housing. Another is killing off a large number of parasites at one time, which may result in inflammation of the gut, causing colic.

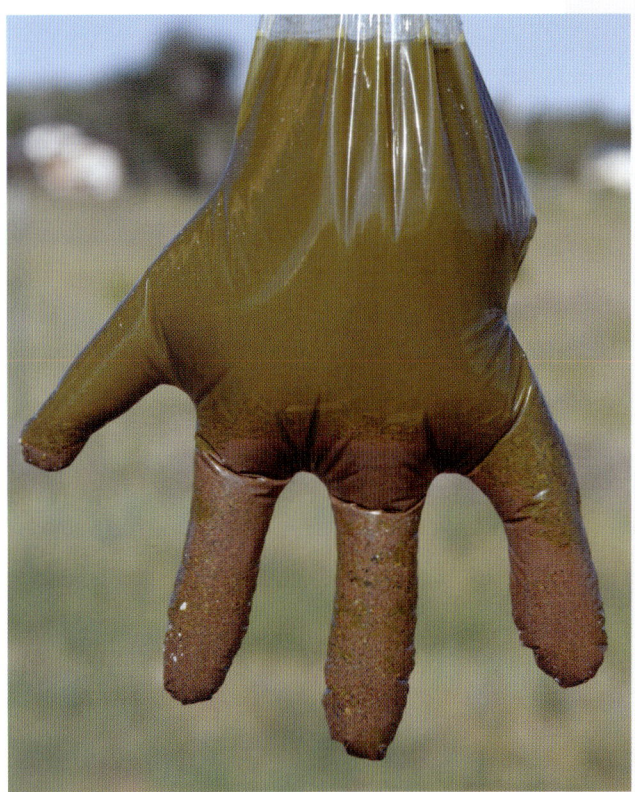

2.11 This fecal sediment test revealed a large amount of sand, which can cause digestive problems.

Coggins Test: In the 1970s, Dr. Leroy Coggins developed a test revolutionizing our ability to identify horses infected with Equine Infectious Anemia (EIA). EIA is also called *swamp fever* and is caused by a virus that is spread by biting flies like horse and deer flies. The disease primarily causes a drop in the number of red blood cells a horse has (*anemia*). Signs include weakness, exercise intolerance, and fever. Affected horses may also have dependent edema, which is swelling of the limbs and lower areas of the body, such as under the belly or in a male horse's sheath. Many infected horses succumb to the virus and die. Although case numbers have decreased with effective surveillance in North America, there is no treatment or

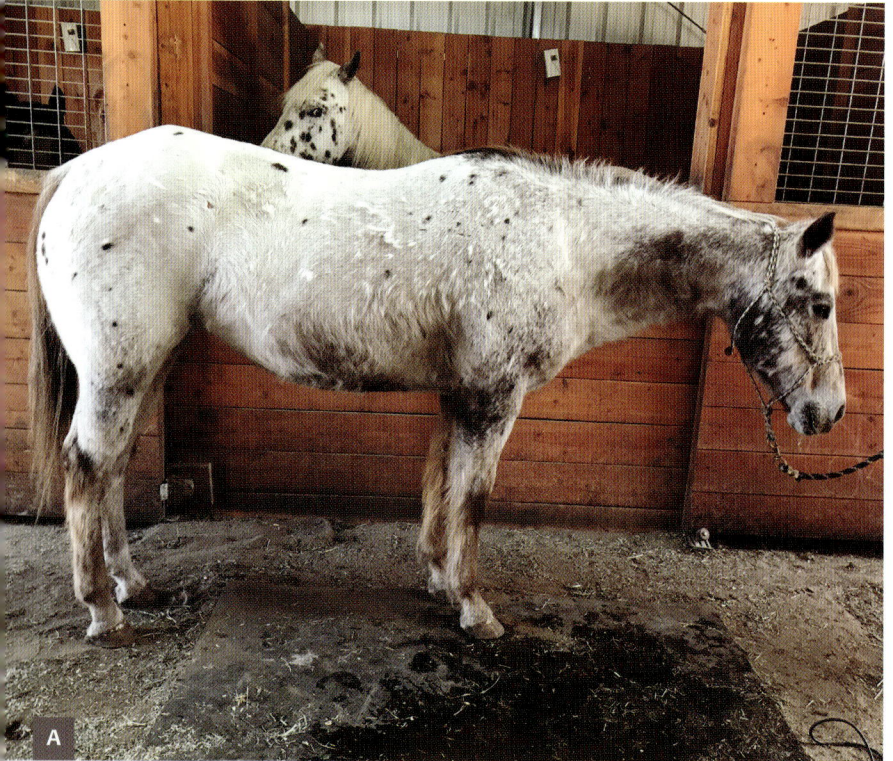

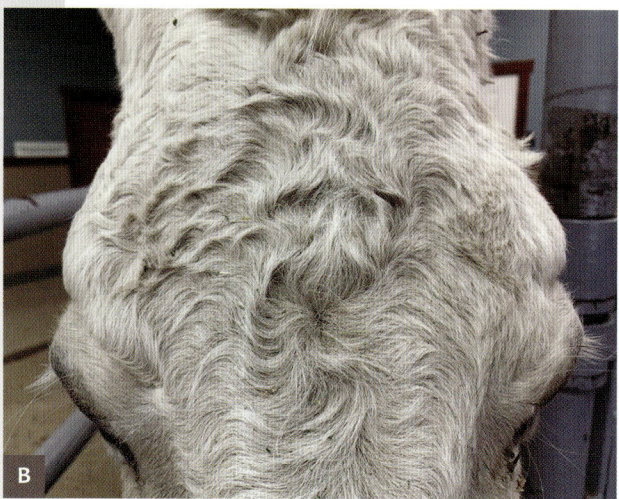

2.12 A & B It's important to identify Pituitary Pars Intermedia Dysfunction (PPID) early so that treatment can commence. Abnormal hair coat on an Appaloosa (A) and fat pads above the eyes on a Peruvian Paso (B) are both common signs of PPID.

cure. Surveillance testing is the only weapon you have to reduce and eliminate the virus from your horse population—and keep your loved ones healthy. Vaccines are in development, but none are yet approved or available in North America.

The Coggins test is the gold standard of testing for EIA. It requires *serum* (the liquid portion of the blood after clotting). The test reveals the presence of *antibodies* (proteins of immunity), which indicates exposure to the virus. U.S. federal regulations require a negative EIA test dated within 12 months for any horse, mule, or donkey being entered into exhibitions, competitive events, sale barns, or moving across state lines, and when ownership changes. A federally accredited veterinarian draws blood and sends it to an approved laboratory. Paperwork accompanies the blood sample and test results and includes horse identification. A multiple carbon copy handwritten form with a hand-drawn likeness of the horse's markings may be used, or the form may be completed electronically with digital photos.

Blood Work: A typical blood work panel includes a Complete Blood Count (CBC) and serum biochemistry profile. Older horses should be tested for Pituitary Pars Intermedia Dysfunction (PPID—see below). Your willingness to obtain information on your horse shows your commitment to working toward health and wellness.

The CBC and chemistry panel are primary screening tests. Abnormal results, whether your horse is sick or not, may lead your veterinarian to recommend further diagnostic specialty tests.

The CBC includes information about blood cells, their numbers, and types. White blood cells are important for immunity. Different types of white blood cells have a variety of functions, including engulfing and destroying microbial invaders like bacteria or viruses. The CBC also evaluates red blood cells, which carry oxygen using a protein molecule called hemoglobin. The CBC screens for anemia by evaluating the size of red blood cells, the number of red blood cells in a given volume of blood, and the hemoglobin content within the red blood cells. The CBC evaluates platelets, too. Platelets are tiny cell fragments that stop bleeding by sticking together when activated, making the initial portion of a blood clot or scab. Too few platelets can be a sign of serious inflammation.

The serum biochemistry panel evaluates proteins, enzymes, and other molecules present in the body. Veterinarians look at abnormal elevations or decreases in these substances, interpreting the health and function of major organs such as the liver and kidneys, and the health of muscles or imbalance of electrolytes.[38]

The biochemistry panel is a good screening tool for every horse, but especially for a thin animal. If there is an underlying disease process, such as kidney failure, you will have a much tougher time working on weight gain. And, you have to ask yourself, how fair is it to keep going with a horse who has a fatal disease that remains unidentified and untreated? Doing blood work helps you make educated choices about what the best, most humane plan is for a horse.

PPID is an endocrine abnormality that results in the imbalance of cortisol, the stress hormone. It was formerly known as Cushing's disease or hyperadrenocorticism. There are a variety of specialty blood tests used to definitively diagnose and monitor PPID, but research is active and recommendations for testing strategies change often.

It is estimated that 20 to 25 percent of horses over the age of 15 have PPID (figs. 2.12 A & B).[39, 40] If your new horse is over the age of 20, or if he shows any signs of PPID, he should be tested. Subtle signs of PPID may go unnoticed, so screening older horses even if clinical signs aren't obvious is important. The classic sign of PPID is a long or slow-shedding hair coat. Horses with PPID may lose muscle over their topline, resulting in a sway back, and have inflammation and pain in their feet (*laminitis*). Affected individuals may also have behavior changes, lethargy, weight loss, abnormal sweating, impaired healing, an increase in infections, and (rarely) blindness.

At the time of writing, there is only one treatment with research support and approved by the Food and Drug Administration (FDA): Prascend (pergolide). Testing and treatment is important because PPID negatively impacts a horse's quality of life. Aside from providing adequate food and water, controlling PPID is the number one thing you can do to improve a geriatric horse's health and well-being.

MAKE TIME TO BOND

Bringing your horse home is an eventful time. Monitoring him in quarantine, managing legal issues surrounding him, and treating underlying ailments will keep you busy. Take time to bond with him and show him how much you love him.

CHAPTER 3

Digestion:
Nutrition, Dentistry, and Colic

This chapter covers three important areas of equine digestion, beginning with nutrition. After I discuss refeeding a starved horse, I will cover forages and basic feeding for all horses. Dentistry is covered because chewing food is the first step in the digestive process. When the digestive system is abnormal and causes abdominal pain, this condition is known as colic.

NUTRITION

Starvation is the most common medical problem seen in rescue horses, and the main reason horses are confiscated for neglect. Horses starve because of three things: a lack of owner knowledge, a lack of financial resources, or because of disease or parasite burdens.[41]

Feeding your starved horse is not a simple task. You must proceed with knowledge, patience, and caution because overzealous nutrition too early can result in illness or even death. After your horse is stabilized, it may take six months to a year for him to be a normal weight. Let's start with the basics: how to determine and document how thin he really is.

BODY CONDITION SCORING

In 1983, Dr. Don Henneke and his colleagues at Texas A&M University published a landmark paper describing a semi-quantitative way of assessing and documenting fat and muscle coverage in horses.[42] The Henneke Body Condition Scoring (BCS) system aims to be objective, is repeatable, and has legal precedents established. With practice, anyone can learn the Henneke BCS system (fig. 3.2).

The Henneke BCS system is useful for monitoring weight changes over time. Therefore, rescue horses should be evaluated and their BCS recorded on a monthly basis. Fat is assessed over the horse's neck, withers, behind the shoulders, along the ribs, and across the loin and tailhead (fig. 3.1). Each location is scored on a scale of one to nine, and then the average is calculated. The assessment should be based on feeling and touching the horse, especially when the horse has a long hair coat.

A healthy horse's BCS is 4, 5, or 6. Horses that score 7 or above are overweight, while 3 and below is malnourished. A BCS of 1 is a state of severe starvation with almost no fat or body reserves remaining.

STARVATION

During starvation, a horse's body initially uses its reserves of fat and carbohydrates for energy. When those reserves are gone, his body must cannibalize its own proteins as a source of nutrition, resulting in muscle wasting and further weight loss. As his body scavenges protein to survive, damage to heart muscle and other internal organs occurs, which can result in permanent dysfunction.

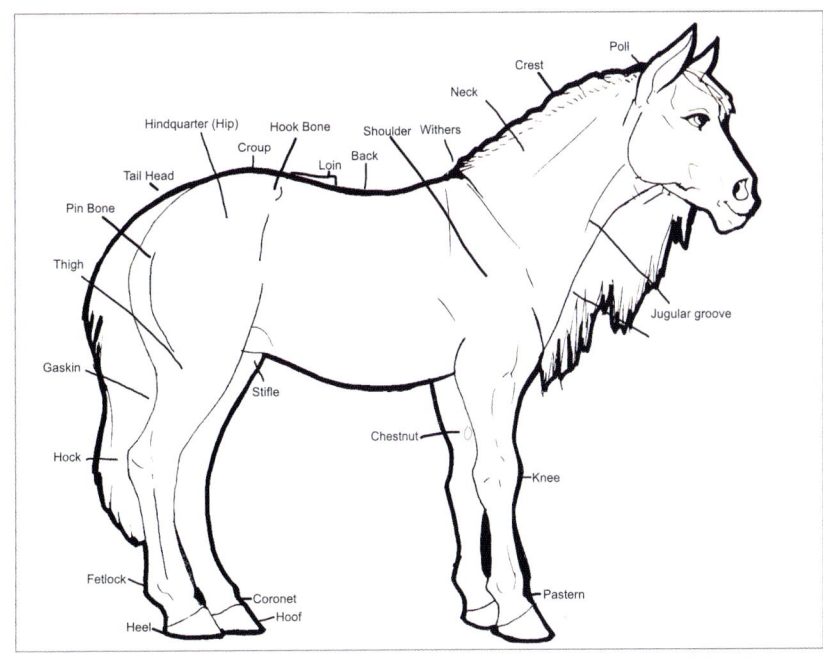

3.1 *Diagram of horse body parts for anatomy and fat assessment.*

Refeeding Syndrome

Refeeding syndrome is a life-threatening metabolic complication that occurs when a starving horse eats too much food too soon. It is not obvious from the outside of the horse when it starts to occur; it is an internal problem. There are many intertwined metabolic abnormalities that occur during refeeding syndrome, so the physiology of all of the changes is unknown to this day.[43]

Refeeding syndrome begins with spikes of soluble carbohydrates (sugars) ingested in the horse's newfound nutrition. His body responds to the sugar by releasing insulin, which carries sugar inside cells so that it can be used for energy. In the case of refeeding syndrome, the body hasn't had access to carbohydrates for so long, it over responds and releases too much insulin. This results in low blood sugar. The animal cannot maintain normal body functions, and although this response is mild at first, it can spiral out of control until the horse develops life-threatening respiratory, heart, and kidney failure.[44]

The thinner the horse is, the higher the risk for metabolic derangements. Complete food deprivation will result in worse metabolic derangements and more intensive, complicated medical care. Horses that have had access to limited amounts of food recover better. When a rescue horse has a BCS of 1 to 3, your veterinarian should be involved in formulating the plan to re-feed him. Signs of refeeding syndrome occur three to five days after being fed, but can be two weeks after the first meal. When the horse has access to large meals too early, his risk is increased.[45]

Safely Feeding the Starved Horse

Small, frequent meals of alfalfa alone are the safest way to feed a starved horse. To determine this, The University of California, Davis has worked with rescue groups to conduct clinical trials using horses with a BCS of 1 or 2. When compared to a diet of grains and

3.2 ORIGINAL HENNEKE BODY CONDITION SCORE TABLE

HENNEKE BCS	NECK	WITHERS	SHOULDERS	RIBS
1: POOR	Bone structure easily noticeable	Bone structure easily noticeable	Bone structure easily noticeable	Ribs protruding prominently
2: VERY THIN	Bone structure faintly discernible	Bone structure faintly discernible	Bone structure faintly discernible	Ribs prominent
3: THIN	Neck accentuated	Withers accentuated	Shoulder accentuated	Slight fat cover over ribs; ribs easily discernible
4: MODERATELY THIN	Neck not obviously thin	Withers not obviously thin	Shoulders not obviously thin	Faint outline of ribs discernible
5: MODERATE	Neck blends smoothly into body	Withers rounded over spinous processes	Shoulder blends smoothly into body	Ribs cannot be visually distinguished but can be easily felt
6: MODERATELY FLESHY	Deposited fat faintly discernible along neck	Deposited fat faintly discernible along withers	Deposited fat faintly discernible behind shoulder	Fat over ribs feels spongy
7: FLESHY	Fat deposited along neck	Fat deposited along withers	Fat deposited behind shoulder	Individual ribs can be felt with pressure, but noticeable fat filling between ribs
8: FAT	Noticeable thickening of neck	Area along withers filled with fat	Area behind shoulder filled in flush with body	Difficult to feel ribs
9: EXTREMELY FAT	Bulging fat along neck	Bulging fat along withers	Bulging fat along shoulder	Patchy fat over ribs

LOIN	TAILHEAD	
Spinous processes projecting prominently	Tailhead, pin bones, and hook bones projecting prominently	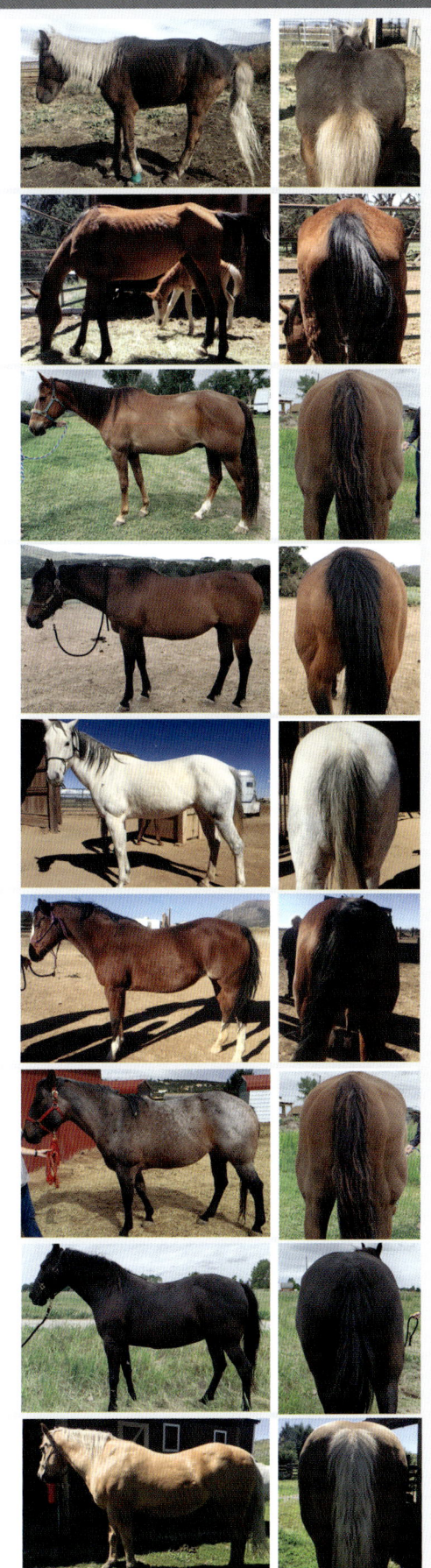
Slight fat covering over base of spinous processes; transverse processes of lumbar vertebrae feel rounded; spinous processes prominent	Tailhead prominent	
Fat buildup halfway on spinous processes but easily discernible; transverse processes cannot be felt; processes of lumbar vertebrae feel rounded; spinous processes prominent	Tailhead prominent, but individual vertebrae cannot be identified; hook bones appear rounded but still easily discernible; pin bones not distinguishable	
Negative crease (peaked appearance) along back	Prominence depends on conformation; fat can be felt; hook bones not discernible	
Back is level	Fat around tailhead feels somewhat soft	
May have slight positive crease (groove) down back	Fat around tailhead feels soft	
May have positive crease down back	Fat around tailhead is soft	
Positive crease down back	Fat around tailhead very soft	
Obvious crease down back	Bulging fat around tailhead	

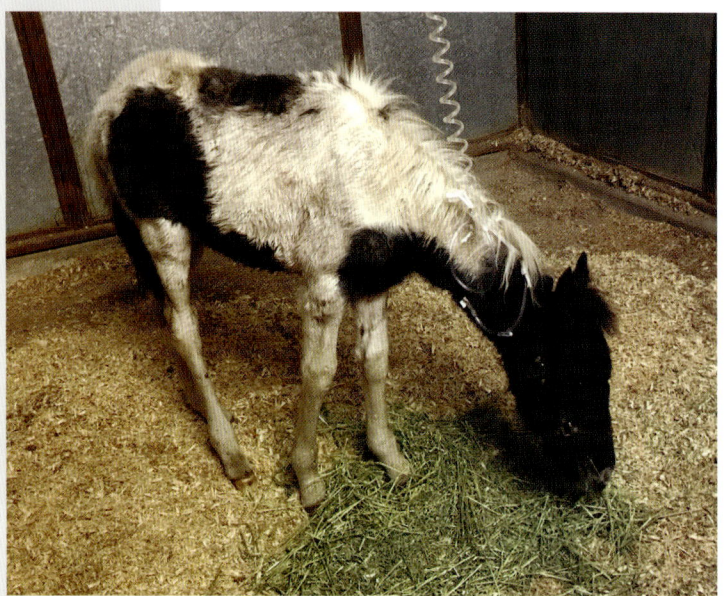

3.3 Refeeding a starved horse with alfalfa. Because of electrolyte abnormalities, in this case, intravenous fluids were required, too.

grasses, the horse's body has a lower peak glucose and insulin response with a diet of alfalfa, reducing the chance of developing refeeding syndrome (fig. 3.3).[46]

For reference, a normal horse should eat 1.5 to 2 percent of his body weight per day in feed (15 to 20 pounds for a 1,000-pound horse). The basis of any horse's diet should be forage or hay.[47]

Feeding Program

Here I have provided science-supported recommendations to re-feed a starved horse. Feed quantities are by weight, so you will need a reliable scale (figs. 3.4 A & B). Also, these numbers are for the average-sized horse who we expect to have an ideal weight of about 1,000 pounds. Feed amounts should be adjusted according to the horse's expected final weight based on his frame.

Starved horses are re-fed beginning with one pound of alfalfa six times daily. It is tempting to feed grain to a starved horse, but this increases the chances of refeeding syndrome and death. Alfalfa is high in protein, which helps to level the blood sugar and insulin spikes that are the problem during refeeding syndrome.

Conventional horse-person wisdom maintains that grass hay is the safest forage, and free-choice access is the best. Research and clinical cases have proven this to be false in the instance of starved horses. While it is hard to resist conventional wisdom, I assure you it is more difficult to watch a starved horse with new access to food lie down and die despite all efforts to save him.

If a horse has not had alfalfa before, there can be some gastrointestinal side effects, such as soft stool or gas production. However, in a truly starved horse who has had little or no access to forage, any feed can result in gastrointestinal side effects. There is a subset of horse owners that ascribe to an "Alfalfa Is Bad" myth. You must abandon this belief in order to properly care for your starved horse.

The purpose of following the feeding plan outlined here is to first reset the horse's metabolic function and mitigate the development of refeeding syndrome. After that has been accomplished, weight gain can occur.

Days One through Three: Feed 1 pound of high-quality alfalfa every four hours for the first three days. The total the horse will eat during this period is 6 pounds per day.

Your horse should be allowed free access to water as well as a salt block during this time. If he is dehydrated as well as emaciated, your veterinarian will make a plan for rehydration.

Day Four to Two Weeks: Gradually increase the amount of alfalfa by about a half pound per day total and begin to decrease the frequency of feeding. Work toward a total of 12 pounds per day divided into three feedings. The three feedings should be eight hours apart.

During the first two weeks, don't expect any weight gain. What you are doing with this feeding program is resetting your horse's metabolic system back to normal so that he can survive and gain weight. It can feel frustrating to not yet be feeding him grain or allowing him free-choice access to his forage, but this is the safest way to ensure that the thinnest horses survive.

Two Weeks to Two Months: Continue to add a half pound of alfalfa per day to your horse's diet. Gradually increase the amount until you are feeding as much alfalfa as the horse will eat. A horse can eat up to 2 percent of his ideal body weight per day. For the average-sized horse, this is about 20 pounds. During this time, you may work to decrease the frequency of feeding to twice daily. Once he is eating all the alfalfa he can, it is safe to gradually add other feed material such as grain or grass hay to the horse's diet (see Other Feeds, p. 34).

Long-Term Plan: Once your horse is approaching a healthy weight—again, this can take from six months to a year—you will be able to adjust to a long-term plan for him based on his ongoing needs and exercise intensity.[48]

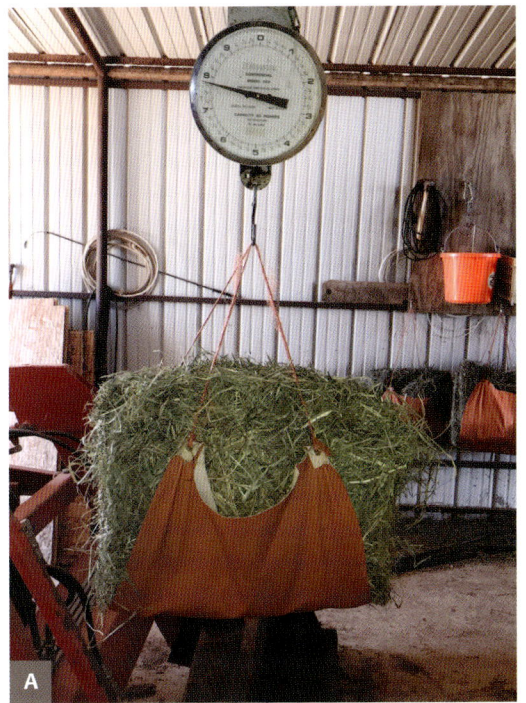

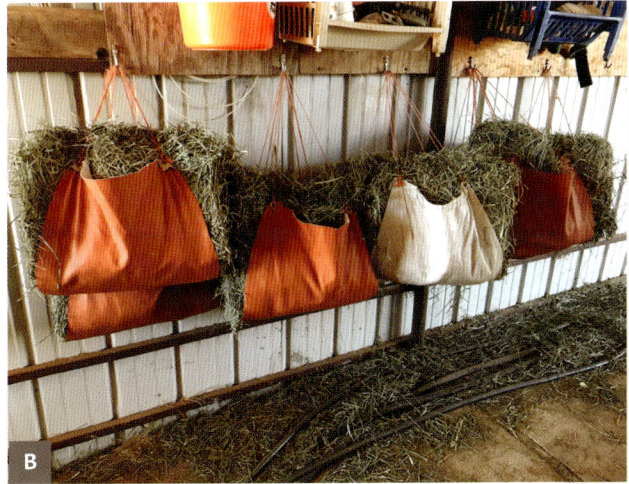

3.4 A & B Weighing out forage and feed is the most accurate way to ensure a horse gets an appropriate amount of feed (A). These hay bags have been efficiently prepared in advance for a week's worth of forage, so that daily feeding is easy (B).

FORAGES

Forage Selection

Ironically, many of the notable food-processing abnormalities observed with refeeding a starved horse are similar to metabolic problems observed with uncontrolled Type II diabetes in humans, which is more or less manifested as *insulin resistance* (IR) in obese horses. IR horses are sensitive to sugar and starches, and have driven forage research and understanding. This knowledge can be extrapolated to helping starved, metabolically deranged rescue horses.

Forage Facts

In the nutrition world, sugars and starches, along with their molecular cousins, fructans, are referred to as *non-structural carbohydrates* (NSC). Determining the NSC and nutrition content by simply looking at hay is impossible; it must be tested. There are a few generalities that will allow you to make an educated guess when evaluating hay (figs. 3.5 and 3.6).

Grains or sweet feeds have the highest NSC content, followed by cool-season grass hays. Cool-season grasses include timothy, orchard, and fescue (fig. 3.7). NSC is lowest

Skinny Surprise

It had taken a long time and significant effort for the authorities to get a warrant and the legal ability to confiscate some thin horses from a farm. There were over 50 horses on the property, and the animals that had a BCS of 2 or less were seized—nearly all of them. Although a rescue organization housed most of the horses, the half-dozen horses in the most critical condition were brought to the veterinary teaching hospital. One horse was so thin he died within a few days of arrival, despite the very best and most aggressive medical care.

I watched an emaciated chestnut mare with a hangdog look lean her butt against the corner of the stall. She was too weak to completely hold herself up. Her chestnut coat had a rough, coarse, unhealthy texture. She grunted every few breaths. The line taking fluids into her vein sparkled as it dripped. She was severely anemic: her red cell count was lower than I had ever seen in a live patient. Despite the fact that every angular bone in her body was visible, she was not interested in her small ration of alfalfa. She looked terrible, and I thought she might die. Even more distressing, her belly stuck out from her body. She was starved, and everyone was shocked to learn that she was maintaining a pregnancy.

Miraculously, she surprised everyone by surviving. After looking for hours like she was dying, she nickered once and began to eat. With further careful rations and care, she improved daily, and her red cell count gradually increased and normalized. The pregnancy was not lost, either.

It took months for the experienced horsewoman who adopted the mare to get her back to a healthy weight. This mare almost lost her life as her body gave all its reserves to keep her baby alive. Ultimately, a small, but otherwise healthy foal was born and survived.

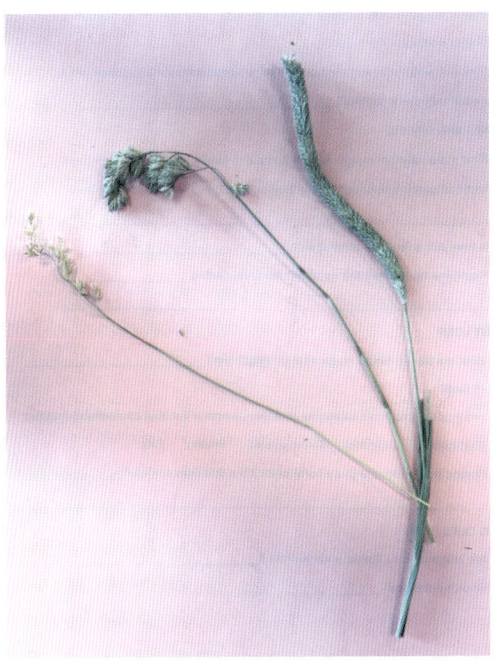

3.7 Seed head types, from left to right: bluegrass-type, orchard, and timothy.

High NSC	Low NSC
Grains or sweet feeds	Legumes (alfalfa, clover)
Cool-season grass hays (timothy, orchard, fescue)	Warm-season grass hay (coastal bermuda)
Young, leafy plants	Mature, stemmy hay or bloomed hay
Cool night with morning harvest	Longer field drying time
Plant stress (drought, freezing) for cool-season grasses	Plant stress (drought, freezing) for warm-season grasses

3.5 Factors Affecting Non-Structural Carbohydrates

Feed	NSC	Calories per Pound
Legumes (alfalfa and clover)	9–15%	900–1050
Grass hays	7–18%	825–900
Oat hay	22%	850
Timothy	12%	800–950
Sweet feed	10–20%	1500–1800
Equine senior feed	17%	1200–1700
Oil or fat	N/A (0)	1900 calories per cup

3.6 Nutrient Content of Forage

in alfalfa (a legume) and coastal bermuda (a warm-season grass hay). Other factors that affect the NSC levels in hay or forage include plant type and maturity, harvest conditions, and local farming practices, which are influenced by geography and weather.

For most horses, a high-quality, easily digestible, nutrient-dense hay is needed. If a plant is overly mature when it is baled into hay, horses won't eat it because excessive indigestible fiber makes it unpalatable (for example, coarse straw).[49]

Alfalfa is the forage of choice for refeeding a starved horse: its caloric content is high because of its high protein content, but the sugar content is low. Additionally, it has high levels of electrolytes such as calcium, magnesium, and phosphorus, which can help ameliorate some of the

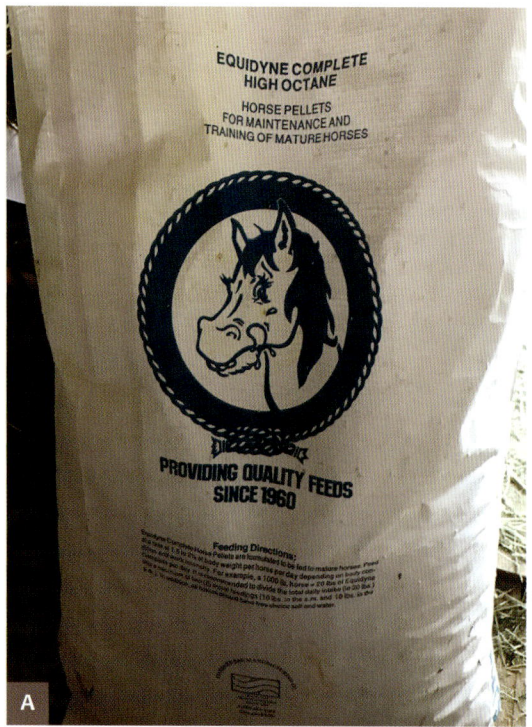 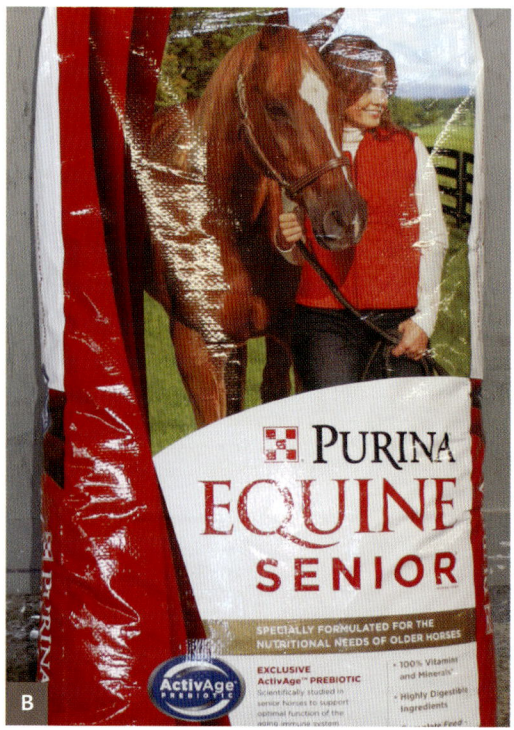

3.8 A & B *Two examples of complete feeds that can be used when a horse is unable to eat grass or hay forages.*

metabolic derangements seen in refeeding syndrome.

If a horse cannot chew hay or forage, another form of roughage must be provided. Alfalfa is available in pelleted and cubed forms, as are some grasses. It is best to feed these soaked or wet because if pellets are swallowed too quickly, *choke* (where the esophagus becomes obstructed or clogged with inadequately chewed food) may occur.

OTHER FEEDS

Grains

Grains for horses are bagged and include some combination of oats, corn, barley, or beet pulp. They may be textured (sweet feed) or processed into pellets. Under no circumstances should you feed grain to your horse until at least three to four weeks into the refeeding recovery period. When you do feed grain, you should start with half a cup three times a day. All feeding changes should be gradual and cautious. If you feed grain or weight-gain supplements too early, it can impede the return to normal metabolic function, resulting in death.

When ready, a 1,000-pound horse can eat up to 10 pounds of grain in conjunction with 10 pounds of hay. Never exceed more than 50 percent of the ration as concentrated feed (grain). The higher the amount of grain that is fed, the higher the risk of colic, ulcers, and metabolic problems, so stay well below the 50 percent mark.

Complete feeds are also available. These are bagged or packaged products that include a grain component, as well as a high-fiber or roughage content. Equine senior feeds are usually made as a complete feed. Complete feeds include necessary roughage, and are designed to be fed alone. Mixing these products with other grains, such as plain oats, will violate their carefully balanced and fortified vitamin and nutrition ratios.

Choosing which grain to feed is important. An equine senior product is best for elderly horses that may not be able to chew or extract nutrients from hay efficiently. Find out how many calories per pound your feed is. Because of the higher roughage content, some complete feeds are not very calorie-dense, and might not be enough for weight gain in a thin horse.

Feeding Fats

Horses do not have a gallbladder. The purpose of the gallbladder is to store digestive enzymes produced by the liver, known as bile. Bile is released into the small intestine when a meal is eaten, and breaks down fats. Since horses have a relatively small stomach and mainly eat low-fat plants in a slow grazing manner, the gallbladder became an unnecessary appendage for them. A horse's liver has a duct that leads straight to the small intestine, which releases tiny amounts of bile as it is produced.

The lack of bile limits the ability of the horse to digest fats. Forages contain 3 to 4 percent fat, although with an adjustment period, horses can tolerate up to 20 percent of their dietary calories from fat. However, UC Davis research showed that fat supplementation in the initial refeeding period did not improve horses' recovery.[50]

Beyond the refeeding period, fat supplementation is useful for increasing weight gain, particularly if a horse has trouble chewing forage. Any horse who has trouble maintaining his weight (a *hard keeper*) needs a diet high in digestible fiber and fat.

Many weight-building supplements are commercially available, and nearly all are based on some type of fat. Liquid oils such as canola, rice bran, flaxseed, soy, corn, or mixed vegetable oil can be top-dressed on sweet feed or pellets and fed to horses. Begin with one teaspoon twice daily, and over the next four to six weeks, work up to one half cup twice daily. A cup of these oils is about 1,950 calories—more calories than a pound of sweet feed. You may choose to use a particular oil based on cost, palatability, and omega-3 to omega-6 fatty acid ratios. Horses need more omega-6 than omega-3 fatty acids, but the omega-3 oils are more important for their beneficial properties, such as immunity, joint health, and anti-inflammatory effects.

Use of Probiotics

Horses are dependent on symbiotic microbes to digest cellulose (the fiber portion of forage). Starvation changes the bacterial population of the gut, which within the horse can result in malabsorption and/or diarrhea. Stress can also result in certain bacterial diarrheas. Probiotics may help stabilize or restore digestive health.

There are a number of probiotic products out on the market today. Only one microbe (a member of the yeast family), *Saccharyomyces boulardii*, has been studied. Most equine probiotics contain *S. boulardii* as well as several other live cultures.[51]

LONG-TERM WEIGHT CHANGES

A normal, mature horse needs a minimum of 15,000 calories per day, and one in hard work may need up to double that amount. When you are trying to add weight to your horse, 20,000 calories per day is suggested. A mare in late gestation or lactation also requires more calories to meet her needs—in the range of 25,000 to 30,000 calories per day (fig. 3.9).

If you want to increase your horse's BCS by one point in two months, he must eat 6,000 extra calories per day. This amount is about four pounds of concentrated feed per day. Alternatively, increase hay intake by six to seven pounds, or pasture intake by six hours per day.

What all this information boils down to—realistically—is that it can take six months to a year of aggressive feeding to get a horse back up to a normal weight.

Monitor His Weight

To avoid discouragement, keep a diary of your horse's condition. This can be as simple as recording his BCS and weight each week on a note card that you keep in your feed room. Weekly monitoring by using a weight tape is even better and will allow you to realize that your horse is gaining weight before your eye notices. The weight tape estimates a horse's weight based on the measurement of the circumference at the girth. You can purchase a version of this specially marked tape measure from feed or tack stores or online suppliers. The tape is placed around the horse, behind the withers and elbow, right where your saddle and girth would go. Then, you line up the end of the tape and read the number (figs. 3.10 A–C).

OTHER CONSIDERATIONS FOR REFEEDING RESCUE HORSES

When you are working with an impoundment rescue or horses that have been confiscated for neglect, you may be legally

3.9 Simple Example Rations

Forage	Grain	Oil	Total Energy
Orchard grass, alfalfa mix 17 lbs x 900 cal/lb = 15,300 cal	n/a	n/a	15,300 cal
Grass hay 16 lbs x 850 cal/lb = 13,600 cal	Sweet feed 4 lbs x 1,700 cal/lb = 6,800 cal	n/a	20,400 cal
Included in complete feed	Equine senior complete feed 16 lbs x 1,250 cal/lb = 20,000 cal	n/a	20,000 cal
Alfalfa pellets 15 lbs x 950 cal/lb = 14,250 cal	Sweet feed 4 lbs x 1,700 cal/lb = 6,800 cal	2c = 3,900 cal	24,950 cal

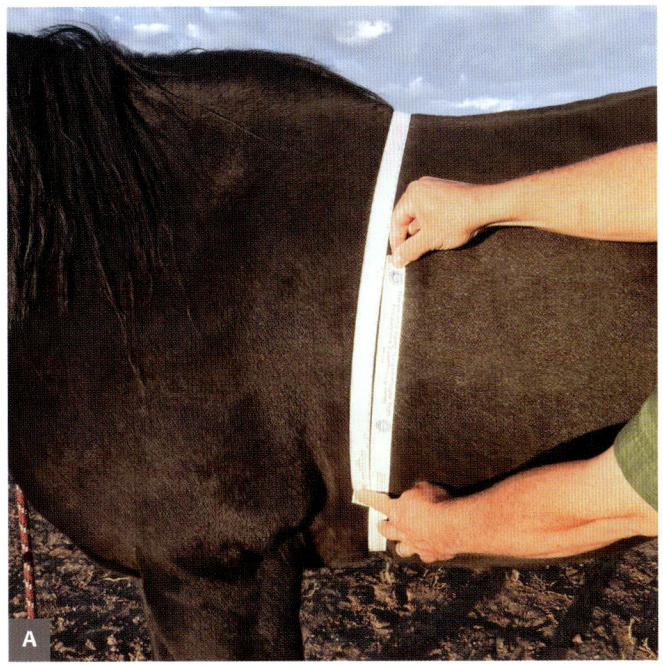
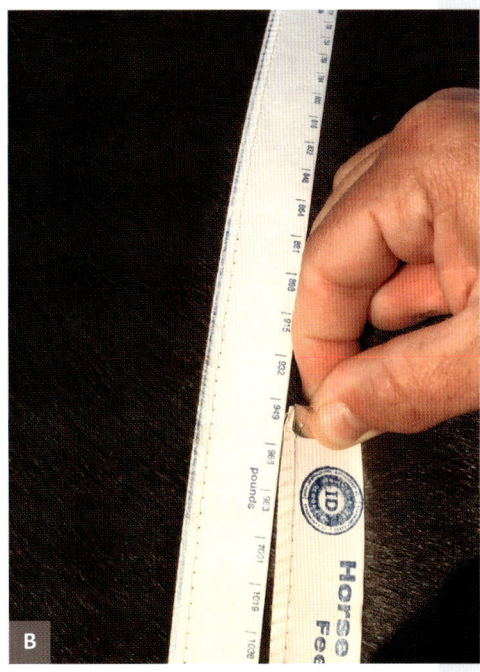

bound to provide only "regular and ordinary" care. Proving that the horse can recover with ordinary and available food supports legal cases of neglect for prosecution, preventing rescuers from resorting to exorbitant and life-saving diagnostics, procedures, or treatments. Proof that the horse was neglected will be what prevents the former neglectful owner from legally acquiring any other horses in the future. The law in this case may be at odds with medicine. This is difficult to adhere to but is the best option we have for ensuring that a neglectful owner is convicted, and preventing them from owning and neglecting many other horses in the future.

It's also important to realize that the gut, like other tissues in the body, may not function properly after extreme starvation. Damage that occurs during starvation may be permanent. Scarring of the digestive tract

Date	Ari	Nina	
	13.3	14.2	
10/8/15	910	1130	
12/16/15	950	1100	
5/1/16	1130	1250	TOOK AWAY SLOW FEEDER
5/10/16	1130	1250	
5/19/16	1015	1190	
5/30/16	1015	1130	
6/10/16	960	1130	
7/4/16	960+	1130	
7/22/16	970	1125	GOT THE SCALE -1 WK AGO
8/1/16	960+	1100	5 LBS EACH
8/8/16	960	1100	5 LBS Ari 6 LBS NiNA

3.10 A–C Using a weight tape to monitor a horse's condition as he improves is important. The correct location of the weight tape is around the horse, just behind the elbows and over the withers (A). This close-up view shows how to read the number in pounds (B). Recording the values allows you to more easily observe trends over time (C).

Part I: Caring for Horses in Need—37

is termed *intestinal fibrosis*. Intestinal fibrosis results in malabsorption (a decreased ability to absorb nutrients). Chronic malabsorption in horses is known to occur after surgical removal of small intestine (a treatment for some types of colic), chronic inflammatory bowel disease, certain bacterial infections, infection with some intestinal parasites, or intestinal *lymphosarcoma* (a cancer).

Veterinarians involved in rescue will tell you that every starvation case is unique.[52] It is critical that you as the rescuer understand the importance of refeeding appropriately. Weight gain can take a long time, just like starvation took a long time. As I stated previously, we expect the horse to metabolically stabilize in the first two weeks but not to gain weight. Real weight gain can take months, and a return to normalcy can take a whole year. This may mean that the horse is always a "hard keeper" who needs special attention and close monitoring.

Psychological Effects of Starvation

Not having enough food is a significant source of mental stress. In the 1940s, Ancel Keys conducted a landmark "Starvation Experiment" at the University of Minnesota. Keys documented the psychological effects of starvation on humans: subjects became depressed, listless, unable to concentrate, socially withdrawn, and apathetic.[53]

Science does not yet fully recognize or understand the psyches of domestic or wild animals. For the sake of argument, let's assume horses experience the world in a way that affects their senses, feelings, emotions, and thought processes. Starvation has negative psychological effects on horses. "In some cases underweight horses may display abnormal behavior in relation to eating, such as aggression during feeding time or *pica* (the ingestion of inappropriate material such as hair, dirt or gravel, or wood). These psychological conditions may not resolve, despite a return to optimum body condition." Pica has been associated with parasites, ingestion of too few calories, and deficiencies of protein, salt, phosphorus, or micronutrients.[54]

A horse who has gone through a state of starvation may never behave "normally" at meal times. He may exhibit anxiety and emotional duress associated with the chronic state of hunger that he experienced.[55]

Extra Winter Care for the Emaciated Horse

A thin horse who has a BCS of 3 or less may have trouble in the cold. Horses are cold-adapted and will grow a heavy protective hair coat as needed. A blanket may help your horse if he has a BCS of 3 or less, and it is exceptionally cold for your area. Studies show that a horse's natural coat is best for optimal thermoregulation,[56] but without an adequate layer of fat, a rescue horse will struggle to maintain his body temperature during particularly cold temperatures.

If used, blankets should always be clean and dry. They should be removed and the horse inspected and groomed daily. A blanket or heavy hair coat can mask weight loss or weight gain.

DENTISTRY

Traditional horse-person lore purports that an old horse is also a thin horse. Good horse care requires you to abandon this mythology. If your horse is aged and has dental disease to the extent that he cannot chew

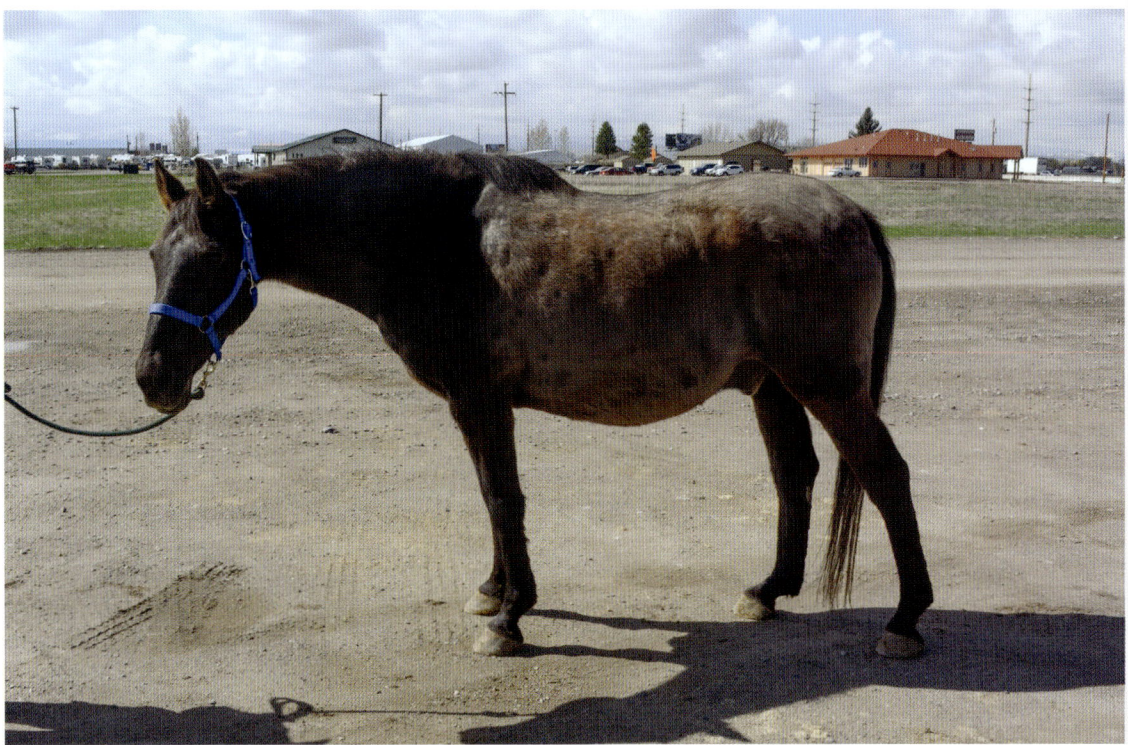

3.11 This horse is in his thirties and has been well-fed. Despite missing some teeth, his weight is appropriate. Old age is not an excuse for a thin horse.

regular hay, there are complete feed options that will meet his needs. Fortified grains and dietary supplements are available to modern horse owners. Age is no excuse for caloric deficiency—horses should be maintained at a healthy weight at every age (fig. 3.11).[57]

Poor dental health can be a reason for weight loss because chewing food is the first step of digestion. A horse must chew his food well in order to digest it. Absorption of nutrients is inversely related to particle size—smaller particles have a larger overall surface area for the same amount of ingesta (food). The larger the surface area, the more absorption can occur from that particle.[58]

Horses' grinding teeth are *hypsodont* where the root of each tooth, which brings in the blood and nerve supply, is relatively

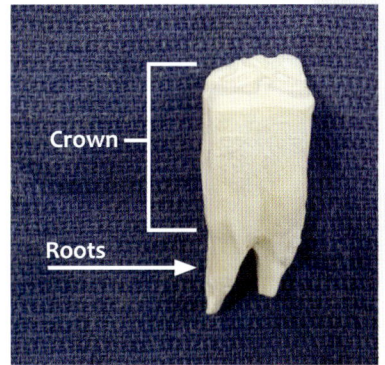

3.12 A hypsodont horse tooth showing the short root and the relatively long crown. This tooth is from an older horse, and the long crown is even more exaggerated in a young adult horse.

small compared to the oversized crown (fig. 3.12). The long reserve crown sits below the gum line within the jaw and sinus cavities. The reserve crown erupts as needed when the exposed crown is worn down. The tooth has many ridges of alternating hard enamel folded with softer dentin, which form the grinding surface. The horse moves his jaw from

Part I: Caring for Horses in Need—39

side to side to break down forage—I think of it as a built-in cornmeal grinder.

Each upper and lower molar pair should line up perfectly. As they grind away at the forage, they are worn away. The wear is countered by continual eruption, so that each arcade of teeth remains flat and functions as a large grinding surface working in concert.

Trouble occurs when the teeth don't match up perfectly or horses are fed lots of concentrate with little forage, causing abnormal wear. Tooth alignment seems to have a lot to do with genetics. We maintain tooth health by removing any mismatched tooth areas that are not ground away by the opposing tooth (figs. 3.13 A–D) in a process known as floating (fig. 3.14).

Uncared for teeth can be a source of discomfort for the rescue horse and a reason

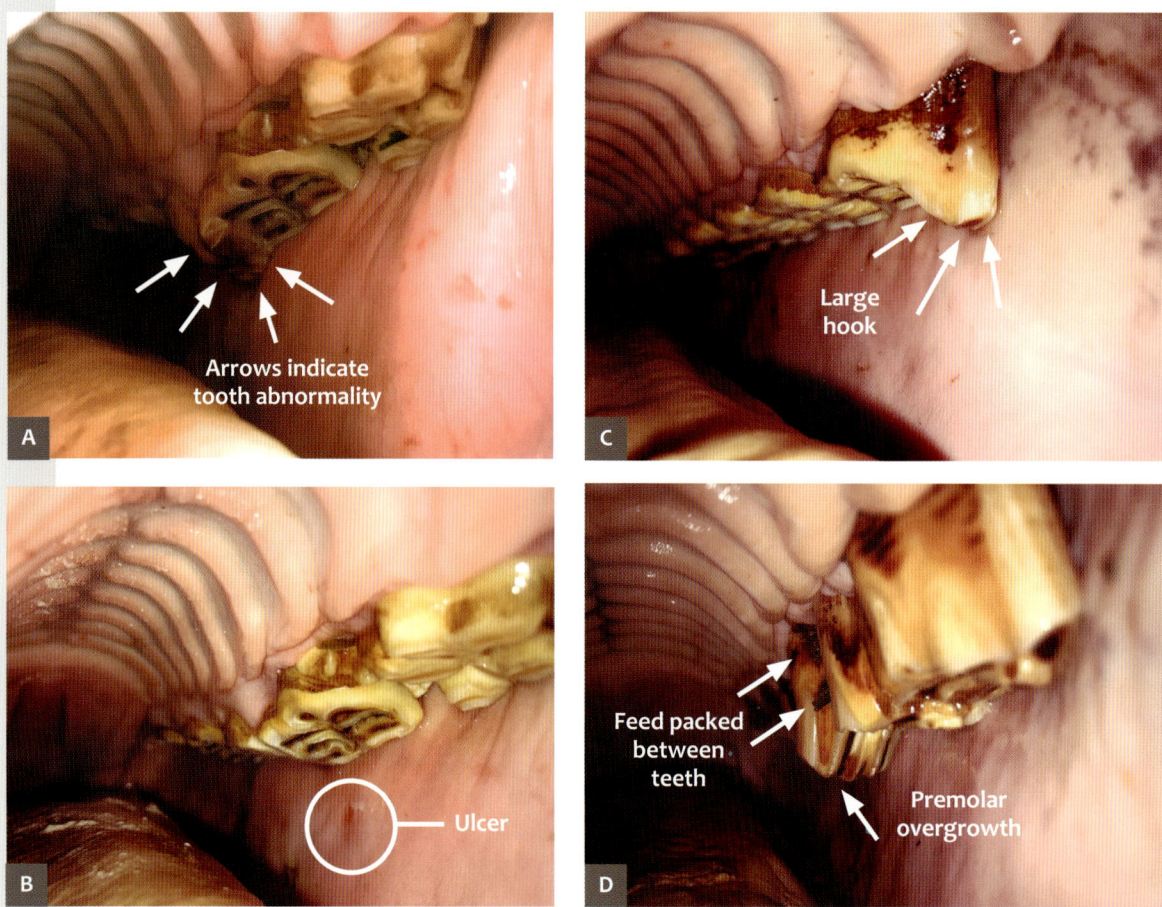

3.13 A–D An abnormal tooth in a young horse that has led to misalignment and abnormal wear (A). The same tooth after being "floated." There is an ulcer on the horse's cheek where the sharp point had been rubbing (B). An abnormal "hook" on a premolar that has resulted from teeth that do not align perfectly (C). An abnormally overgrown premolar in a geriatric horse (D). This horse was unable to chew forage. After correction, his hay consumption improved, but he will need access to concentrated or complete feeds to maintain a healthy weight into his golden years.

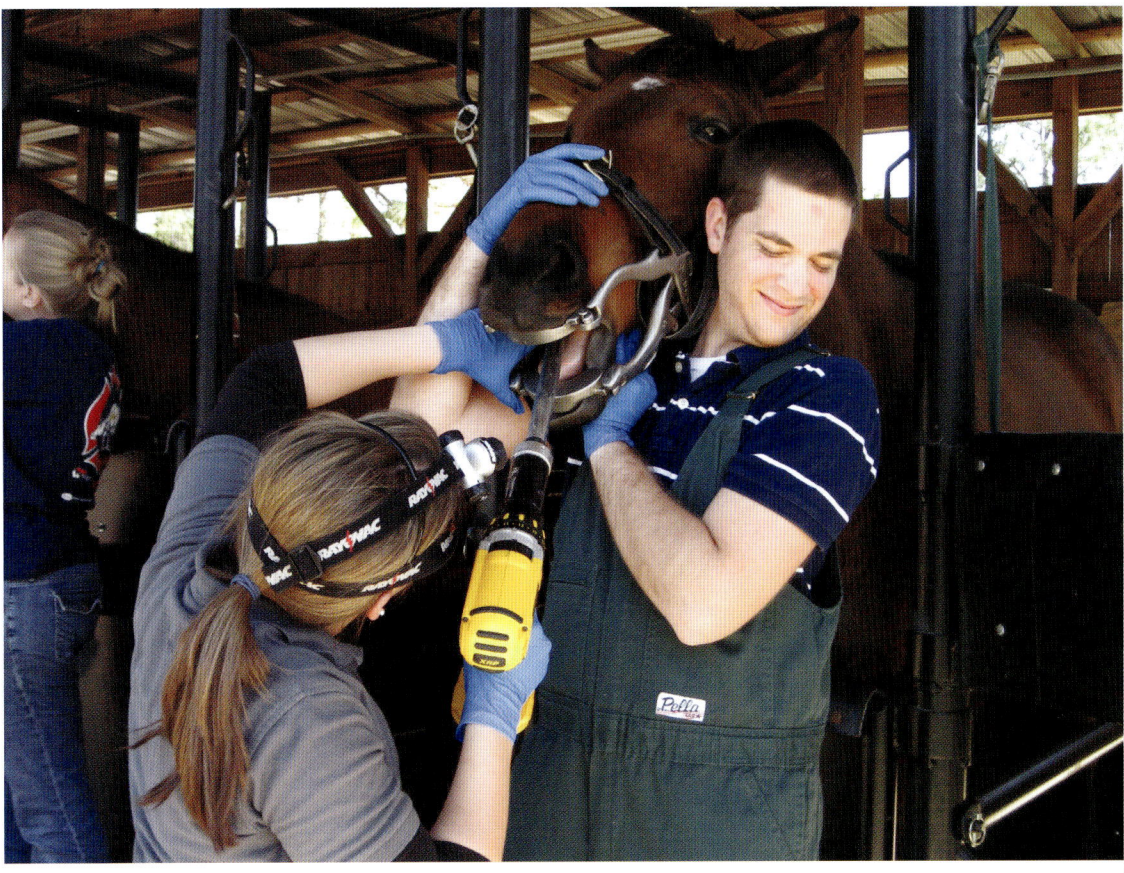

3.14 A horse's teeth being floated.

he isn't digesting his food. Unfortunately, there is a limited amount of tooth that can be removed in one float procedure without causing harm. If your veterinarian cannot correct all problems, she may suggest floating the horse again in a few months; otherwise, annual dental examination is recommended (fig. 3.15).

Although the horse's teeth are continually erupting throughout his life, at some point the tooth becomes fully erupted, and the hard grinding enamel wears smooth. These horses are referred to as *smooth-mouthed*, and this was historically considered the kiss of death (fig. 3.16). A smooth-mouthed horse succumbs to starvation even when hay is in front of him at all times.

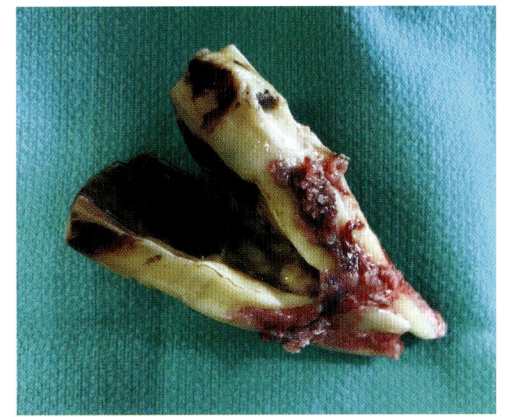

3.15 A broken first molar from a rescued horse. This horse had right-sided nasal discharge because of a sinus infection due to the loss of tooth integrity. Although it had been going on for four years, after the abnormal molar was removed the infection and nasal discharge resolved completely.

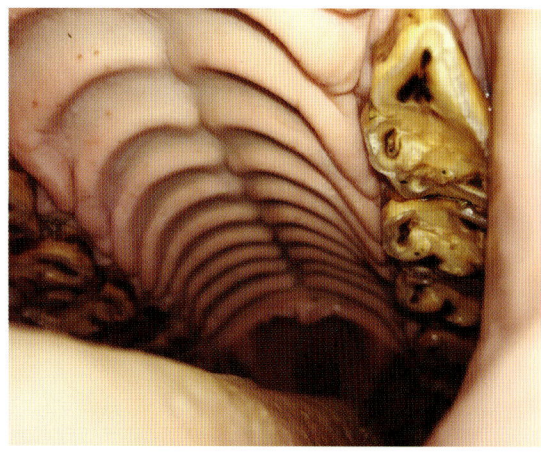

3.16 *Smooth teeth that are at the end of their wear life. This horse will not be able to grind forage.*

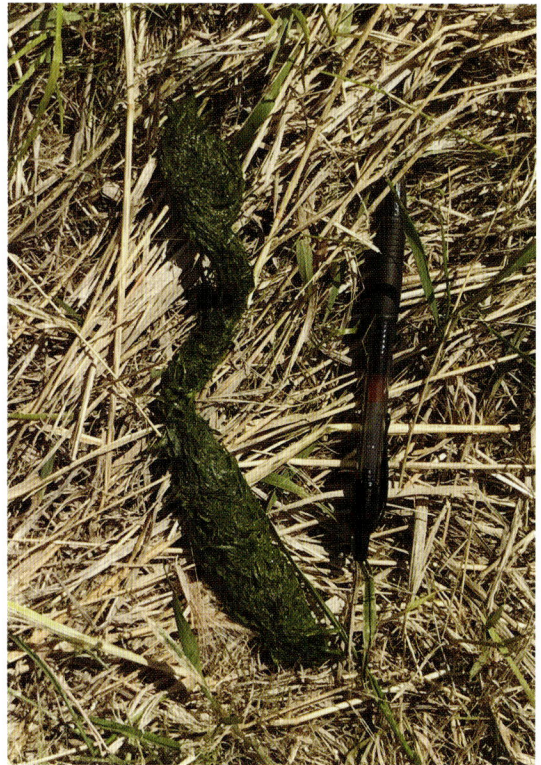

3.17 *A fresh quid (wad of unchewed forage) from a smooth-mouthed horse.*

Horses that chew abnormally may *quid*. A quid is a bit of semi-chewed forage that the horse does not swallow, but rather, spits out (fig. 3.17). When a horse cannot chew hay and is quidding, he should be given other feed that requires less chewing. Available options include pelleted forages such as alfalfa, timothy, or combinations. Complete senior feed rations often contain beet pulp as the fiber, and are vitamin and mineral fortified in a way that hay or alfalfa pellets aren't. Oils, as discussed above, can be added to increase easily digestible calories. For a horse who cannot chew, pellets and complete feeds should be soaked before feeding.

Some of the most heartbreaking horses are those that choose not to eat the pelleted feeds. The old adage, "You can lead a horse to water, but you can't make him drink" seems to apply here. If the opportunities are provided, but the horse does not maintain his weight at a minimum BCS of 4, euthanasia should be considered. When horses do choose to eat the pelleted feeds, many live well into their thirties and some into their forties—a significant feat with no functional teeth. The Remus Memorial Horse Sanctuary in Britain apparently knows how to keep geriatric horses well fed. They had a mare, Orchid, who lived to be 50, and a gelding, Shayne, who held a world record and lived to 51 (fig. 3.18).

Cost is a factor when maintaining a horse who needs a complete feed ration. It can cost hundreds of dollars per month to feed horses with unusable teeth. These horses may be unaffordable.

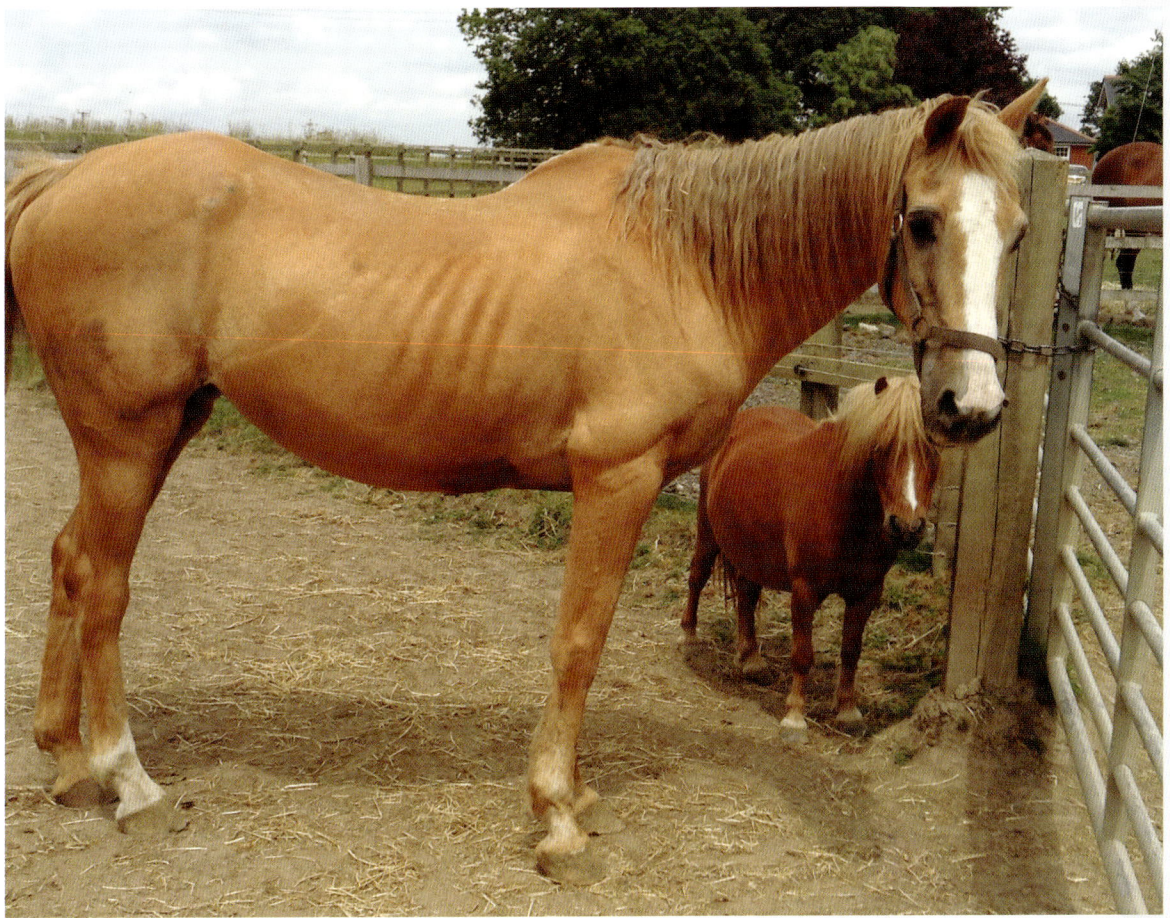

3.18 Orchid, a horse who lived to be 50 years old.

OTHER REASONS FOR WEIGHT LOSS

Caloric deficiency is by far the most common reason for weight loss in horses. Teeth play a role in the development of malnutrition, but there are other illnesses that contribute to a horse having an abnormally low BCS. These include digestive deficiencies (such as ulcers of the colon or stomach), kidney or liver disease, and infections. Parasites can also be a factor.

The problems listed above are not identifiable from the outside of the horse, which is one reason why having blood work done at intake is so critical (see p. 24). The results of the blood work may strongly influence how a horse is rehabilitated. For example, a horse with kidney disease should not be fed alfalfa. And, no matter how much you feed a horse with peritonitis (infection of the abdominal cavity), he isn't going to gain weight until the infection is treated. He is going to feel ill and not eat, even when food is offered.

A horse with a tumor or cancer can experience extreme weight loss—called *cancer cachexia*. Even with blood work, it may be difficult to identify this particular internal problem, but the horse will not respond to the prescribed feeding program as others have. This is one reason why starting with a guideline and standard is important. Of course, the program should be tailored to each horse. Knowing where you started and what to expect helps you know when and where to tweak the nutritional program. Close monitoring and record keeping will help you and your veterinarian identify a horse who is underperforming when it comes to expected weight gain.

If end-stage organ failure is an underlying reason for a horse being unable to maintain his weight, an ethics question arises. How long do you let the horse continue in a state of starvation with no real cure for the organs that aren't working? The answer must be decided on a case-by-case basis, with caretakers' and veterinary input.

Signs of Colic

- Lying down repeatedly or rolling
- Pawing
- Kicking at belly
- Flank watching
- Sweating
- Stretching out or posturing to urinate
- Painful grimace
- Decreased or absent appetite
- Depression or lethargy
- Abnormal consistency or volume of feces

Gastric Ulcers

The only way to know for sure if a horse has an ulcer in his stomach—a gastric ulcer—is if a gastroscopy (looking into the stomach with an endoscope or miniature camera) is done. The endoscope must be 3 meters (9 feet) long to reach the horse's stomach.

There are behaviors that may raise your suspicion that your rescue horse has a gastric ulcer. Sometimes the horse will begin to eat grain, and then appear to be uncomfortable and stop eating the grain. Some horses will exhibit chronic, low-grade, repeat episodes of colic. A few horses will exhibit pain when being tacked up.

Travel, stress, use of non-steroidal anti-inflammatory medications, stall confinement, and twice-daily feeding of high levels of high-starch feed contribute to ulcer formation. Treatment is with omeprazole (Gastroguard® or Ulcerguard®).

COLIC

Colic is a general term for abdominal pain, and there are a multitude of specific disease processes that result in colic. Most of these disease processes involve the digestive tract.

Signs of Colic

Signs of colic vary. The severity of the underlying problem may change the magnitude of the colic signs. Factors about the horse also influence the intensity of signs—some horses are more sensitive than others and display a more conspicuous pain response. Horses that do this may be young, a sensitive breed (Arabians and Thoroughbreds, for example), or flighty, nervous individuals. Cold-blooded breeds like Clydesdales or other draft horses, stoic breeds like

Tennessee Walking Horses and Quarter Horses, or older horses might not express colic signs as strongly.

Signs of colic may include repeatedly changing position from standing to lying down, or lying down and being unwilling to get up. A horse may also be rolling, kicking at his belly, watching or looking at his flank, or stretching out (which sometimes can look like he is trying to urinate, but can't). Most horses have a decreased appetite, and some are lethargic or depressed. Some horses will exhibit a wrinkled lip and nostril flare that is characteristic of pain. Signs that your horse has a more severe problem include a lack of response to Banamine® (flunixin meglumine, a pain-relieving medication discussed further in chapter 5—p. 77), and violent rolling, especially if he has damaged the skin of his eyelids or head while trying to rid himself of pain. He needs veterinary attention immediately if you see any of these signs.

Generally, it is a good idea to monitor fecal output closely. A decrease in fecal output can forewarn of an impending episode of colic, and when your horse's stool is either abnormally dry or turns to diarrhea, these are also signs of problems within the gastrointestinal tract. Although horse lore says that when a colicking horse defecates, the trouble has been resolved, this isn't always true. Signs of colic pain should be attended to no matter what is happening with the poop.

Types of Colic

The two most common types of colic are *gas colic* and *impaction*. Impaction in horses is similar to constipation in humans. An impaction occurs when the material in your horse's gastrointestinal tract moves more slowly than usual, leading to a backup. In horses, the obstruction is usually in the large colon, which is before the 10 to 12 feet of small colon that leads to the rectum. However, impactions can occur in other areas as well.

Many risk factors for colic cause a decrease in gut motility. This gastrointestinal movement slows if the horse becomes dehydrated: The horse's body tries to restore a normal blood volume by extracting more water from the gastrointestinal contents. This results in thicker, dryer feed material, which is more difficult to move through the digestive tract.

Electrolytes are also important to the normal muscle contraction that is responsible for gut motility. The two most important electrolytes for the contractility are calcium and potassium. The horse will lose these electrolytes and others (sodium, chloride, and magnesium) through sweat. Finally, the horse may experience changes in motility related to changes in exercise or feed.

Impaction Colic: About 4 to 10 percent of horses colic each year,[59, 60] and newly re-homed horses have an extra high risk. Risk factors for their development of impaction colic include: abrupt changes in feed, a change in housing or daily exercise levels, electrolyte deficiencies or imbalances, stress, and long hours of travel with consequent dehydration. Horses that travel drink less water than normal, even when available to them during the ride.

Gas Colic: Gas in the colon causes horses to experience severe gas pain, just as humans sometimes do. Gas colic can occur after a change in feed, travel, or a change in the weather. Most of the time, controlling the

Hobby Horse Rescuer

During my veterinary training, I spent a few weeks as a guest at a university's surgical facility. I will never forget the case or the people who owned this rescue horse. The long-yearling filly was a lovely palomino, but she was thin, with a BCS of 3. Her people had owned her for such a short period of time, she didn't even have a name yet. She was lying in the stall where anesthesia was induced before horses were moved into the surgical suite. We could not subdue her pain enough to keep her standing. While lying on the ground, the filly suddenly started kicking all of her legs quite violently. She was in agony.

I accompanied the surgeon responsible for the case as she talked to the owners. They appeared to have no idea what they were doing—they did not have the appearance of horse people. Sandra wore jeans and a nice shirt, with practical hiking shoes, but her husband was dressed in a tailored suit and tie. Their daughter was still dressed in a cheerleading outfit from a school event earlier that evening and did not seem interested in the horse. The dire situation was explained to these people, but I wasn't sure how much they understood. Sandra said she had rescued the palomino and intended to give the filly whatever she needed. She said to go ahead with surgery. I wondered if she had any idea about horse handling and if she would be able to care for the horse's medical requirements after surgery.

The filly was anesthetized and moved into the operating room. After several hours of work, about 20 gallons of pea-sized gravel was removed from her gut.

As the filly recovered, Sandra visited her in the hospital daily. One day Sandra brought a thick scrapbook filled with brightly colored paper, photographs, and decorations. It contained images of horse after horse that Sandra had rescued and re-homed. She had helped dozens of horses, and she knew a lot more about rescuing horses than I initially gave her credit for.

Sandra explained that when she developed empty nest syndrome after her son left for college and her daughter entered high school, she decided that rescuing horses would be her hobby. This wasn't the first time she had taken a horse to surgery, either. Sandra had the financial resources and time to pursue whatever entertainment or hobby she wanted to, and she was dedicated to helping one horse at a time, and then finding permanent homes for each one.

The filly fully recovered, and Sandra's devotion still inspires me.

pain until the gas passes is all that can be done. Walking the horse keeps the intestines moving, allowing the gas to be expelled.

Preventing Colic

Hydration: Keeping your horse well hydrated is the single most important factor in preventing colic. Maintenance of hydration may be difficult on long trailer rides, but every attempt should be made to offer water. Even a warm horse should have access to water to replenish fluids lost through sweating. At a minimum, make sure your horse has access to water before setting out and immediately upon arrival.

Many people try to entice a horse to drink unfamiliar water by using Gatorade or Kool-Aid powder, or adding apple juice. The water can be flavored at home for a few days before using the same flavor when traveling. While this process is helpful for some horses, it is labor-intensive, and may not be possible in all settings.

Probably the most helpful tactic to encourage drinking is to get the horse comfortable and relaxed in his surroundings. This may mean adding a buddy horse to the pen next to him, or just waiting a few hours for him to acclimate to the new location. Of course, any water you offer should be clean and fresh.

Avoid Sudden Changes in Feed: To minimize abrupt feeding changes, offer as similar a forage as possible to what your horse was previously eating. It is safe to skip grain completely as your horse settles in.

If your horse refuses to drink and has a reduced fecal output, feed a soaked replacement roughage, such as alfalfa pellets. Depending on availability, grazing on fresh green grass for a few minutes can be helpful. You may consider adding some flax seed or other type of oil to his ration to help keep things moving smoothly.

Access to electrolytes is important. A salt block should be provided, but loose mineral is better absorbed and utilized by your horse's body.

Veterinary Evaluation and Treatment of Colic

With an unhandled horse, treatment is challenging. This is one reason why halter training your rescue horse is so important.

The standard basic colic workup includes pain medication, tubing the horse, and doing an examination *per rectum*. Sedation helps facilitate these diagnostic and therapeutic procedures.

Pain control is primarily through administration of Banamine®, which can be given either in a vein or orally. Additional medications or sedatives may be used by your veterinarian.

Fluids and a cathartic may be administered through a stomach tube. Common cathartics include Epsom salts, electrolytes, mineral oil, or the surfactant DSS (dioctyl sodium sulfosuccinate). You may be familiar with DSS because it is marketed for human use as stool-softener capsules.

The stomach tube also is considered a diagnostic procedure. Horses can't vomit, so if there is pressure in an overly full stomach, the contents may be expelled via the tube. The odor, consistency, and color of the stomach contents can be informative about the type of colic the horse has.

Examination per rectum allows your veterinarian to palpate the reachable portions of the gastrointestinal organs. If abnormalities are present, they can be more specifically addressed.

Further Treatment and Management of Colic: After diagnostics and treatment, your veterinarian will advise you how to modify your feeding regimen until your horse is fully recovered. You may be told to hold off feeding your rescue horse until he defecates. As part of the effort to get the guts moving, you may be asked to walk or exercise your horse to increase gastrointestinal motility.

Most colics (90 to 95 percent) are caused by an impaction or gas and, with basic first-line treatment, will work themselves out in about 12 to 72 hours. There are more serious causes of colic, and referral for further evaluation and medical treatment for these horses can be in the thousands of dollars if the horse is in the hospital.

A portion of that cost is further diagnostics, such as ultrasound, blood work, and assessment of a sample of fluid from within the abdomen. The most serious problems require surgery, but this occurs in 5 percent or fewer cases of colic.

UNDERSTANDING IS CRITICAL FOR SUCCESS

A horse who is starving due to calorie deficiency can actually die if fed improperly, especially if it is too much and too soon. Understanding forage types and a feeding plan is critical for success. Dental care is important for maintaining the horse's ability to eat and digest food, although other factors and illnesses can play a role. Colic is common in horses that have been re-homed due to travel and changes in diet and housing.

CHAPTER 4

Germs and Worms:
Vaccination and Parasite Management

Routine, preventive care for horses includes parasite management or deworming and vaccination to prevent illness. I'll jump right in and talk about current guidelines.

PARASITE MANAGEMENT AND DEWORMING

When a horse has trouble maintaining weight, one of the first things that people tend to blame is internal parasitism, or "worms." It is rare for an adult horse to have enough parasites to truly be the only source of weight loss. Horses' immune systems have been developed over millennia to deal with internal parasites and keep them at bay—or at least keep their numbers to a minimum. Compared to free-ranging horses of eons ago, horses in our modern era are kept in smaller areas and are more likely to be exposed to large numbers of parasite eggs. Just as bacteria can be resistant to antibiotic drugs, parasites develop resistance to dewormer medications.

There are three reasons to evaluate the quantity of parasite eggs in feces. First, a neglected horse should be appropriately dewormed so that his newfound nutrition goes to his body and not to the parasites. The second reason to check for internal parasites is to prevent a horse who is shedding a large number of parasite eggs from contaminating clean paddocks and pastures. He should stay in quarantine until his fecal egg count is sufficiently low.

Thirdly, if you work with a rescue organization that is trying to prove a case of neglect, documenting fecal egg counts is useful. If the horse is thin *without* parasites, it shows that the horse did not have access to adequate nutrition. If an entire group of horses has abnormally high fecal egg counts, it shows that basic medical needs were not attended to.

Parasite Management

Before *anthelmintic* (anti-parasite) drugs were available, the only way to combat intestinal parasites was manure and pasture management to reduce exposure. When *levamisole* became available in 1966 and *ivermectin* in 1971, they seemed a miracle cure. However, over a couple of decades, it was clear that dewormers did not kill all the parasites. Some individual worms were not susceptible to the anthelmintic used. These worms were resistant and survived.

Veterinary medicine has tried (and

failed) to prevent resistance from happening: administration of a low dose of dewormer medication in the form of daily flavored pellets was recommended for a period of time. The thought was that if we killed all the worms, none would exist to become resistant. This approach quickly selected for worms that survive despite administration of these chemicals.

Scientists devised another tactic to prevent parasite resistance: *rotational deworming* schedules. It was thought that if some worms were not killed by Dewormer A, they could then be killed the next time around using Dewormer B, or Dewormer C. It was only a few years before it was noted that parasites were resistant to multiple dewormers.

Scientifically, we have come full circle and now veterinary medicine recommends manure and pasture management as the mainstay of internal parasite control. These strategies reduce the exposure an animal has to parasite eggs. This is critical for ensuring that internal worm numbers (a horse's *parasite burden*) are minimized. Dewormers should be reserved for when they are necessary.

Toxicity and Environmental Concerns

Parasite resistance is not the only reason to avoid use of chemicals; there are also toxicity and environmental concerns.

Toxicity to other animals commonly occurs after the medication passes through the horse. For example, farm dogs that eat horse feces may ingest toxic levels of ivermectin. Those that are highly sensitive to ivermectin include Collies, Australian Shepherds, Sheepdogs, and related breeds. In susceptible individuals, toxicity causes twitching, seizures, blindness, and other neurologic problems, which in some cases progresses to death.

Another serious problem of parasiticides is toxicity to natural, beneficial insect populations and water-dwelling animals. Experiments have shown suppression of insects in,

4.1 A & B *Adult intestinal parasites expelled in feces after their host horse was dewormed: Small strongyles from an adult horse (A) and roundworms (ascarids) from a young horse (B).*

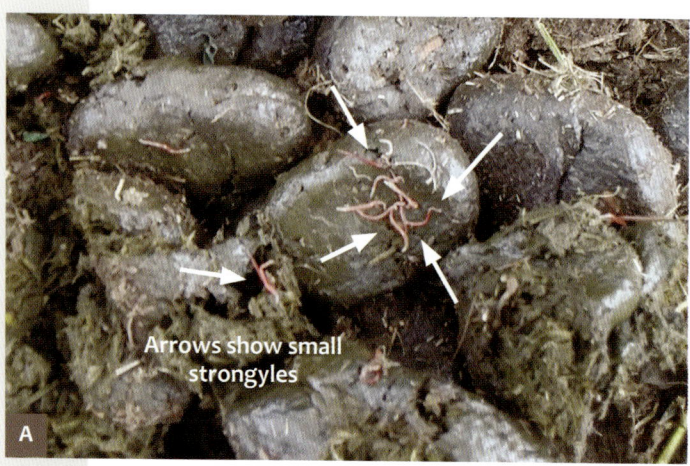
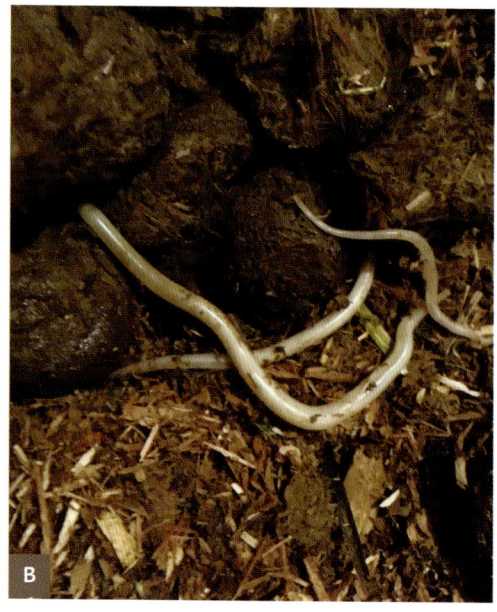

and delayed degradation of, cattle feces after treatment with parasiticides. Dung beetles and other insects are responsible for breaking feces down to keep pastures healthy. In addition to killing insects, dewormers are toxic to many aquatic species including fish, crustaceans, aquatic bacteria, and oysters.[61, 62]

Manure Management

To understand how to manage parasites, you must understand their lives. Intestinal parasites generally have an oral-fecal life cycle. The adult parasite lives happily in the intestine, expelling eggs that are then shed by the host animal in its feces. A horse then ingests the eggs or hatched larvae, which grow internally into adult worms (figs. 4.1 A & B).

Heat, ultraviolet light and desiccation destroy parasite eggs. As I've said, manure management is the single most important factor in effectively reducing parasite populations. Cleaning pens, pastures, and paddocks is critical for parasite control. Manure composting effectively kills parasite eggs: when the temperature reaches 122 to 140 degrees Fahrenheit, eggs become non-viable.[63, 64]

If you have a traditional, green-grass horse pasture that has been used for many years, it may be highly contaminated with parasite eggs, which can survive for years in the right conditions. You can reduce contamination by grazing another species, such as sheep or cattle. Other animals will ingest the eggs, but they will not complete their life cycle in a non-host species. Another way to help reduce pasture contamination is to identify horses who are *high-shedders*. They are 10 to 20 percent of

Modified McMaster's Fecal Evaluation

Here is McMaster's technique for quantifying parasite eggs shed in feces. This test targets strongyles and ascarids (figs. 4.2 A–E):

1 The setup of supplies for the McMaster's fecal egg count: fecal flotation solution, specific measuring (graduated) cylinder, small syringe, and microscope chamber slide with grid (A).

2 The graduated cylinder is first filled to the 26 ml line with fecal flotation solution (B).

3 Feces is used to fill the cylinder to the 30 ml line, thus quantifying the amount of feces used for testing. The mixture is stirred well (C).

4 The syringe is used to fill both chambers on the gridded slide (D).

5 Strongyle eggs within the grid are counted and multiplied by a factor of 25 for the final eggs per gram (EPG) value (E).

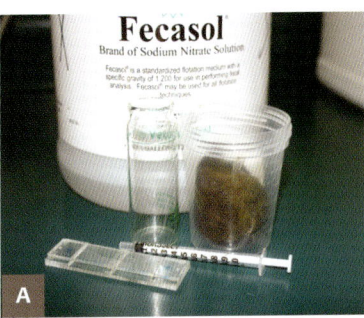
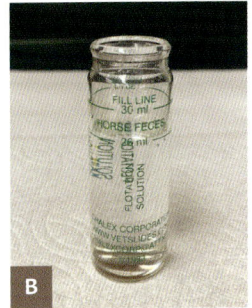
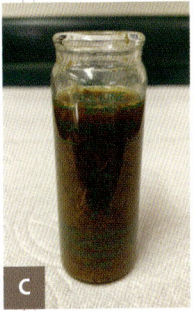
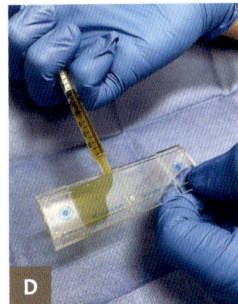
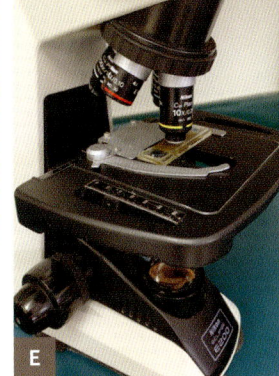

4.2 A–E McMaster's technique for quantifying parasite eggs shed in feces. This test targets strongyles and ascarids.

the horse population, but contribute up to 80 percent of the pasture contamination.[65]

Fecal Egg Count

Your veterinarian will identify horses that shed a high number of parasite eggs by doing twice yearly McMaster's fecal egg counts. This laboratory test quantifies the parasite eggs per gram of feces (EPG). Small strongyles are the most important parasite to manage for adult horses in the United States, although the McMaster's fecal egg count detects other intestinal parasites. Collect a fresh fecal sample from your horse. It can be stored in the refrigerator for up to one week prior to analysis.[66]

In arid climates, fecal egg counts are often zero. Deworming is recommended if the fecal egg count is more than 200 EPG. Horses that are mid-range shedders have 200 to 1,000 EPG, while more than 1,000 EPG is considered a high-shedding horse. Animals with parasites that are the major contributor to weight loss may have 10,000 to 75,000 EPG.

After fecal egg count determination, your veterinarian will guide your deworming for best effectiveness. Directions and dosage on the dewormer label should be followed precisely. Inappropriate dosing is less effective for parasite control and may contribute to resistance.

The McMaster's fecal evaluation can also determine if your horses or farm harbors resistant parasites by determining EPG before and after deworming.

No tool is perfect. The McMaster's test does not reliably detect pinworms (fig. 4.3), tapeworms, or bots. Pinworms lay their eggs directly on the horse's tail hair, which are then rubbed off on to fence posts, tree trunks, or other upright objects. Tapeworms shed eggs only intermittently, so it is uncommon to find them in a fecal sample.

The bot fly lays her eggs directly on the

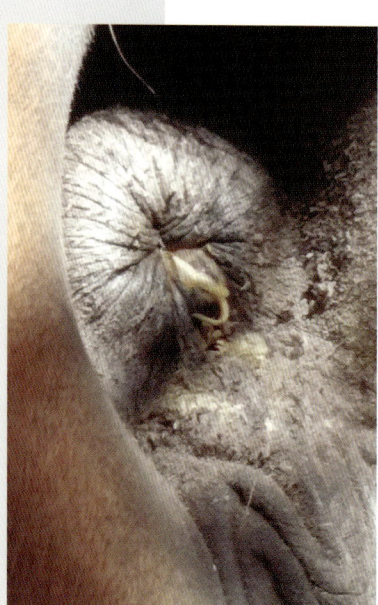

4.3 A pinworm on a horse's anus.

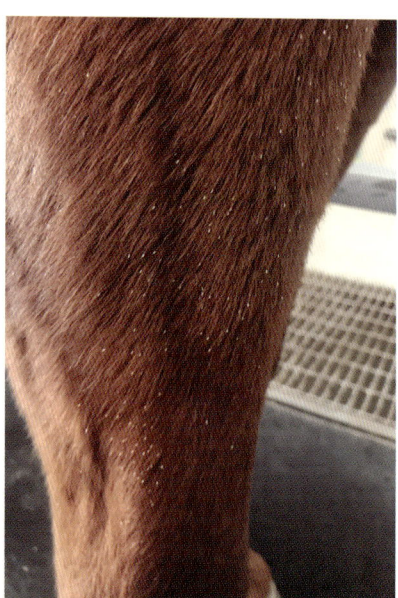

4.4 Typical yellow bot fly eggs on a horse's leg hair.

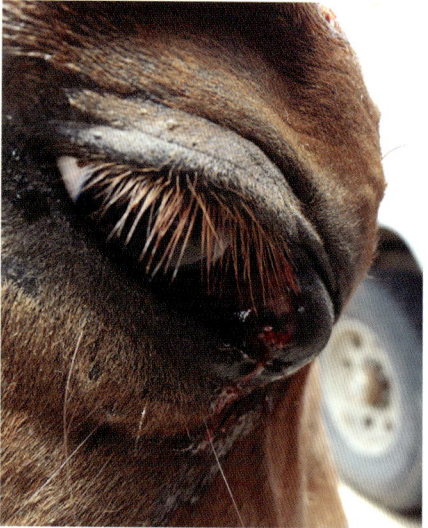

4.5 A horse's eye that has been infested with aberrant *Habronema* larvae. The problem resolved after administration of ivermectin paste.

horse's hair—these are the little yellow nits that you may see on horses' legs in the autumn (fig. 4.4). When your horse scratches his leg with his teeth, he ingests the nits. The eggs sense the warm, moist environment inside the horse and hatch into larvae. The larvae winter over inside your horse's stomach before becoming flies in the spring and repeating the cycle.

Special Cases and Considerations

Some age groups are more prone to parasite problems.[67] Horses less than three years old need a more intense parasite-control program: Younger individuals are more prone to heavy, life-threatening infestations as their immune system is not fully developed to control the parasites.

A heavier worm burden can be present in geriatric adults due to waning immunity. Logically, it follows that older horses with PPID (see p. 25) may have a higher parasite burden because of a compromised immune system.

Habronema are parasitic species prevalent throughout the southwestern United States and are more commonly known as the *stomach worm* (fig. 4.5). Two species affect horses. Aberrant or abnormal migrating larvae can cause skin lesions or conjunctivitis (inflammation around the eye), which is painful. While the larvae of *Habronema* have been identified in fecals, it often is only observed when skin lesions occur during abnormal migration, called *summer sores*. While ivermectin kills larvae, sores or eye problems need further treatment.

Maggots can infest injuries, and ivermectin is a useful adjunct treatment in addition to cleaning and caring for the wounds properly (figs. 4.6 A–C).

Long Ears

Donkeys harbor the *Dictyocaulus arnfieldi* lungworm. This parasitic worm does not typically cause problems for the donkey, but horses that are housed with donkeys in pasture can develop bronchitis or other respiratory signs due to a variation in the parasite life cycle in an atypical host.

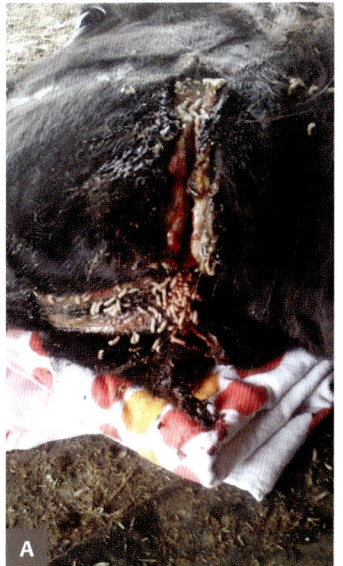
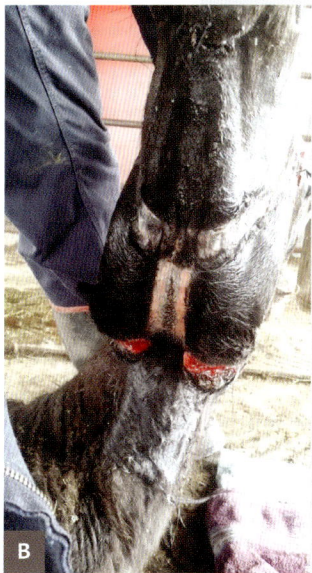
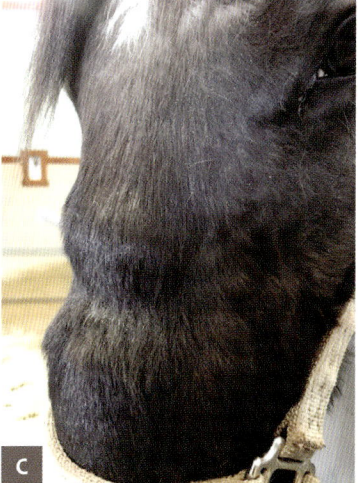

4.6 A–C A rescued horse who had outgrown his halter. He is anesthetized in photos A & B for treatment of the wounds and castration. **The injury is infested with maggots.** Photo C shows the horse a year later, with a permanent bony deformation due to the incident, but a kind attitude and a good home.

Deworming Needy Horses

One troubling point is that deworming is a risk factor for colic. When it comes to an emaciated horse, the first thing he needs is acclimation to a normal nutritional intake. Even if he is a moderate shedder, it may be appropriate to wait until his system adjusts to his new plane of nutrition before deworming.[68] If the fecal egg count is high, deworming him is appropriate, but watch him closely for signs of colic.

As mentioned, deworming horses on a rotational basis is not supported by current science. Overusing dewormer medications is a harmful source of environmental toxicity. Parasite resistance to dewormers is a common problem, making manure and pasture or paddock management critical for modern parasite control.

Fecal egg counts and veterinary consultation should be used to develop an appropriate deworming strategy for each individual horse. It will take into consideration the horse's age, climate, possible parasite exposure, and any special circumstances.

ECTOPARASITES AND SKIN CONDITIONS

External parasites that live on the horse's skin or haircoat are referred to as *ectoparasites*. Many ectoparasites are *vectors* for (carry) diseases. In the United States, major vectors include mosquitos, stable flies, horse flies, and deer flies. In addition to carrying diseases, the bites from these insects can cause local irritation and allergic reactions. Control is through manure management and use of fly spray.

Neglected, unhealthy horses are highly

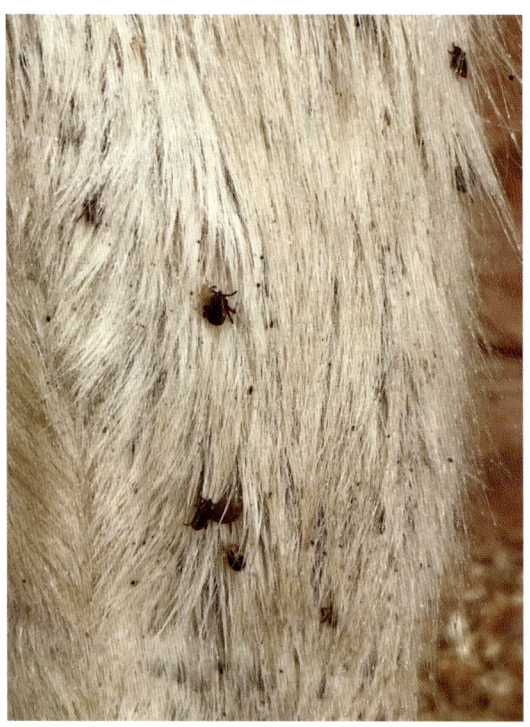

4.7 *Ticks on a severely infested filly. Thousands of ticks were on her, and while the largest ones were removed manually, she was also treated with topical permethrin (fly spray) to kill the remaining ones (this is why her hair is wet in the photo).*

susceptible to harboring ticks and lice and may arrive at your barn carrying large pest populations. Few well-cared-for horses have problems with these parasites. The parasites are a vicious cycle: The unhealthy horse will have a large population, and the enormous population will sap the host horse of nutrients and energy. One reason this happens is because a thin horse needs and will grow a significantly longer hair coat, which shelters the parasites. Also, horses self-groom by rolling, which takes energy a skinny horse may not have.

Reducing the parasite burden helps restore health to an unthrifty horse. *Pyrethrin* or *permethrin* fly spray kills ticks and lice. Their numbers should also be controlled by removing as many as possible by hand or with a comb (fig. 4.7).

Other Skin Conditions

When talking about animals' living conditions, I often think of my veterinary school professor that explained to our class that M.U.D. stood for *manure, urine,* and *dirt.* A poor environment can result in *mud fever* or *scratches* (fig. 4.8). Long-term exposure to moisture destroys the barrier function of the skin, rendering it susceptible to infection. Bacteria invade (*Dermatophilus congolensis* and *Staphylococcus spp,* sometimes with a fungus). Treatment consists of cleaning the area, keeping the horse in a dry place, and applying topical antimicrobial ointments.

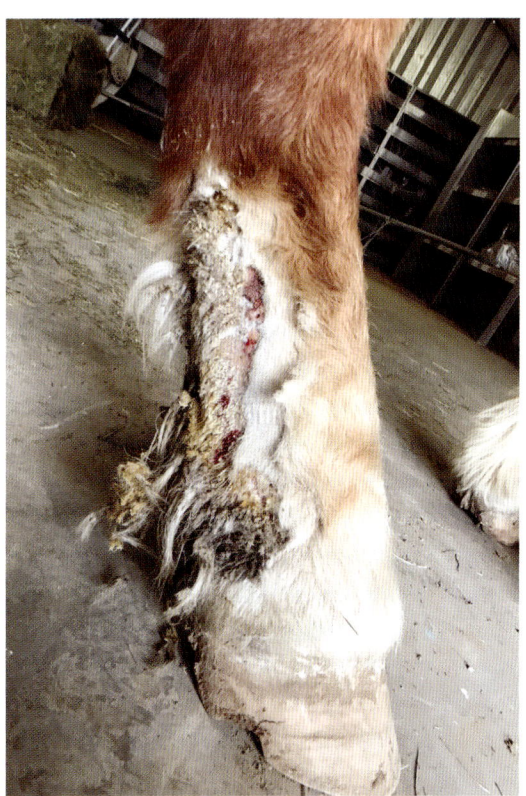

4.8 A severe case of mud fever.

D. congolensis also commonly infects skin over the horse's back and rump, causing scabs, crusting of skin, and hair loss. In this case, the condition is called *rain rot.* Although healthy horses can be affected by rain rot, a long hair coat, lack of shelter, and poor immunity can contribute to the problem in poorly kept horses. It's unusual, but humans can be infected if basic handwashing and hygiene is ignored.

A similar-appearing problem is ringworm, which is actually caused by fungus that causes circular areas of hair loss with crusts around the edge. It is also very itchy. The fungus can be spread by direct contact or by fomites, especially blankets and brushes. Various antifungal sprays or creams are effective treatments. Humans can also get ringworm.

Finally, it should be noted that a dirty haircoat does not insulate well, so unkempt horses must burn more energy to stay warm in cold weather.

VACCINES

We can prevent a large number of devastating diseases with routine vaccination (figs. 4.9 and 4.10). However, the horse's immune system must work to respond to the vaccine and build antibodies.[69] An emaciated horse with a BCS of 1 or 2 cannot be expected to mount an appropriate response.[70] Wait until he gains muscle and strength: If his weakened immune system cannot respond, he might as well not have been vaccinated, leaving him vulnerable to disease. While adverse reactions to vaccines are uncommon, for a horse who is teetering on the edge of health, the benefit may not override the risk until he has gained weight.

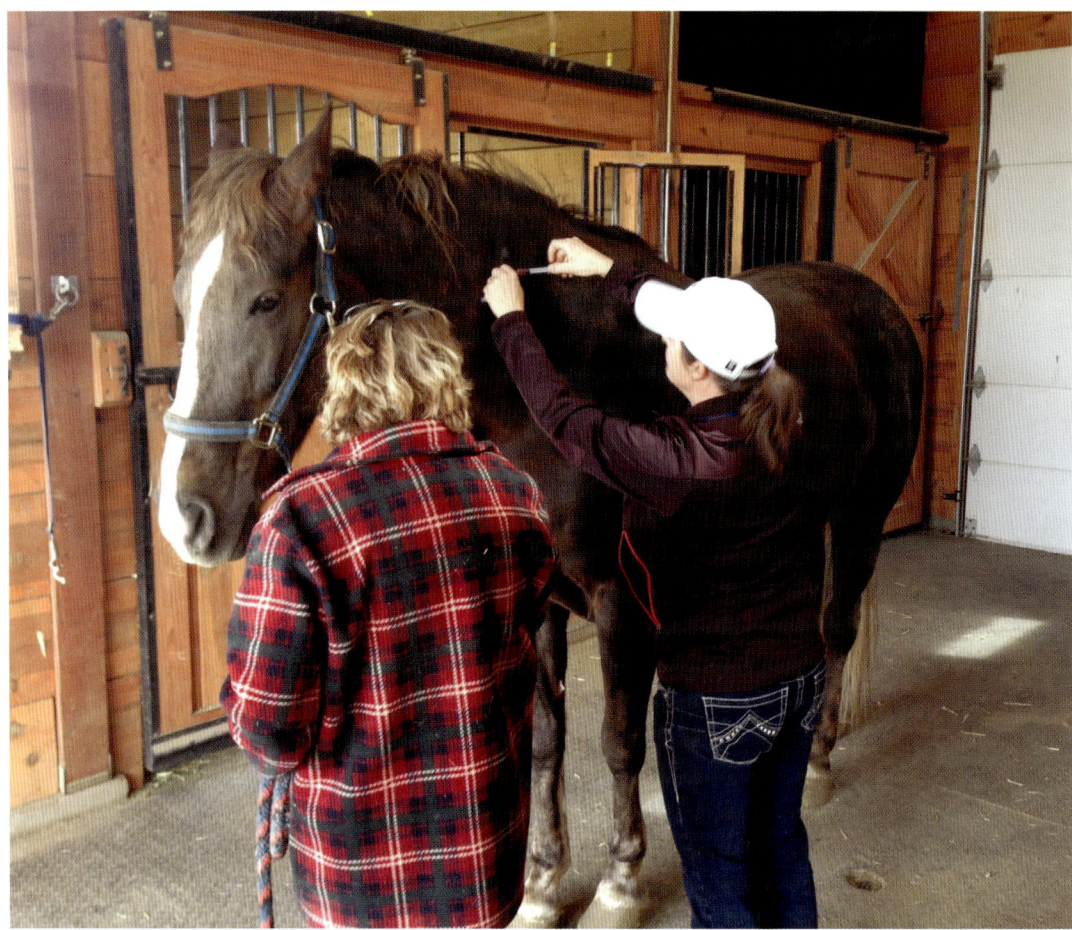

4.9 I am vaccinating this horse to protect him from rabies.

A horse with a BCS of 3 or more and an increasing plane of nutrition can and should be vaccinated.

Annual core vaccine recommendations per the American Association of Equine Practitioners (AAEP) include tetanus, Eastern and Western equine encephalitis (EEE and WEE), West Nile Virus (WNV), and rabies. Vaccination against respiratory diseases (rhinopneumonitis, influenza, and strangles) are based on risk, such as show or travel, or stables that have horses coming and going frequently.

After initial primary immunization, boosters should be administered at two to four week intervals to maximize immunity. Aside from vaccinating your horse, make sure that your established group of horses is fully protected prior to bringing any new horse home.

Most vaccines in horses are injected into muscles of the neck. Occasionally, the pectoral muscles at the base of the chest or the large muscle groups over the croup or rump are used. Some of the respiratory vaccines—strangles and influenza—are formulated as modified live vaccines that are administered *intranasally* (in the nose).

Tetanus

Horses are exceptionally susceptible to tetanus, caused by the bacteria *Clostridium tetani*, which is found ubiquitously in the soil.

C. tetani is anaerobic, and survives only with no oxygen—such as in damaged, necrotic tissue. It does not survive in normal, healthy, oxygenated tissue. *C. tetani* releases a neurotoxin that is absorbed by the peripheral nerves, and ascends to the spinal cord. The neurotoxin causes violent muscle spasms, especially if the animal is stimulated by loud noise. As the bacteria multiply and release their toxin, the local area near the wound is affected first. The next muscle groups affected are those of the face and

4.10 Vaccines

DISEASES OF THE NERVOUS SYSTEM

Disease	Causative Agent	Other Animals Affected	Signs	Vaccine Type	Duration of Immunity
Tetanus	*Clostridium tetani* bacteria	Horses are the most susceptible, but any mammal can be affected	Tetanic (stiff) paralysis	Core; killed bacteria, intramuscular	Three or more years
Rabies	Rabies virus	All mammals, including humans	Neurologic—drooling, muscle problems, 100 percent of infected animals die	Core; killed virus, intramuscular	At least three years for the majority of horses.
Sleeping Sickness	Eastern, Western, and Venezuelan encephalitis viruses	Mammals, including humans, and birds, reptiles, and amphibians	Neurologic—lethargy, seizures, gait abnormalities	Core; killed virus, intramuscular	+/- one year
West Nile Fever	West Nile virus	Mammals, including humans, and birds	General illness; neurologic—tremors, seizures, coma	Core; killed virus, intramuscular	One year

DISEASES OF THE RESPIRATORY SYSTEM

Disease	Causative Agent	Other Animals Affected	Signs	Vaccine Type	Duration of Immunity
Rhinopneumonitis	Equine herpesvirus	n/a	The equine "common cold"; also abortion; rarely neurologic disease	Recommended intramuscular	Four to six months
Influenza	Equine influenza virus	Horses, dogs possibly share a variant	Respiratory illness—cough, nasal discharge	Recommended killed virus, intramuscular; modified live virus, intranasal	About six months
Strangles	*Streptococcus equi equi* bacteria	Horses, many non-diseased carriers	Pus in the guttural pouches; sequela of purpura hemorrhagica	Optional killed bacteria, intramuscular; modified live bacteria, intranasal	One year

jaw—hence the name *lockjaw*. About 80 percent of infected animals succumb to the disease: the paralysis results in the victim being unable to breathe. Animals that recover do not develop protective immunity, only the vaccine provides that.

Tetanus is the foundation of every combination vaccine available for horses. There is also a vaccine for tetanus alone. Standard of care is annual vaccination, but if a horse has surgery or an injury and has not been vaccinated in the last six months, a booster is usually administered.

Rabies

Rabies is a virus that is able to infect any mammal, including humans. There are 20 to 40 confirmed cases of rabies in horses annually in the United States. Wild animals such as skunks, raccoons, and bats harbor the virus. Exposure is via infected saliva through a bite or exposure to a mucous membrane, such as your horse's gums.

Rabies causes neurologic signs: an abnormal gait or staggering, fever, depression, tremors, paralysis, increased sensitivity to stimulation such as touch, and convulsions or seizures. Horses with rabies are sometimes taken to the veterinarian for increased salivation. Unfortunately, this sign then results in an oral examination, which is how humans are exposed.

The vaccine is given in the muscle and provides excellent immunity.[71] Every unvaccinated horse that contracts rabies will die.

Mosquito-Borne Viruses That Affect the Nervous System

Eastern, Western, and Venezuelan Encephalitis: This group of viruses, spread by mosquitoes, causes encephalitis, or inflammation of the encephalon, which is just a fancy word for the brain. These diseases are important because each virus is also capable of infecting a wide range of species, including birds, reptiles, amphibians, and humans. All three viral diseases have been researched by the U.S. government biological weapons program.

Signs of disease are mainly neurologic problems, including fever, increased sensitivity to light, and head-pressing (humans have headaches). Dullness and lethargy can occur, and this is why these diseases are referred to as *sleeping sickness*.

Cases of Eastern encephalitis occur in the humid, eastern area of the United States. There are about 100 to 300 cases in horses per year in horses and 3 to 15 in humans. About half of animals with the disease do not survive. The vaccine in horses lasts about a year, although there seems to be a gap in coverage toward the end of that time, so some horses in high-risk areas are vaccinated twice a year. WEE is typically less severe, with 70 to 80 percent of horses surviving.

West Nile Virus: This is also a mosquito-borne viral disease that causes encephalomyelitis—inflammation of the brain and spinal cord—resulting in neurologic signs. Both horses and humans are susceptible to the disease, although wild birds are the main culprit for harboring and spreading the virus throughout North America.

Horses may have a fever and lethargy or other nonspecific signs of systemic illness, and can recover. Signs of infection specifically in the nervous system are twitching of the muscles of the horse's head, shoulders, and neck. Horses may also have abnormal movement, toe-dragging, stumbling, inability to stand, seizures, coma, or death. Horses with neurologic signs are less likely to recover. The vaccine, given in the muscle, is quite effective.

Respiratory Diseases

Herpes/Rhinopneumonitis: Nine variants of the equine herpesvirus (EHV) have been identified. The most common sign is like our common cold—large amounts of mucous production, fever, cough, and general malaise. Herpes is particularly dangerous, though, because variants of the virus are also known to cause abortion in mares, or, rarely, neurologic infection and disease in any horse.

Several modified live and killed virus vaccines are available to be given intramuscularly. An exception to the BCS guideline of 3 or more is a pregnant mare—she should be immediately vaccinated to help prevent abortion.

Horses with respiratory illness from EHV almost always recover, but horses with neurologic disease have a guarded prognosis.

Influenza: There are many variants of the influenza virus. Like in humans, influenza infecting horses causes a respiratory infection that is typically self-limiting, but occasionally life-threatening. Vaccines are moderately effective, and should be administered to horses once or twice yearly, depending on risk factors (travel or contact with other horses). There is both an intramuscular and an intranasal vaccine formulation.

Strangles: Strangles is a scary-sounding problem caused by the *Streptococcus equi*

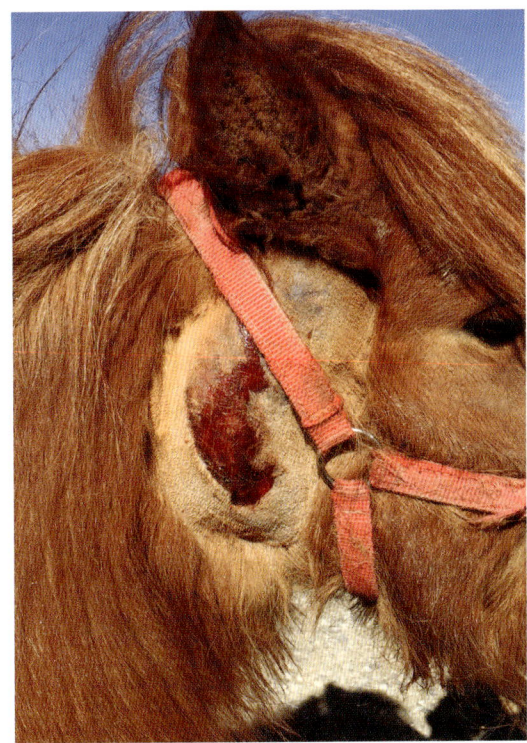

4.11 *An abscess in one of the common locations where strangles occurs.*

ssp. *equi* bacteria. It infects the back of the horse's throat, particularly within specialized structures called the *guttural pouches* (similar to the *eustachian tubes* of our ears). The bacteria produce pus and swelling, resulting in respiratory noise and restricted air flow—hence the name *strangles*. It is common around the world, and is often seen in horses that come from auctions, where diseases easily spread. It is most likely to affect very young, very old, or otherwise immunocompromised horses (fig. 4.11).

There is a killed intramuscular vaccine as well as somewhat more effective modified live one that is administered intranasally. Not considered a core vaccine, it is only recommended for young horses or those at a high risk of disease. A possible occasional sequela of either the disease or the vaccine is *purpura hemorrhagica*—an allergic-type reaction to the cells lining blood vessels. Horses that develop this problem have bleeding of small capillary vessels that results in red spots (*petechiae*) on the gums and swelling of the legs, head, and belly. Purpura is difficult to treat and can result in death.

Respiratory Disease in Needy Equines

Rescue horses are at a high risk for developing respiratory diseases. They may travel long distances and be exposed to stress, dust, and disease-causing agents. They often do not have current vaccines. Even if they have received proper vaccines, rescue horses may have a weak immune system due to malnutrition. Because of this, they often do not have good immunity to the contagious diseases they are exposed to at auction houses or in other groups.

There are many types of respiratory illnesses, and there is variation in the severity of each. It can be as simple as a virus where your horse has a runny nose for a few days, a fever for less than 24 hours, and recovers quickly. The worst case scenario is a horse developing *pleuropneumonia* (shipping fever), a serious, life-threatening lung infection. Recovery can take months, and affected horses may have long-term breathing issues.

Diagnosing Respiratory Illness: The most important factor in successful treatment is early recognition. Screening for early respiratory problems is one of the main reasons to monitor a horse's temperature during the quarantine period. It is also important to watch for coughing, nasal discharge, or general malaise.

At the first sign of a problem, contact your veterinarian. After a thorough physical examination that includes listening to the horse's lung sounds, she may use a variety of diagnostic tools to help identify your rescue horse's specific problem. These may include a rebreathing bag, where a plastic bag is placed over the horse's nose for a few minutes to increase his respiratory depth. It is a test of normalcy, and helps bring out subtle problems. Your veterinarian may also run blood work or ultrasound the chest to assess the lung surface.

Treating Respiratory Illness: Treatment of respiratory disease will be specific to your horse's problem. It is likely to include anti-inflammatories and antibiotics. The good news is that with early intervention, the majority of horses make a full recovery. The bad news is that pleuropneumonia can be one of the most expensive problems to treat.

Vaccines are critical for preventing disease in your rescue horse. It is crucial that the horse be vaccinated only when he is healthy enough to mount an immune response to develop immune protection from disease. Follow your veterinarian's recommendations for vaccination of both your new and established herd.

CHAPTER 5

Keeping Them Moving and Sound:
Hoof Care, Lameness, and Wounds

A portion of the definition of "unwanted horse" refers to one that is unable to do his job, and unaddressed or unrecognized lameness is a major reason for poor performance in racing and competition horses. *Lameness* is a change in the way a horse moves because of pain and is very common in rescue horses. The pain can range from mild, manageable arthritis to an excruciating, crippling, and life-threatening joint infection.

Many horses have some degree of lameness. Individuals, rescue groups, and sanctuaries should understand that lameness can adversely affect a horse's ability to get to food and water or defend himself in a group. It can also be a reason that a horse objects to training requests (for example, he may buck when asked to canter because it hurts to canter).

Before you can determine if the horse you are about to rescue is or is not lame, you'll need to understand "normal" foot anatomy, and since rescue horses frequently have neglected feet, you'll want to know what to do to restore hoof health—topics that are covered in the pages ahead. In addition, options for managing arthritis, the most common cause of lameness, are presented.

Finally, a horse with a chronic, incurable lameness is often suffering, and rescuers should recognize when that is the case. The lameness can affect his attitude and outlook, making him cranky or mean. It is cruel to allow a horse to live with an untreated, severe, long-term lameness. A horse that has such a lameness may lie down and, at some point, be unable to rise (more on this in chapter 8—see p. 122). Being able to differentiate treatable neglect from other, more sinister sources of pain is vital as you select a horse to help.

FOOT ANATOMY

The horse's foot is a complicated and dynamic structure. Understanding the anatomy is critical for understanding problems (fig. 5.1). The word "hoof" as it will be used here specifically refers to the hard, horny portion of the foot and is synonymous with the terms *hoof horn*, *hoof wall*, and *hoof capsule*. Other structures of the foot (such as bones, tendons, and ligaments) are contained within the hoof capsule.

The front of the hoof is the *toe*, the sides are the *quarters*, and the projections in the back are the *heel bulbs*. The bottom of the foot is the *sole*, and the wedge- or V-shaped area within it is the *frog*. The frog has more moisture content than the sole and hoof capsule do. The line between the hoof wall and the sole is the *white line*.

The hoof capsule is made of an insensitive but flexible protein tissue, *keratin*, which is also the main structural component of your fingernails and hair. The keratin of the hoof is arranged as millions of tiny moisture-retaining hollow columns (think of them as microscopic straws) called *horn tubules*. The hoof wall meets the horse's skin and hairline at the *coronary band*, a structure akin to your cuticle.

Pain and Attitude

The little bay mare with the high white socks and a blaze face, Lefty, was very important to her family—the daughter Susanna rode her, and the mare was her best friend.

When Lefty had a puncture wound that went straight into her joint, the ensuing infection was crippling. She was barely touching her right front toe to the ground when she hobbled into the hospital. We took her straight to surgery. The arthroscopic procedure—putting a miniature, sterile camera-on-a-stick into the joint—involved flushing the joint with several liters of fluid at a high pressure, pushing out all the infection. We also used the arthroscope to evaluate the cartilage and joint capsule. Other specialized instruments were used to remove any abnormal tissue from the infected area.

Three days later, Lefty should have been sound. But, there I was, helping our technicians catch and hold her for a simple follow-up antibiotic medication. The mare was mean, and I couldn't imagine her being ridden by a child. In fact, when Susanna visited, Lefty pinned her ears. Lefty had been a difficult and impatient individual since the day she entered our hospital. She seemed dangerous, and nobody was allowed in her stall alone. I wondered if Susanna's parents were being irresponsible by letting their daughter be with the mare.

On the fourth day, we determined that the joint had some residual infection. Lefty was not as lame as she had been on the first day, but her foot was still bothering her. This development was unusual, but a second arthroscopic procedure was needed. After flushing the joint again, and observing no further abnormalities in it, Lefty was bandaged and recovered from general anesthesia.

The following morning, Lefty was like a whole new horse. She nickered when people walked by. She greeted us happily at the front of her hospital stall with soft nuzzles and willingly submitted to the bandage changes and medications she needed.

When Susanna visited later that day, I saw the bond the two shared, and I finally understood what had happened. The pain of the infected joint was so severe it affected everything about the mare. Lefty was a lesson to me: She was actually a kind horse, but her agony had made her into a beast. She was an extreme example of how pain and illness can negatively affect behavior and attitude.

Within the hoof capsule is the *coffin bone*, which is covered by tiny projections of sensitive tissue called *lamina*. These sensitive laminae have millions of tiny ridges which engage and fit in between the insensitive laminae that line the interior of the hoof capsule (fig. 5.2). The interdigitation (interlocking) of the sensitive and insensitive laminae hold the foot together.

Other vital structures within the foot are the *navicular bone*, the *coffin joint*, and supporting ligaments of each. Finally, the *deep digital flexor tendon*—one of the most important structures of the horse's leg—attaches to the bottom of the coffin bone within the hoof capsule.

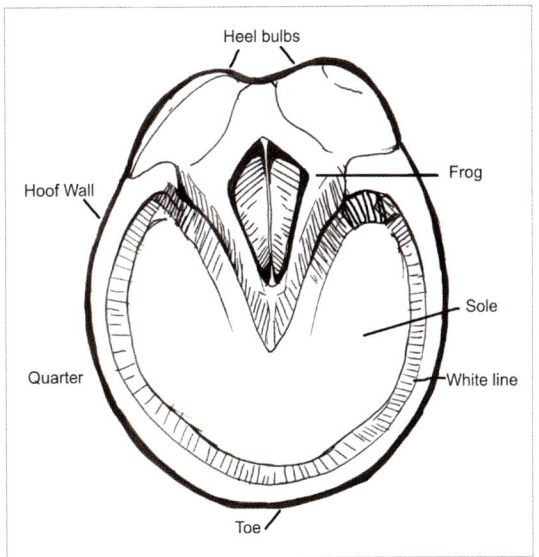

5.1 Diagram of the bottom of horse hoof showing relevant structures.

ROUTINE HOOF CARE

The horse's feet should be evaluated and picked or cleaned out on a regular basis. Although some horse-care manuals recommend hoof cleaning and grooming daily, I have observed that many horses do not have this frequent handling. At a bare minimum, you should pick his feet each time he is ridden or groomed.

Just like our keratin-based fingernails constantly grow and need trimming, your horse's hooves grow continually and will need regular, scheduled trimming. The recommended interval for this is between four and eight weeks, depending on the growth rate and any problems the horse may have. A growing youngster grows foot faster, and during his early and fast growth period should be trimmed every four weeks. Trimming can be used to help correct leg growth abnormalities.

Once the fast rate of growth has slowed down, every six weeks is an appropriate

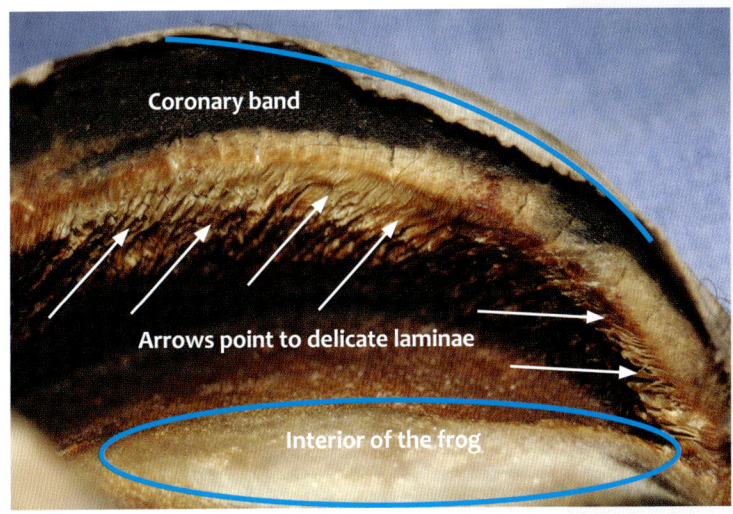

5.2 A photo of an anatomical specimen demonstrating the insensitive lamina lining the hoof.

schedule for horses that are two years or older. Horses' feet do grow more slowly in winter, but that does not mean you can neglect to trim them throughout the entire season. They should still be attended to every six to eight weeks. If a horse is barefoot and there is normal, active wear on the foot, you may be able to safely extend your farrier visit by a week or two. Horses that are wearing shoes don't wear their feet off, and should be a on a six-week or shorter schedule. Because of the frequency of this routine procedure, you will need to have a good relationship with a farrier and train your horse to accept hoof care.

Long Ears

Compared to horses, donkeys' feet are more upright, and have a narrower, oval shape. Mules have something in between the donkey and the horse foot. The naturally more upright foot of these species is normal, and no attempt should be made to change their natural hoof angle. Upright hoof growth is one reason it is said that mules stay sound and are more surefooted than a horse (fig. 5.3).

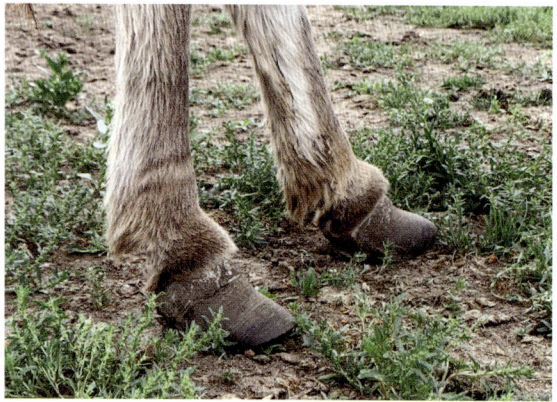

5.3 A donkey with moderately overgrown feet. Although the overgrowth has resulted in extreme stress on her joints and ligaments, you can still see that genetics affect hoof growth. Donkeys are more upright than horses, and her hooves have a narrower, more upright shape than a horse's despite being overgrown.

Factors Affecting Hoof Structure and Growth

Genetics, environment, and nutrition all affect the quality of hoof growth. Nutrition is the factor you can control the most.

How Nutrition Affects Hoof Growth

The body of a horse with an energy-poor diet is going to expend its energy maintaining essential organ and life functions. Hoof growth is a secondary need that is likely to suffer.

The hoof capsule is made primarily of keratin protein. Amino acids are the building blocks of protein, and *methionine* and *lysine* are the two most critical to hoof growth. A horse with a protein deficiency is metabolically unable to produce the keratin of the hoof.

Biotin is the most widely known vitamin relevant to hooves. It is a water-soluble substance and is made by microbes in the horse's digestive system. Some horses' hooves benefit from biotin supplementation.

Minerals and electrolytes derived from the horse's diet must be balanced. Substances important to hoof growth include zinc, calcium, phosphorus, and selenium. The actual amount of calcium and phosphorus as well as their ratio to each other will influence hoof development.

High-quality hoof growth depends on fats as well. They function as a barrier that prevents microbial invaders from entering and compromising the hoof.

The effects of diet change on hoof growth may begin to manifest in a few weeks, and will be initially visible as a *growth ring* at the top of the hoof. In four to six months, the new, healthy hoof will replace the entire old, unhealthy hoof from the top

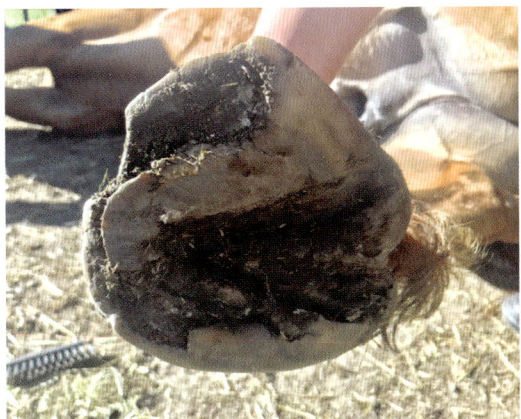

5.4 This horse was confiscated for neglect. His rear foot is being trimmed while he is anesthetized because he was not trained and had never had his feet handled.

down. Overall, it is more important that the horse gets enough energy, protein, and fat with an appropriate vitamin and mineral content in the diet.

Genetics Affect Hoof Growth: How much growth, the general shape tendency, and the number of the horn tubules of the hoof are highly influenced by genetics. The more densely the horn tubules of the hoof are arranged, the stronger the foot. Most stock horses and Mustangs grow good, dense, tough hooves. Some Thoroughbreds have notoriously thin hoof walls and/or thin, sensitive soles.

Environment Affects Hoof Growth: If your rescue horse has been in unsanitary conditions, such as standing in mud or years' worth of manure, his feet may be suffering the consequences.

Normal hoof growth is counteracted by the abrasive nature of the footing horses are designed to be traveling over. When footing is constantly wet and soft, the hoof will not

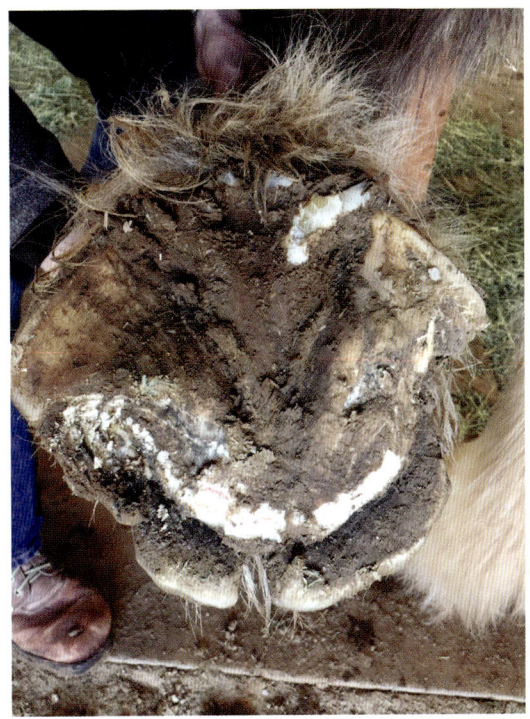

5.5 The environment affects hooves. Here is a draft horse's foot that is overgrown and dirty from standing in unsanitary conditions. This horse had multiple hoof abscesses and thrush.

experience normal wear. It will grow and, if not trimmed, will fold over and sometimes crack or break in unnatural and painful ways (fig. 5.4).

Excessive moisture of mud and manure also soften the hoof wall, increasing susceptibility to bacterial and fungal infections of the hoof such as *white line disease* or *thrush*. White line disease is a fungal infection that can degrade the white line at the bottom of the foot, and work its way up between the layers of hoof wall, destabilizing it. Thrush, a mix of bacterial and fungal microbes, creates a foul odor and erodes the frog. Both infections are painful, but can be treated by removing abnormal tissue and applying topical antimicrobials (fig. 5.5).

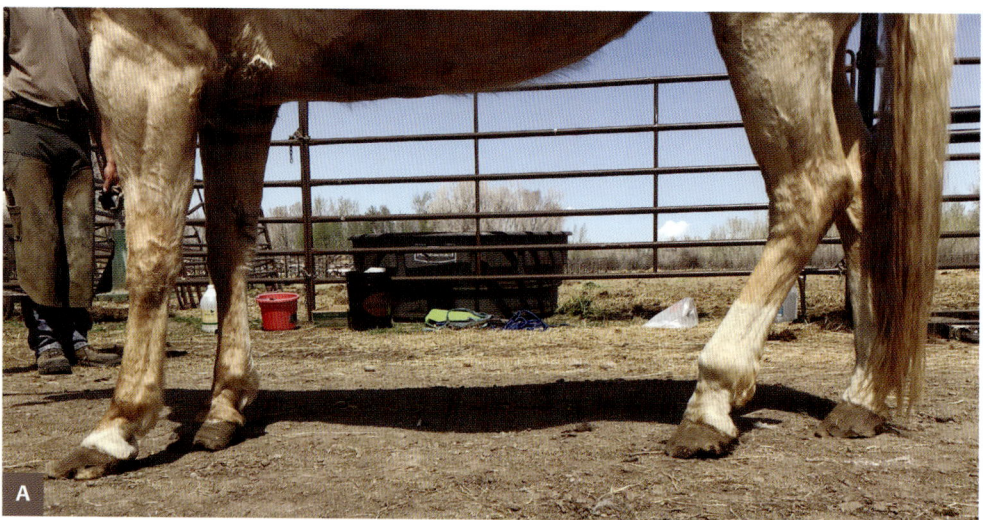
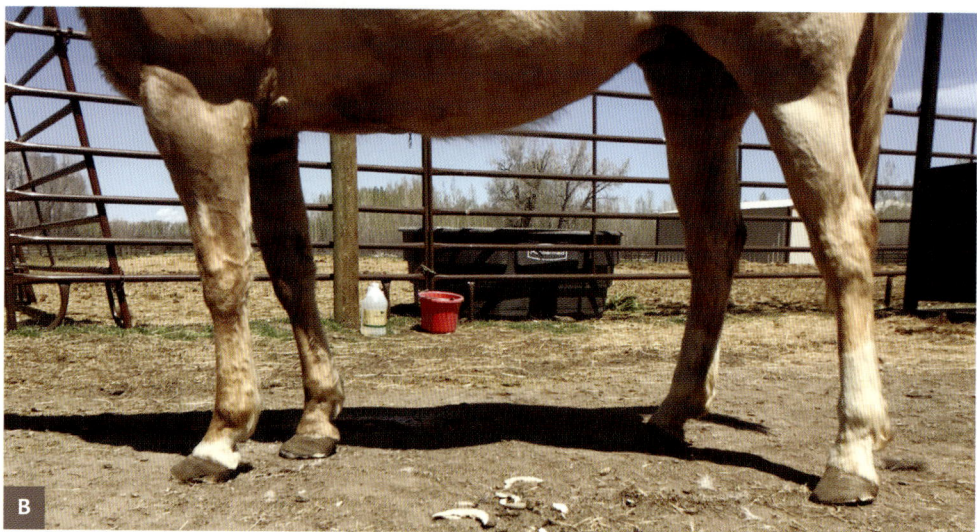

5.6 A & B This mare confiscated for neglect had overgrown feet (A). After she was trimmed, her stance and comfort improved from less stress on joints, tendons, and ligaments (B).

RECOGNIZING LAMENESS IN RESCUE HORSES

Many horses have a subtle or mild lameness, while others can have severe and obvious problems. Recognizing and treating lameness is important. When you are rehabilitating your horse, if he has pain, training will be more difficult. It's also important if you intend to help and re-home your horse. It is more difficult to find a good home for a lame horse. Even if he is not ridden and his sole purpose is as a grass-guzzling companion, it is critical to address lameness for your horse's overall comfort and to maintain a good quality of life. It's especially important to educate your eye to detect lameness if you are getting horses from auctions or so-called "kill pen" markets. Horses that aren't performing due to lameness are more likely to end up in these markets.

There are two main things for you to look at in order to learn more about a horse's soundness: how he moves and what his feet look like (figs. 5.6 A & B). In a rescue situation, you may not have the opportunity to watch him move very much, but you should be able to at least glance at his feet, which can reveal a lot about his past history and the way he moves. Looking at the shape of his hooves and recognizing problems early will help you meet his needs (figs. 5.7 A–C).

Evaluating the Feet of a Rescue Horse

Hoof Neglect: Many rescue horses have suffered from hoof neglect and simply need a good trim. There may be several reasons for this situation. If the former owner was unable to provide adequate food, any other necessary care—like the farrier or veterinarian—was also unaffordable. A horse may be poorly behaved or untrained, making it difficult to keep up a regular schedule of trims. An older horse may be cranky during trims because arthritis makes leg and foot manipulations painful.

Mismatched Hooves: A horse who has a moderate to severe chronic lameness in one limb will have feet that are noticeably mismatched.

When the hoof hits the ground three factors affect the impact: the horse's weight, his speed, and the degree of shock absorbency of the footing. The force of impact the foot absorbs causes the hoof to flex. This movement influences hoof growth. In the lame horse, the hoof of the

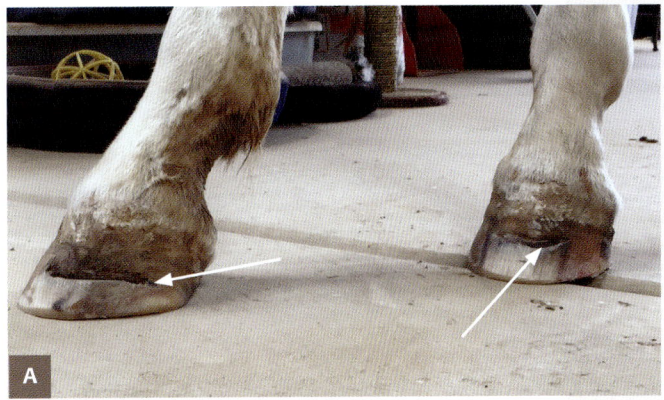
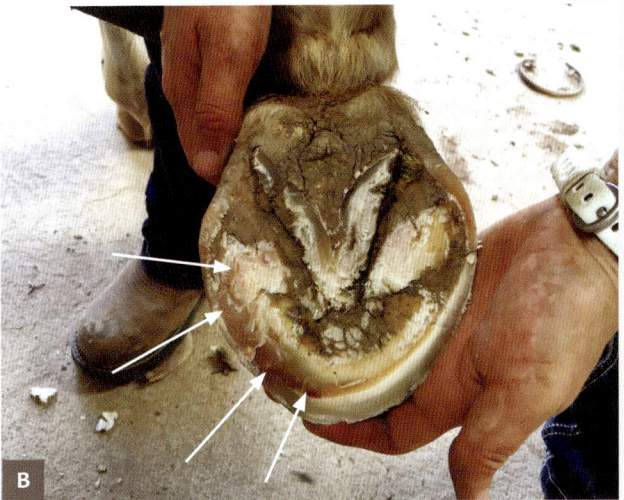
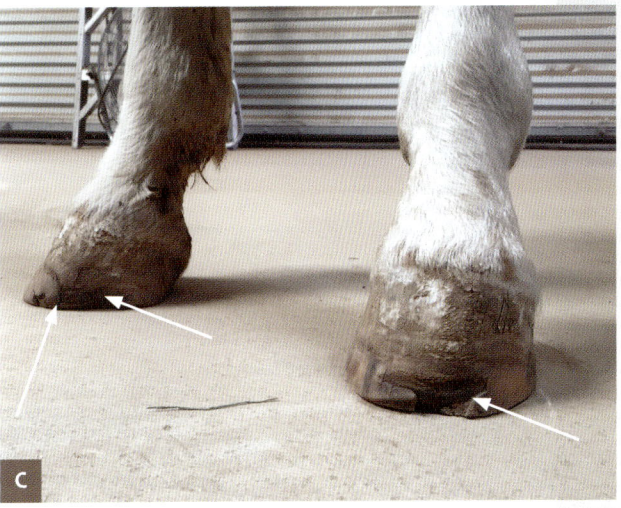

5.7 A–C *The hoof of a rescued horse who sustained an unknown illness or injury. All four feet had similar areas of damage at the same level (A). The abnormal hoof during a trim. Not only is it discolored, but the texture is abnormally hard (B). Here, the damaged hoof tissue has nearly grown out and all new growth is normal (C).*

sore leg chronically absorbs less impact and will grow more narrow and upright because of fewer concussive forces. Conversely, the opposite foot may chronically bear more weight and the hoof becomes flattened and wide as a result.

For example, a chronic right forelimb lameness will result in the horse bearing less weight on that hoof. The right front hoof will be smaller and upright. The left forelimb must compensate and bear more weight, which will result in a hoof that is wide and flat due to the increased impact it sustains.

That said, there are other reasons for a mismatch. Many horses have naturally mismatched hooves, so an otherwise normal horse with a minor mismatch is probably not cause for alarm. The greater the difference between the feet—particularly in a horse who has not had proper trimming or care—the more likely there is to be a serious, long-term, underlying problem.

Club Foot: A club foot in horses refers to an abnormally upright foot (figs. 5.8 A & B). The angle of the hoof wall and the pastern will not match. A horse may be born with this as a congenital problem, or it can be acquired later in life through injury or abnormal growth. One or both feet may be affected, but usually one is worse than another.

In a congenital club foot, the problem originates from the angle of the coffin bone. The abnormal exterior shape actually occurs from within, with the coffin joint causing the aberrant growth of the hoof. X-rays of the foot are necessary for accurate assessment and diagnosis. Unlike cases of

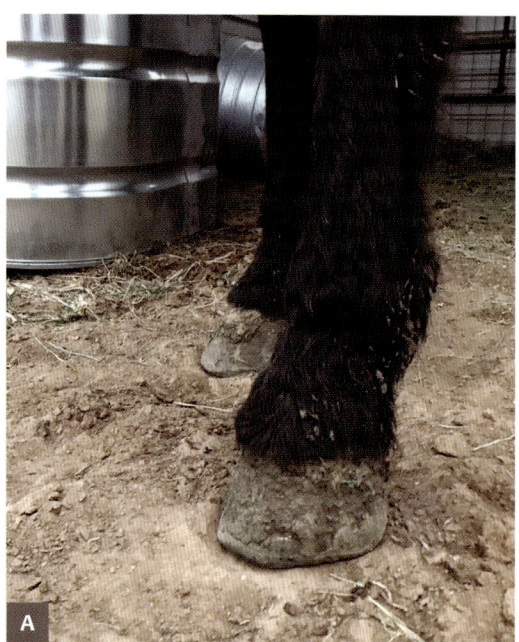
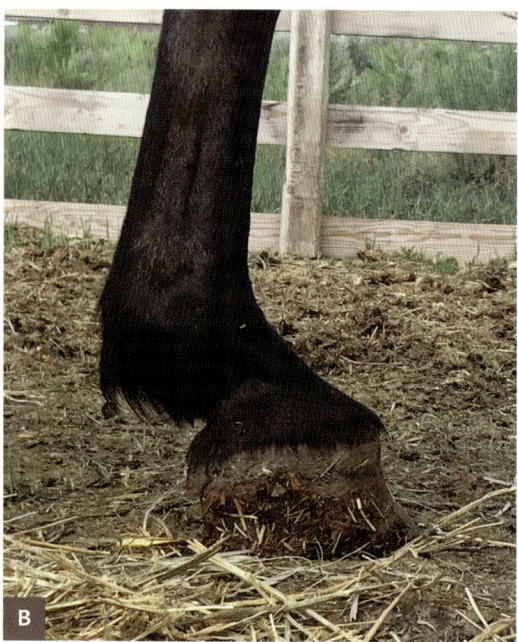

5.8 A & B Two examples of club foot horses in poor conditions: A gelding with a moderate club foot who was confiscated for neglect (A). A mare with a severe club foot. Notice that the angle of the hoof wall is different from that of the pastern. The hoof wall also has a "dished" shape, typical of a club foot (B).

lameness causing an upright foot, a congenital club foot's uprightness is not caused by a decrease in weight-bearing.

Club-footed horses are graded on a scale of 1 to 4, with 4 being the worst. Most horses with low-grade club foot are not lame. A young horse's conformation abnormality can be corrected by trimming to adjust the angle of the coffin bone and foot. For more severe cases, a surgical procedure to release ligaments can help. The older a horse, the less likely it is that surgical correction is successful. Without surgery, if a farrier trims the hooves to match, the resultant stretch on the tendons and ligaments in the leg of the more upright foot will make the horse quite sore.

Laminitis: A horse with chronic laminitis will have the classic "ski" shape to his feet or growth ridges growing down from the coronary bands, called *laminitic rings* or *fever rings* (fig. 5.9).

Monitoring Movement

The most straightforward lameness to diagnose is a forelimb lameness in one leg. Lameness is most visible at the trot, a gait that should be perfectly even and a left-to-right mirror image of itself, or bilaterally symmetrical. Lameness is more difficult to detect if it occurs in both forelimbs or both hind limbs at the same time because the gait may remain symmetrical despite the pain the horse has.

Forelimb lameness is easier to detect than hind-limb lameness because the horse's head will "bob" up and down as he moves. Normally, the head should be carried level as he moves. The head bob occurs when a lame horse reduces the weight carried by his painful leg. When watching the head bob, remember "down on sound": The horse's head goes up when the lame leg hits the ground, and goes down when the sound leg hits the ground. Even skilled horse people and veterinarians can miss subtle lameness issues.

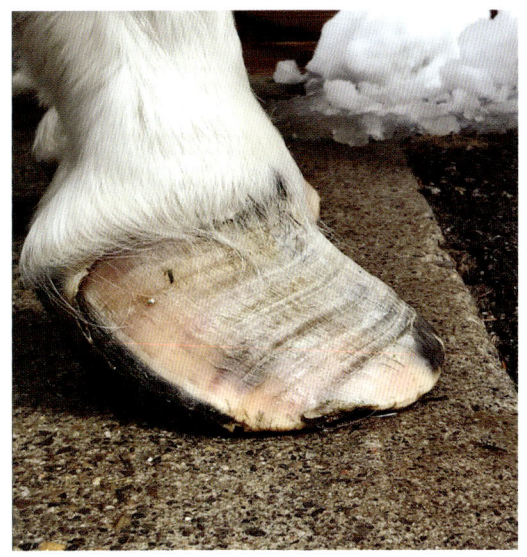

5.9 A foot with chronic active laminitis, resulting in abnormal hoof growth rings.

When you are able to watch a rescue horse move out, you will have a better idea of what breed he is (he may not trot—he may amble, fox-trot, four-beat, rack, or do something else), and you will be able to further assess his comfort level and adoption potential. The more you know about the horse before taking him home, the better you can help him. When the horse is weak and thin, you may not be able to perform this movement assessment.

WHEN TO SHOE

I would like to quote a good article from The Horse Network (horsenetwork.com): "It is true that wild horses, in nature, do not wear shoes. That is an indisputable fact. Wild horses also get eaten by coyotes and die from diseases and injuries modern veterinary medicine can easily treat. Sometimes you take the good with the bad. They wore their feet down wandering the plains all day, which is tough to replicate on most farms unless you have a lot of land."[72]

If a horse remains comfortable, functional, and sound without shoes, that's great. If he isn't able to achieve this, shoes will be necessary. There is no "one size fits all" answer to the necessity of shoes. There are entire books that address this issue—the textbook *Equine Podiatry* by Andrea Floyd and Richard Mansmann covers this topic in depth.[73] Here, I embark on a brief discussion of shoeing with respect to neglected horses. It is necessary to protect a horse's hoof when hoof wear exceeds hoof growth, when the horse experiences pain

Bobbing Bobby

Brenda is a soft soul who rescues horses to use in a non-profit, mental health hippotherapy program for her psychiatric clients. She has taken several horses through the ups and downs of rehabilitation, and has become experienced with equine rescue.

Brenda buys horses out of feedlots that are known to sell to buyers who take loads of horses to Mexico for slaughter. On one occasion, she selected a tall, skinny, lanky, middle-aged bay horse with a kind eye, and a minor cut on his left hind leg. She brought Bobby home and started feeding and working with him, improving his halter-training skills.

I evaluated the wound: it was all the way through the skin, but Bobby was not lame. It would heal fine with the treatment plan we made. I noticed that he had several scars. I told Brenda this was worrisome, because some horses don't pay attention to where their feet and legs are in human-made enclosures. They don't take care of themselves and can really get into trouble.

Bobby was still wearing a bandage on his left hind when he came in with a cut directly over the fetlock on his right front. He was in pain, bobbing his head up each time the right front foot stepped on the ground, even at the walk. The wound had entered the joint. The horse was too thin to safely undergo general anesthesia for proper treatment of the infected joint. Besides, Brenda's group was a non-profit that also needed to look after half-a-dozen other horses, and take care of the needs of their human clients. They didn't have the thousands of dollars it would take to treat the infected joint properly. If they used all their money on Bobby, they would not be able to take care of others. Brenda and I decided together that euthanasia was the best option for Bobby.

With her kind nature, and positive attitude, Brenda still was glad she had brought Bobby home. Before I euthanized him, she explained that she was grateful to have given Bobby a few weeks of good meals and kindness, and to know that he did not experience an excessively long trailer ride or unkindness in his death.

or lameness, or when the horse has either a temporary or permanent abnormality from injury or aberrant growth.

When Wear Exceeds Growth, Shoes are Necessary

Some horses don't grow enough good foot due to their genetic predisposition. Some horses have the ability to tolerate rocky terrain, but most need some foot protection when the footing is rough. A rescued horse may need shoes due to poor hoof growth that occurred during times of illness, poor nutrition, or stress.

Factors that influence the wear rate of hoof wall include the frequency and duration of riding and the terrain. If you are riding your horse six hours a day, three to four days a week on rocky terrain, your horse is highly likely to need shoes. If you ride him for an hour in an arena twice a week, and then go out on a trail with good footing once a month, your horse probably won't need shoes.

Hoof boots can be a useful, temporary alternative to shoes. These afford the foot the protection your horse needs, while helping decrease the overall expense of hoof care.

You now know that the foot moves with each step, so you might be wondering how nailing a hard, unbending metal horseshoe to the foot affects the normal, dynamic hoof. The majority of movement occurs behind the quarters, especially through the frog and heel bulbs. Traditional shoes, nailed on cranial to (forward of) the quarters, allow normal dynamic hoof expansion to occur, and often you can see normal wear in the shoe where the hoof has rubbed it (figs. 5.10 and 5.11).

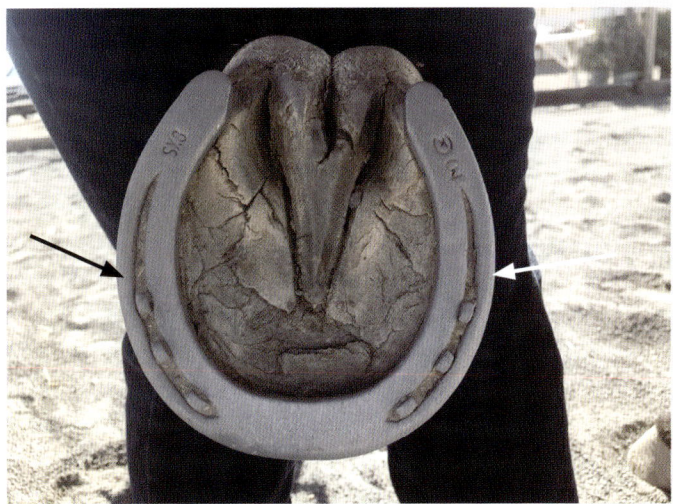

5.10 Location of shoe nails forward of the quarters so that the heels can still expand and contract with normal movement.

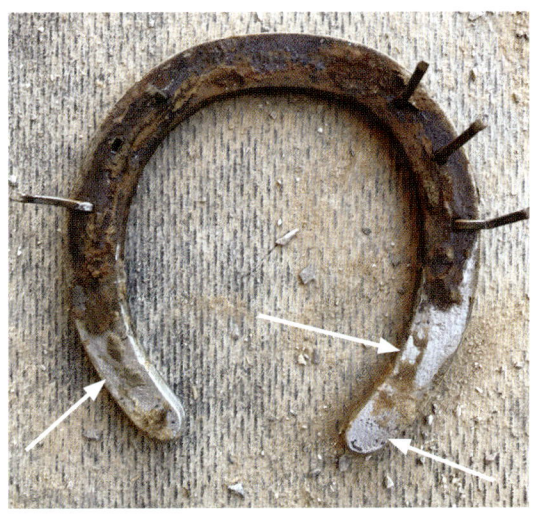

5.11 Top (inside) of a freshly removed horseshoe showing silver-colored wear marks where heels have continued to move.

When the Horse Experiences Foot Pain, Shoes are Necessary

It is inhumane to ask the horse to continue working through pain, and pain can cause your training efforts to fail. A horse with pain in one limb may exhibit a head bob as discussed above. When both front feet are painful, the horse will exhibit a short, choppy stride, and may be reluctant to move out. Shoes support the foot and protect it from the terrain, making the horse comfortable. If the horse has problems with the angles of his feet that result in pain, a wedge shoe can change the angle and enhance his comfort.

When shoes alone don't alleviate pain, sensitive horses may benefit from a pad for further protection of their sole. Technology has improved since the historic first use of leather pads (fig. 5.12). While the shoe protects the hoof wall, the pad covers and protects the sole, and can absorb impact because it is made of a softer, flexible material. Pads can also come in a wedge shape to help change the angle of the foot. Pads are nailed to the hoof between the shoe and the hoof wall. Leather pads are still available today, and they can change with the absorption of moisture, but are more breathable than rubber or plastic pads. Pour-in pads come in various densities, and conform perfectly to the bottom of the foot. Modified pads may also be used specifically to reduce the build-up of snow in the shod horse's foot during the winter.

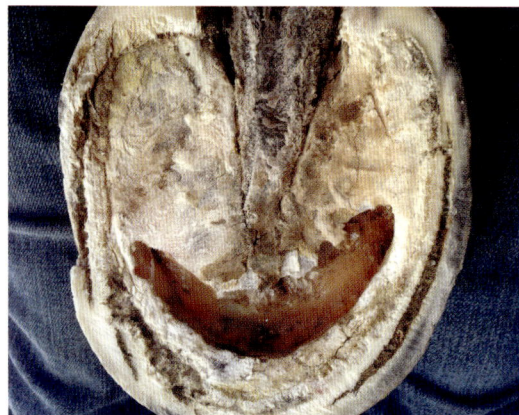

5.13 *A hoof abscess after the extent of abnormal sole tissue has been removed. It will need a shoe and pad for protection as the hoof grows back in.*

Shoeing Horses with Abnormalities

Abnormalities may require a shoe to correct. For example, a horse who has had a previous sole abscess needs protection until the sole regenerates (fig. 5.13). This protection may include both a shoe and a pad.

Shoes are the traditional, time-tested solution to foot protection and stability. However, they are expensive when compared to barefoot trims. Many people use shoes on the front feet only but leave the hind feet barefoot.

The traction provided by a metal shoe in some terrain is not as good as that of a bare hoof. To overcome slippage problems, rim shoes, borium, or screw-in studs may be used to add traction. A rim shoe is designed for the edge to catch debris or dirt within the rim, adding additional traction. Borium

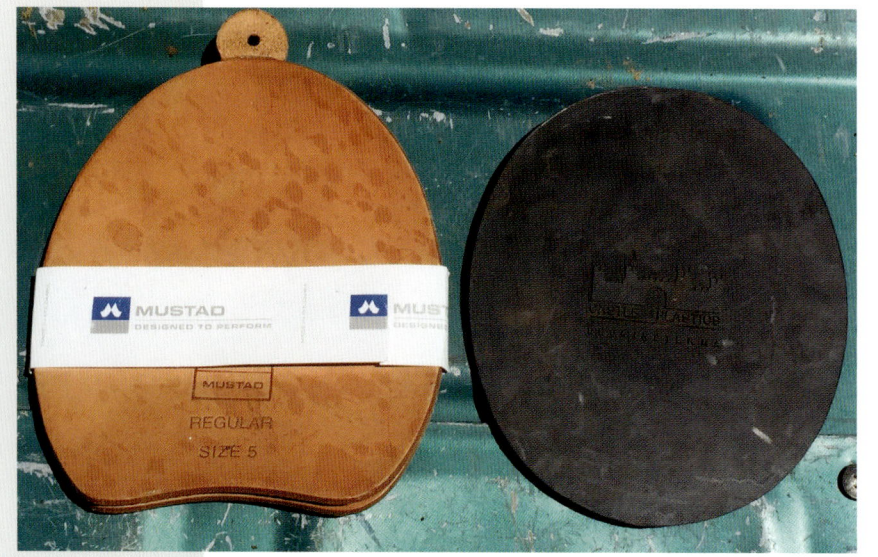

5.12 *When needed, pads are trimmed to size based on hoof and shoe shape, then nailed on between the hoof and the shoe to provide protection to a horse's soles.*

5.14 A–C *Shoe designs used for traction: New and used rim shoes (A), a shoe with an orange snow pad and borium welds (B), and an old shoe with a snow pad (red arrows) and borium-impregnated screw-in studs (black arrows) for additional traction (C).*

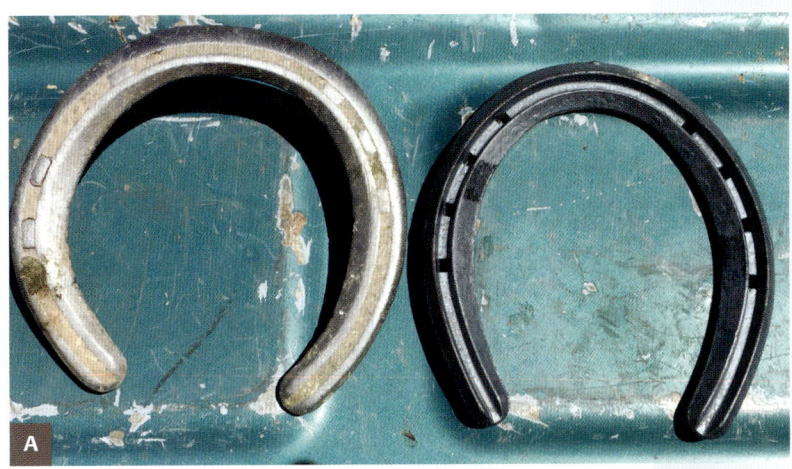

is welded to the bottom of the shoe to roughen the surface (figs. 5.14 A–C).

CAUSES OF LAMENESS

There are many causes of lameness. Common ones include injury, hoof abscess, laminitis, and arthritis.

Injuries That Damage the Hoof

The coronary band is where hoof growth originates. When the coronary band is damaged, the hoof may grow with a ridge, crack, or scar—just like damage to a cuticle can result in abnormal fingernail growth. If the crack is deep, it can be painful for the horse, just like a crack in your fingernail can affect the sensitive tissue underneath and be painful for you.

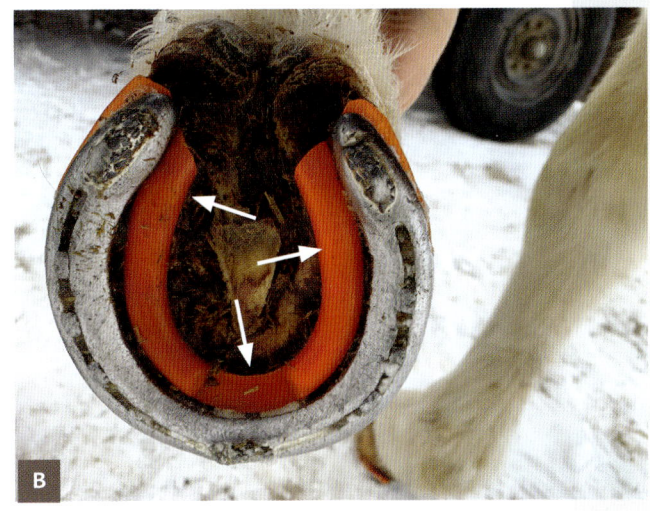

Your first goal is to keep the horse comfortable, and manage the instability so that the crack grows out or disappears (figs. 5.15 A–D). The second goal is not always possible because a horse with a scar at his coronary band will always have abnormal hoof growth. Coronary band scars in horses are common, and most farriers are adept at trimming and shoeing the horse to maintain his comfort. One of the things a farrier may do is *float* the area under the crack, meaning the hoof wall is rasped in such a way that a small portion may not actually be touching the ground. Impact on the cracked

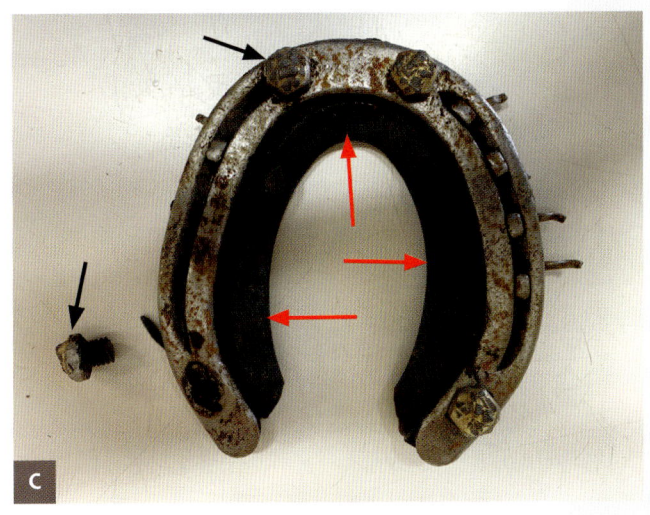

Part I: Caring for Horses in Need—73

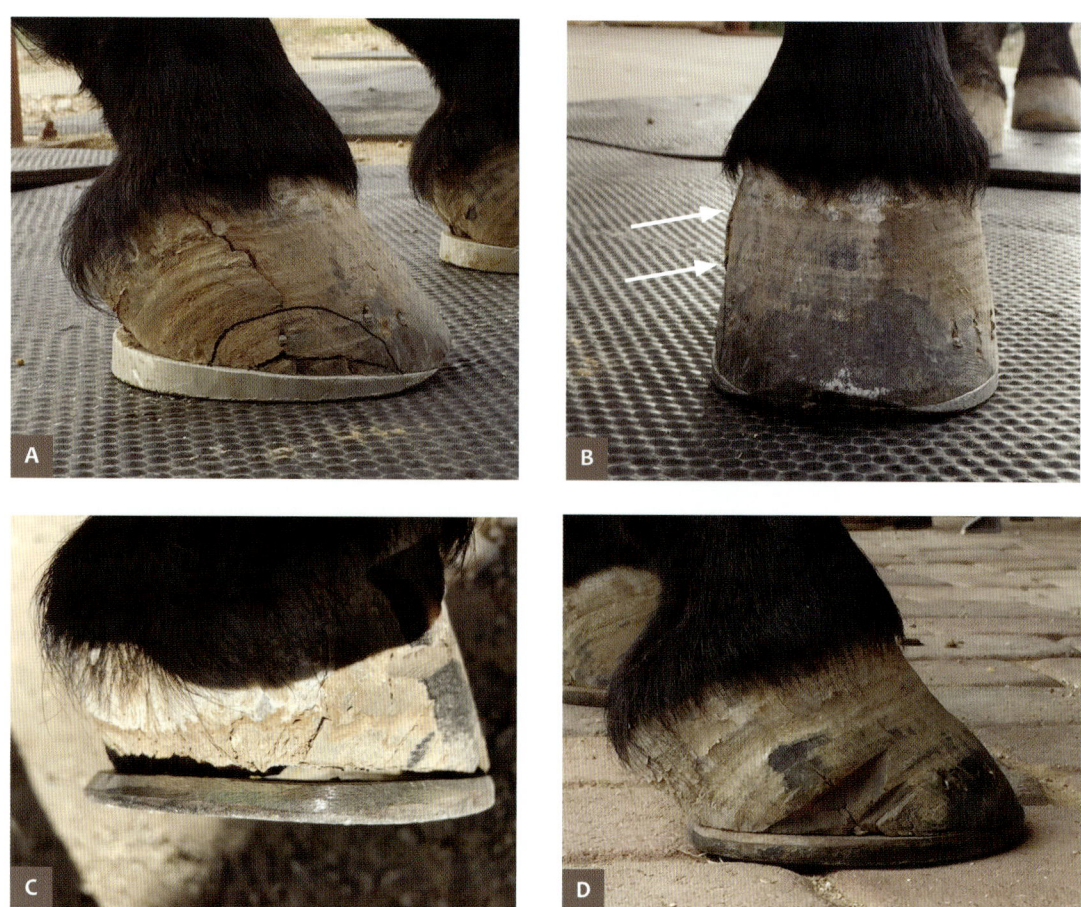

5.15 A–D An abnormality such as the quarter crack shown in photo A can be the impetus to shoe a horse. The black marker indicates an exaggerated way the hoof wall could be removed or "floated" to restore normal balance. The imbalance in the hoof in photo B is evident when viewing the horse's hoof from the front; the crack bulges out. In photo C we see a view of a hoof that has been "floated" to help restore balance. The same quarter crack about three months later is shown in photo D, nearly grown out. The horizontal groove was made with a hoof rasp and is a marker to help monitor hoof growth.

area may be transmitted to the sensitive coronary band, which is the primary way these cracks can cause pain. Also, continued impact will keep propagating the crack, so floating it will minimize that effect. You should be aware that shoes may be needed to help normalize growth of a damaged hoof (fig. 5.16).

Hoof Abscesses

A hoof abscess is a common cause of lameness in horses. It can be scary. Your horse may be totally normal at breakfast and be severely lame by dinner. Swelling of the lower leg can occur.

The hoof abscess is an extremely painful, localized infection, a lot like an ingrown toenail, except that the horse only has one toenail (his hoof), and it bears all of his weight. Bacterial infection invades the horse's foot in between the insensitive sole and the sensitive tissue underneath. This causes severe inflammation and a buildup of pus and pressure.

Treatment is aimed at establishing and maintaining an exit path for the pus. This may involve soaking your horse's hoof for several days. Your veterinarian or farrier will identify the location of the abscess and pare out sole as needed to get to healthy, non-infected tissue and allow the pus to drain.

Once drainage is established, antibiotics are not usually necessary. In fact, most antibiotics given by mouth don't reach the infected tissue in a concentration high enough to kill the bacteria. Occasionally, there are other factors that warrant antibiotic use (fig. 5.17).

Due to the pain and inflammation, a non-steroidal, anti-inflammatory drug (NSAID) may be used to help quell inflammation and relieve pain. This will help the horse feel better and restore the inflamed hoof tissue to normal homeostasis.

Laminitis

Laminitis is inflammation of the laminae that hold the foot together. Laminitis may occur acutely for many reasons, including shock due to *sepsis* (bacteria in the bloodstream), as a result of carbohydrate overload, after ingestion of a toxin, or as a result of insulin resistance. Equine metabolic syndrome (EMS) results in decreased blood flow to

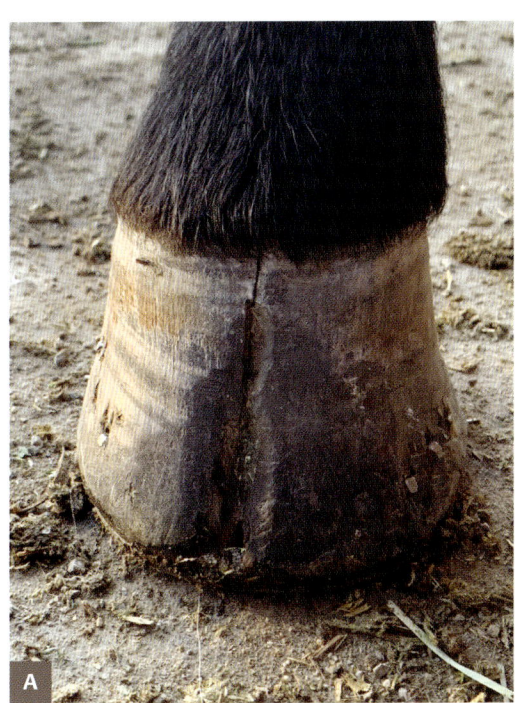

5.16 A coronary band scar in conjunction with hoof imbalance has resulted in a significant, deep and painful toe crack on this foot.

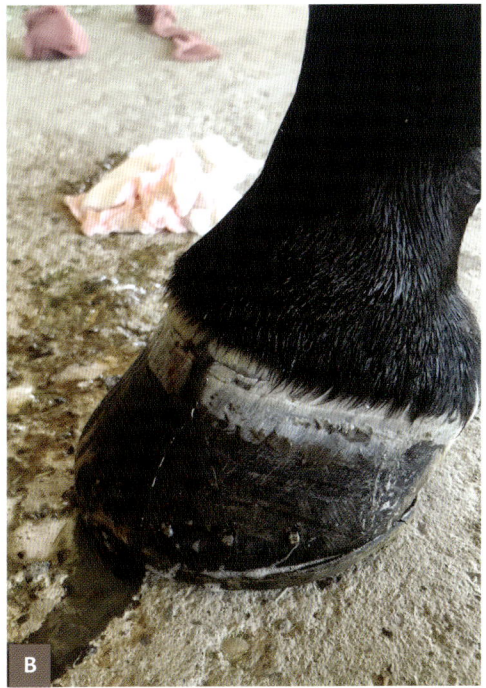

5.17 This hoof abscess (pus in the foot) has established drainage at the coronary band.

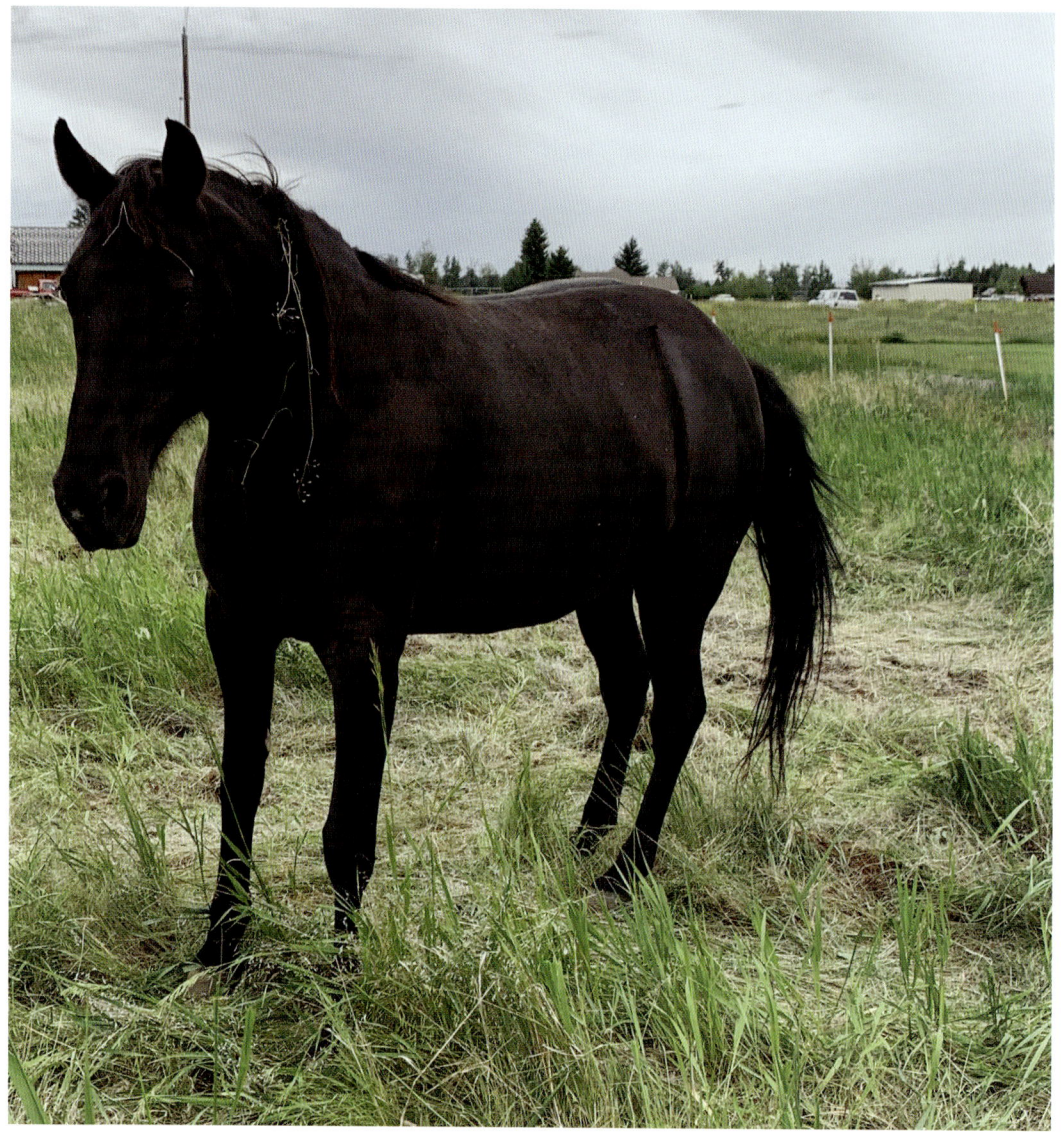

5.18 *The stance typical of laminitis. This horse is painful in her front feet and is rocked back over her haunches, trying to relieve the pain in her front limbs.*

the hoof, which causes a lack of oxygen to tissue, and it becomes diseased or inflamed. Research is still expanding our understanding of laminitis. It is one of the most painful conditions horses endure (fig. 5.18).

Sometimes laminitis becomes chronic. A hoof with chronic changes because of laminitis will have divergent hoof growth rings. Your rescue horse may need special care or have dietary restrictions, so being aware of this problem is critical for good management.

Chronic Generalized Arthritis

Aside from a plethora of specific lameness issues that occur in horses of any age group, the most common lameness issue in older rescue horses is chronic, generalized arthritis. Arthritis is inflammation of joints. Horses with arthritis can have multiple joints affected, which are painful and inflamed due to accumulated damage from injury and use. This problem plagues older humans, dogs, cats, and horses. There is no cure, but there are a variety of management options. Treatment regimens are highly individualized and based on the patient's response.

The three main tools we have for managing arthritis are: 1) non-steroidal anti-inflammatory drugs (NSAIDs), 2) disease-modifying osteoarthritis drugs (DMOADs), and 3) steroids injected directly into affected joints. The points below are not comprehensive, but are summaries of the broad categories themselves.

Non-Steroidal Anti-Inflammatory Drugs:
Like all drugs, NSAIDs each have a generic pharmaceutical or chemical name as well as a brand name. NSAIDs, such as phenylbutazone (sold under many brand names, but nicknamed "bute"), flunixin meglumine (Banamine®), and firocoxib (Equioxx® or Previcox®) are the most effective tool for managing arthritis pain. These drugs modulate nerve-mediated pain signaling.[74]

NSAIDs can have adverse effects on the gastrointestinal tract (GI), especially at high doses.[75, 76] They reduce blood flow to the digestive organs, which can result in ulcers of the stomach or colon. Ulcers are painful, resulting in signs of colic, loss of appetite, and weight loss. GI side effects are much more likely to occur if more than one NSAID is administered in a 48-hour period. Stress and other factors contribute to ulcer development. Bute also has adverse effects on kidneys.

Bute is the least expensive, and perhaps most effective, NSAID for equine orthopedic pain. Although many horses tolerate this drug with no sign of problems, bute is also the NSAID that can have the most severe GI effects. The dose range is 1 to 2 grams once or twice daily; 4 grams is the absolute maximum dosing for an average-sized horse. Higher doses and longer duration of usage increase the risk of GI side effects. Bute is available in four formulations: injectable, tablets, powder, and paste. The injectable medication is harmful to tissue when injected outside the vein, so it is administered by veterinarians, but not dispensed. In oral formulations, the drug is extremely bitter. Even the flavored powders may have to be mixed with additional sweeteners such as Karo® syrup or applesauce to make them palatable enough for your horse to willingly eat.

Empirically, bute is used for orthopedic pain and Banamine® for GI pain. In experiments comparing the two drugs, there is no discernable difference between the two.[77] If a horse has short-term orthopedic pain, such as a hoof abscess, Banamine® will work fine in a pinch to relieve his pain and quiet the inflammation. Banamine® is available as an injectable drug and an oral paste. Like bute, the injectable drug is harmful to tissue when given outside of the vein. It should never be injected into muscle because an abscess caused by *Clostridium spp.* bacteria can occur (fig. 5.19). These abscesses are difficult to treat, and can be fatal due to the toxicity of the bacteria. If paste is not available, the injectable medication can given by mouth, because it is absorbed orally.

The third common NSAID, firocoxib is

available as an injectable formulation, paste, and tablets. In pharmacology studies, its efficacy is equal to or better than bute.[78]

Disease Modifying Osteoarthritis Drugs: Disease modifying osteoarthritis drugs (DMOADs) aim to help the joint maintain normal joint fluid composition, reduce cartilage damage, and thereby decrease inflammation. Adequan® is the most research-backed and expensive therapy in this section. It is a polysulfated glycosaminoglycan—a big word for a tiny molecule found in joint fluid. While we don't know everything about how it works, research has shown that it is absorbed from the site of intramuscular injection, and is attracted to areas of inflammation. So, inflamed and painful joints that need it the most will get it. It should be started as a loading dose—one injection every four days for seven doses (28 days), then once monthly thereafter.

There are other, injectable polysulfated glycosaminoglycans on the market. As of this writing, Adequan® is the only one approved by the FDA for use in osteoarthritis.

Glucosamine is in many oral joint supplements. Manufacturing and storage conditions can greatly affect the amount in a supplement. Research shows that when used daily, glucosamine results in a decreased need or dosage of NSAIDs, although it is not usually well absorbed or very helpful in horses.

Hyaluronic acid (HA) comes in a variety of brands, and is commonly used for joint injections (see below). There are also formulations (Legend®) for IV administration. HA is a component of joint fluid and helps maintain lubrication and cartilage health.

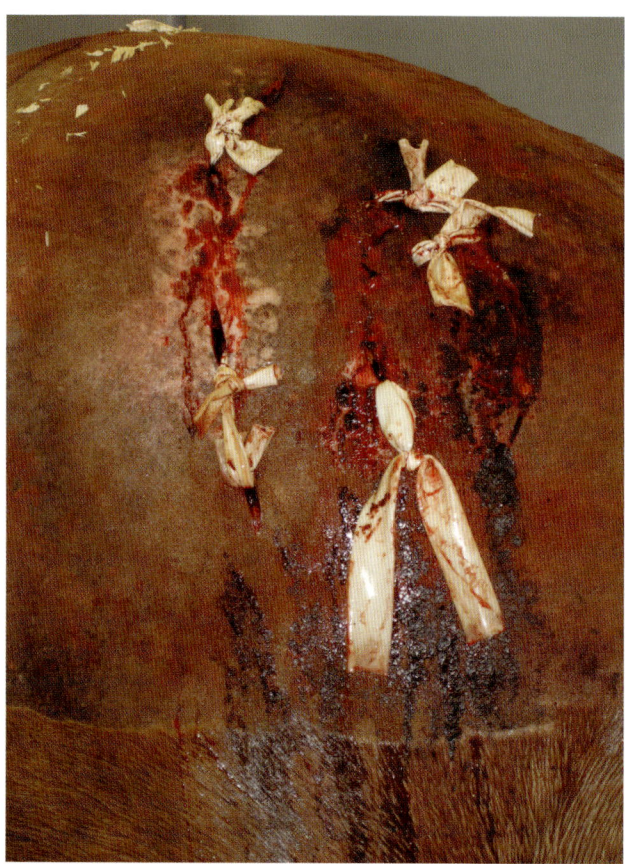

5.19 A Clostridial abscess as a result of an injection of Banamine® (flunixin meglumine) in the muscle.

Steroid Injections: Understanding facts regarding joint injections for your horse is critical, because there are many myths and legends that circulate among horse people regarding this therapy. Modern steroids are potent anti-inflammatories that reduce the pain of arthritis, maintaining joint health and the horse's quality of life. These injections are akin to a "cortisone shot in your knee" that physicians administer to people. However, when administered repeatedly into a joint with an underlying, treatable problem (such as a bone chip), steroids can merely mask the pain resulting in long-term damage. It is important to assess the joint structure with X-rays prior to injection.

In horses, we aseptically prepare the skin over the joint. There are a variety of protocols used, but all result in a decrease in the bacterial population on that area of skin. Veterinarians wear sterile gloves and use aseptic technique to perform the injection. Contamination of the joint can result in infection, a rare but serious complication. This is reported to occur at a rate of two to eight in 10,000 joints.[79]

In addition to the steroid, some larger joints will accommodate injection of HA. Finally, many veterinarians also inject an antibiotic to help prevent the complication of infection.

The cost for joint injection depends on what area of the country you are in, the joint that is injected, and the drugs that are used. This treatment is not typically within the budgetary range of most rescue groups, as an acceptable level of comfort can often be obtained with daily NSAID use and periodic Adequan® injections. The discussion is included here for the sake of thoroughness. If you ride your needy equine, you may find joint injections are necessary from time to time to maintain soundness.

WOUNDS

Some horses have lived in inappropriate housing, such as a small area with poorly maintained fence or the use of unsafe, make-do materials, like pallets held together with baling twine. Horses kept in this type of enclosure are more likely to sustain wounds or lacerations, especially on their lower limbs (below the hocks or knees). Injuries can also occur when horses have rough rides during shipping or fall down because of weakness. Horses unaccustomed to being handled or not trained to load in trailers may panic, which can result in traumatic injury.

If you are looking at a horse to rescue who has a longstanding wound, keep the following in mind: a horse with a chronic wound who is not lame generally carries a

5.20 Arthritis Treatment

NON-STEROIDAL ANTI-INFLAMMATORY DRUGS (NSAIDS)

Treatment	Dosing Notes
Phenylbutazone (bute)	IV injection, oral (paste, flavored powder, tablets), mainly used for orthopedic pain
Flunixin meglumine (Banamine®)	IV injection, oral (paste only), mainly used for colic pain
Firocoxib (Equioxx® or Previcox®)	Injection, oral (paste, tablets), used to treat orthopedic pain, especially long-term

DISEASE-MODIFYING OSTEOARTHRITIS DRUGS (DMOADS)

Treatment	Dosing Notes
Adequan®	Injection in the muscle	Attracted to all inflamed joints, good scientific support
Glucosamine	Oral	Poorly absorbed, may interfere with metabolic disease, weak scientific support, many formulations available (choose a high-quality one)
Hyaluronic Acid	IV or in the joint

OTHER

Treatment	Dosing Notes
Joint Injections	Only by your veterinarian, may last four to six months, only targets a specific joint

better prognosis than one whose wound has caused a lameness. Horses with cuts that invade or expose deeper structures such as joints are less likely to heal and may remain lame even if the wound heals (fig. 5.21). A severe, chronic wound may take a year to heal completely. A malnourished horse will have a delay in healing due to a lack of nutrients to serve as building blocks for tissue repair. The cost of bandaging is considerable. The tolerance and trainability of the horse to accept treatment is also a major consideration. If you can't touch him, it's going to be impossible to bandage his leg in a safe manner.

Wound Evaluation

If you acquire a horse who already has a wound, call your veterinarian for an intake examination. She can help you manage the wound. Wound depth is a critical factor for recovery. Anytime you discover a wound on one of your horses, you should try to evaluate and describe the wound as follows:

- Pull the skin apart. A full-thickness wound will have a gap with red tissue underneath showing. A partial-thickness wound is superficial and will not have a gap when you manipulate it.

- Walk the horse several strides and determine if he is lame or sore on his injured leg. Wounds that cause lameness need more intensive veterinary care to heal.

- Look closely and see if a flap is present or if a section of skin seems to be missing.

- Determine if the wound is near a joint.

- As you inspect the wound, if you can see muscle, bone, tendon, or other underlying structures, it is a deep wound that will need extensive treatment.

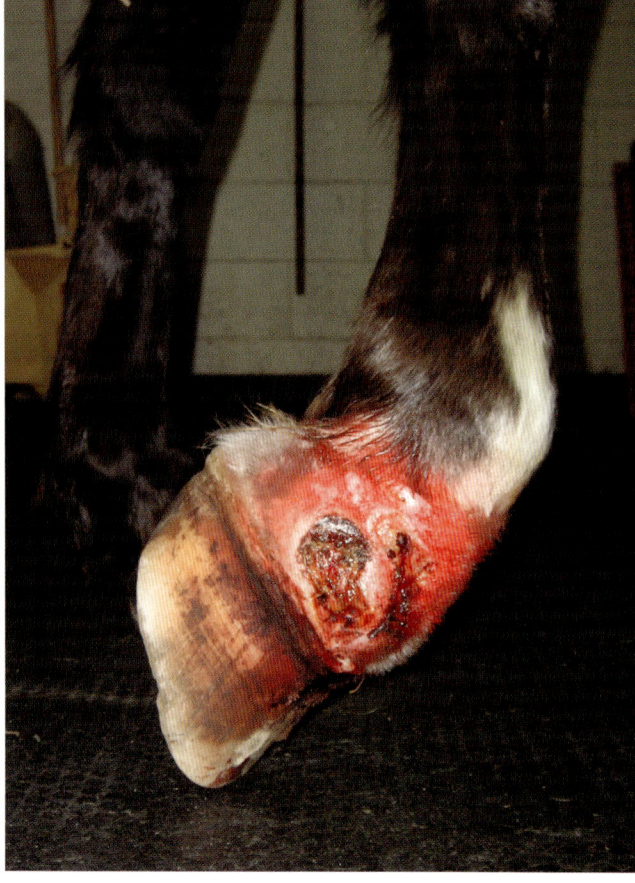

5.21 *A severe longstanding joint infection in the pastern as a result of a wound. This horse was non-weightbearing on this leg. He was humanely euthanized due to a grave prognosis for recovery.*

If possible, you should evaluate the whole horse, as well:

- His temperature should be between 99.5 and 101.5 degrees Fahrenheit. This may increase with agitation, infection, or inflammation.

- A normal horse's pulse should be between 32 and 44 beats per minute. A wounded horse's heart rate may be increased due to pain, shock, excitement, or a high body temperature.

- His respiratory rate should be 8 to 16 breaths per minute at rest. This parameter increases with a hot environment, pain, lack of oxygen, or stress. Pulse, temperature, and respiration will all also increase with exercise.

- Checking his gum color is also a good diagnostic tool. His mucous membranes should be moist and pink to pale pink (not relatively red, white, purple, or yellow). When you press your thumb or finger to the tissue and blanch the color out, the capillaries should refill and re-color in less than two seconds. A severe wound that has resulted in excessive blood loss, or one that has entered his chest cavity may drastically change these vital parameters.

Consult your veterinarian for any wound your horse sustains. Talk to her before you administer medication to your horse or apply topical treatments to the wound.

Wound Treatment

First of all, provide first aid. You must stay calm because losing your head over the sight of blood will not help your horse. Consider your own safety: If you are alone, ask a friend or family member for assistance while you wait for your veterinarian to arrive.

All items in your first-aid kit should be unused, clean, and in date. Because many horse owners have experienced wounds first hand, there is a fair amount of fear and hype regarding first-aid kits. Most of the time, you are going to need something relatively straightforward, like a basic bandage.

A basic kit contains a thermometer, some selection of bandage material, and a pain-relieving medication. You should be familiar with each item in your kit and know how to use it.

Move your horse to a clean, dry, and safe area. If there is blood running out of the wound, apply some absorbent material such as cotton gauze, and apply a bandage tight enough to stop the hemorrhage. If your veterinarian is on the way, this may be all you can do. Cleaning a wound may cause bleeding to resume.

When the wound is dirty and you do clean it, keep in mind that many wound-cleaning agents and techniques can harm tissue. Scrubbing causes physical damage. Many antiseptics are toxic to the healthy, healing tissue and will slow wound healing or damage the cells within the fresh wound. If you are considering a topical medication, a rule of thumb is if you wouldn't put it in your eye, don't put it on a wound. Thorough rinsing is helpful and appropriate. In veterinary medicine, we have a saying, "The solution to pollution is dilution."

Full-thickness wounds that are stitched up and treated properly from the beginning heal faster and are more likely to result in full return to function—even when the sutures don't stay in. Your veterinarian may prescribe anti-inflammatory pain medication and an antibiotic. She may also update your horse's tetanus vaccine.

Sometimes suture lines will pull apart due to tension, infection, or poor healing. However, the tissue underneath has had the benefit of being covered and protected by skin for the initial healing stages.

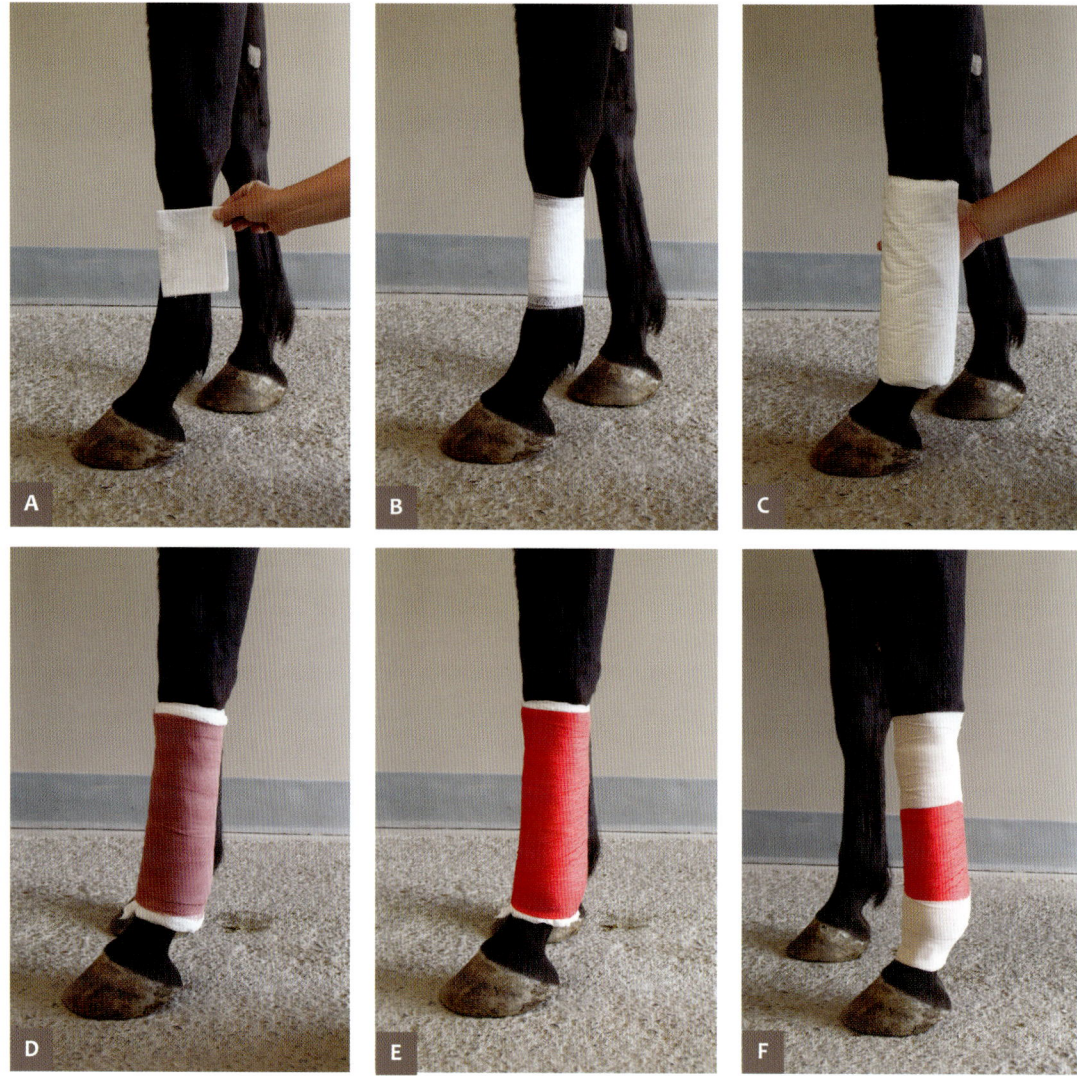

5.22 A–F *Steps for bandaging a leg: Start with a nonstick pad, such as a Telfa™ pad (A). Use rolled gauze to hold the pad in place (B). Follow with an absorbent padding layer (C) and a brown gauze compression layer (D). Your final steps are Vetrap™(E) and a final layer of Elastikon™.*

Bandaging

A bandage for a leg wound will begin with a non-stick layer, such as a Telfa™ pad. The Telfa™ may be held in place with cast padding or roll gauze. A layer of absorbent padding, such as quilt batting or cotton is next. Padding provides pressure and protection to the wound and the leg. The third layer compresses the absorbent padding layer.

Vetrap™ or a similar product can be used alone or on top of non-stretch rolled brown gauze. This final layer holds everything in place and protects deeper layers of bandage. A bit of the absorbent padding layer should be visible on both the top and the bottom of the layer. Avoid applying Vetrap™ or a constricting layer directly to the skin—it can cause damage if left on for more than a couple of hours. Finally, Elastikon® can be used at the top and bottom to keep debris out and to help hold the bandage in place. When you apply this bandage, roll tendons on the back of the leg to the inside. This is the natural direction they lie, and rolling with their natural location can help avoid damage caused by pressure (figs. 5.22 A–F).

It is not necessary to apply topical ointments or creams. Most substances delay healing. If it is colored, don't use it because it's bad for the tissue (for example, scarlet oil, strong iodine, *nitrofurazone,* or *ichthammol*). The least harmful over-the-counter medications for wound therapy are *Vetricyn®* or plain triple antibiotic ointment (for example, *Neosporin®*). Your veterinarian may provide you with safe and soothing *silver sulfadiazine* (SSD) or another topical product for a specific purpose.

Extensive or Deep Wounds

Complicated wounds are those that did not heal with sutures, or a wound that invades a vital structure. First of all, it can be difficult to differentiate these wounds from a superficial or non-complicated wound—especially at first glance. A large, gaping, bloody wound that involves only muscle and skin may heal extremely well. Conversely, a seemingly small and minor puncture can result in a serious joint infection. This is why it is important to consult with your veterinarian for any wound (figs. 5.23 A–C).

The deepest wounds may expose internal organs—parts of the body that should remain sterile. If a wound enters the chest cavity, cover it to ensure that air (and dirt, debris, or contamination) cannot enter. If the abdominal cavity has been compromised and intestines are open, the horse

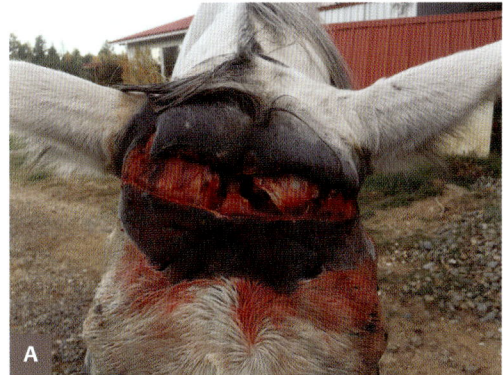

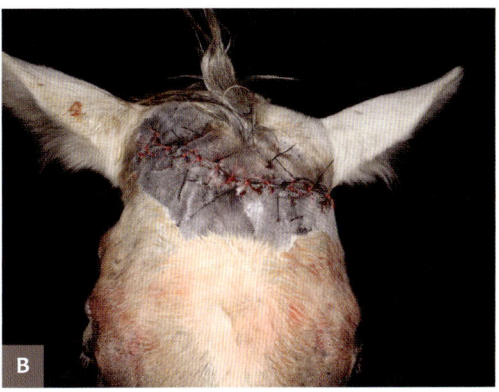

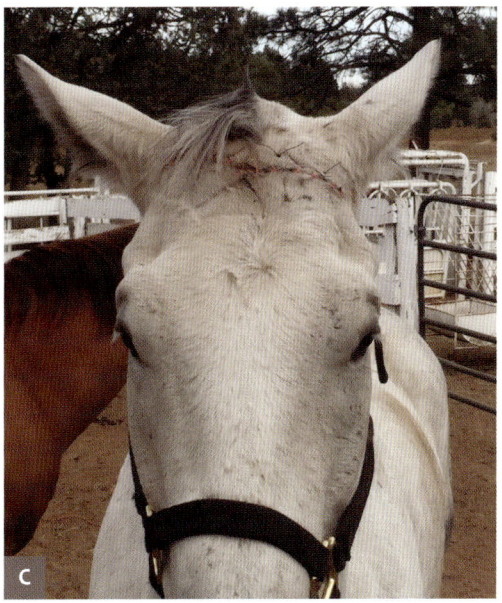

5.23 A–C *This serious-appearing wound had several small bone fragments in it—here it is pictured after it has been clipped and cleaned (A). Fortunately, the bone over the brain was intact. The same wound, after repair (B) and fully healed (C), just two weeks later with no complications.*

will not survive and should be euthanized immediately.

Deep wounds can be difficult and expensive to treat. If a deep wound enters the abdominal cavity and the digestive tract is torn or damaged, the horse's odds of survival are unfortunately nearly zero. Because deep wounds require extensive treatment, cost is high.

Infected Wounds

Horses live outside and contact dirt and manure, therefore every wound they sustain is considered a dirty wound. An infected joint can result in permanent lameness. If not resolved, euthanasia may be the only option.

There are a variety of treatment options for infected joints. Essentially, two factors influence outcome: how early the infection is diagnosed and the way the infection is treated. What this means is that choosing the ideal—and more expensive—treatment option increases the chances of being able to restore your horse's soundness.

It may not initially be obvious that a joint is contaminated. A horse with this type of wound will not be immediately lame, but as bacteria multiply inside the joint, the pain the horse experiences will increase. It takes two to four days for this type of infection to manifest as a crippling lameness.

The initial trauma may expose bone, damaging its blood supply. When this happens, an area of the bone may die. The body will treat the *sequestrum* (piece of dead bone) as a splinter or foreign material, and the wound will not heal until it is removed.

Trauma may also result in a fracture. Depending on which bone is broken, some treatment options may be available, and your veterinarian can help you determine the best course of action. One of the most common broken bones in horses is the wispy end of a splint bone. Unlike most other broken bones, horses with fractures of the splint often fully recover and are sound.

THE REALITY OF LAMENESS

It is important to recognize lameness and hoof problems, as well as disease conditions—hoof abscesses, laminitis, and arthritis—with respect to rescue horses because you want to improve their quality of life. You want the horses in your care to be comfortable and happy. It may be very sad as a rescuer to bypass a beautiful horse, but if he is one that has an obvious lameness, it is going to be difficult and expensive to care for him. Obtaining a horse with a wound adds a level of complexity and expense to his needs. Know that a lame horse's riding (and therefore adoption) opportunities are limited.

CHAPTER 6

Birth Control:
Managing Mares and Castrating Colts

Many small animal shelters must focus on spay/neuter programs to quell companion animal overpopulation; people involved in equine rescue must also consider the reproductive status of horses. Castration of male horses is routine and the primary way to restrict reproduction in equines. Conversely, the increased risk and high cost of spaying a mare renders it a rare necessity, rather than a routine procedure. You should also consider the less obvious, but perhaps more important, pregnancy status of your new mare or filly. If she is already pregnant, she will need special care throughout her gestation.

CASTRATION OF MALES

Gelding is the horseman's term for castration and is also known as *cutting*. Gelding is the surgical removal of the testes and has been used for hundreds of years to prevent reproduction and undesired, testosterone-associated masculine behavior. Occasionally, horses can develop medical problems associated with the testes, such as tumors, scrotal hernias (where intestine escapes from the abdomen and falls into the scrotum), inflammation, or trauma. Any of these problems can require removal of one or both testes as treatment.

When to Safely Castrate Males: When you acquire a stallion or colt, he should be gelded as soon as possible. However, he should not undergo anesthesia until he has at least a BCS of 4, has completed his quarantine period, and is up to date on vaccines (see pp. 28, 21, and 55). Your veterinarian has to be able to touch your horse to sedate and anesthetize him, so you must make sure he is halter-broke.

Before Castration: Your horse should have an examination to determine that he is healthy, and that both testes have descended into the scrotum. Occasionally, a horse will "retain" a testis and will need a more involved procedure.

Anesthesia

One reason we wait until the horse has attained a BCS of 4 is because he will need strength to recover from *field anesthesia* or tolerate *standing sedation*.

Field anesthesia (fig. 6.1) is administered by a veterinarian using injectable, fast-acting, short-duration drugs. Your horse will be down and unresponsive for about 30

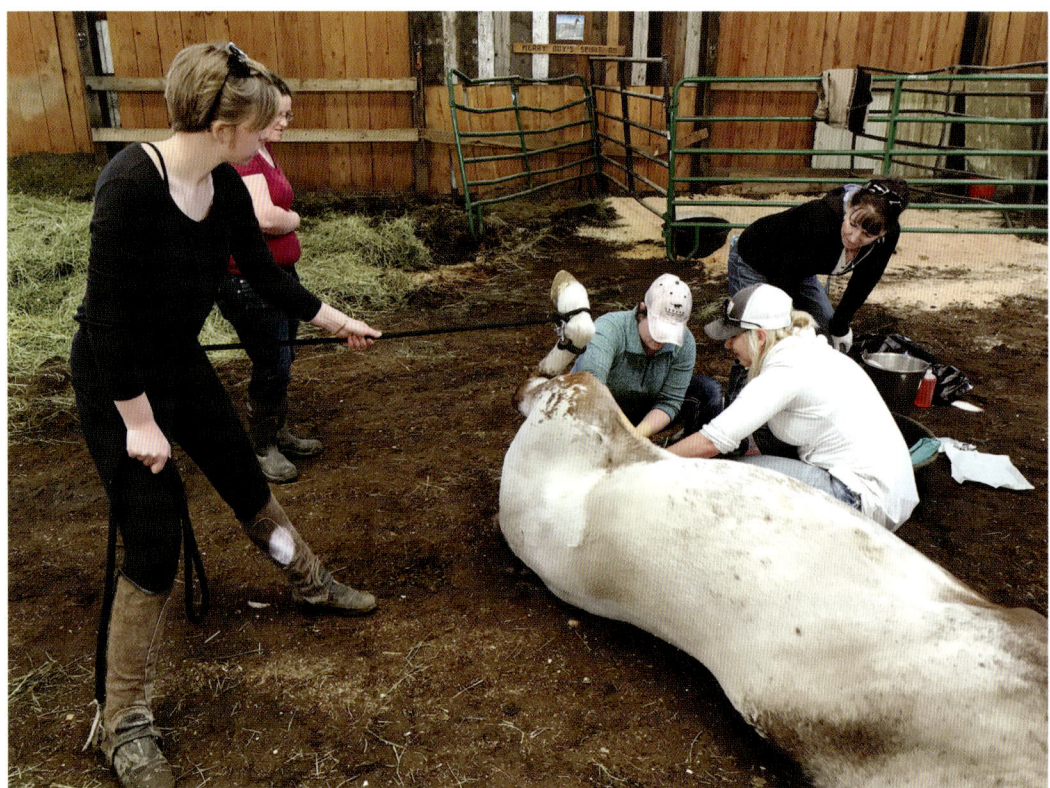

6.1 *A horse being castrated. The EquiSave Foundation in Livingston, Montana, acquired 40 horses when one of their owners passed away. Eight were stallions, and all were castrated in one day with a number of volunteers assisting me.*

to 60 minutes. As a prey animal, the horse has an extreme flight drive, so as soon as any speck of consciousness returns, he will try to stand. He will be uncoordinated and weak from the drugs, and sometimes it will take several attempts to stand up. In the field, horses typically recover from the short anesthetic episode quite well, but we want to make sure your colt is strong enough to do so without problems.

Another reason we wait until he is an appropriate weight is that during anesthesia, blood pressure drops. Because horses are large, their muscles can be crushed by the weight of their body due to the decreased blood flow. If your horse is too thin, muscle damage can happen more easily over pressure points.

A potential complication of anesthesia is pneumonia. Therefore, the horse needs to be completely healthy and through his quarantine period. We want to make sure he isn't harboring a virus or on the cusp of illness before his procedure.

When castration is done with the animal standing but sedated, local anesthetic that desensitizes the area is necessary (fig. 6.2). In order to castrate a standing horse, he must be tall enough for a veterinarian to reach under the belly to perform the procedure, and the horse must be gentle enough for proper restraint. Doing this surgery while the horse is standing clearly carries an extra risk for the veterinarian and also carries an increased risk of some complications (for example, contamination leading to infection) for the horse.[81] Also, if intraoperative complications such as hemorrhage or evisceration occur, your horse will have to be anesthetized to correct the problem.

So, why would a veterinarian choose to castrate a horse standing? Because it takes much less time as she doesn't have to wait for the horse to recover from anesthesia. It also eliminates any risks of general anesthesia for the horse (as long as there are no intraoperative complications).

Routine Castration

The surgical procedure for a routine castration takes 10 to 15 minutes. At the time of surgery, some veterinarians choose to give the colt a dose of antibiotics[82] and/or a dose of an anti-inflammatory pain medication. Your veterinarian will also require your horse to be up-to-date on his tetanus vaccine.

To geld a horse, two incisions are made directly into the scrotum over each testis. Blood flow to each testis is eliminated by crushing the spermatic cord with the emasculator (fig. 6.3). Then the spermatic cord is cut, removing the testis. The emasculators are left in place to maintain the crush for several minutes to ensure that a stable clot forms. The stump of the spermatic cord is inspected for any bleeding before being returned to the horse's abdomen. The process is repeated for the second testis.

Routine After-Care

Your horse will recover from field anesthesia and stand in about 20 to 30 minutes (fig. 6.4). The incision is left open and will

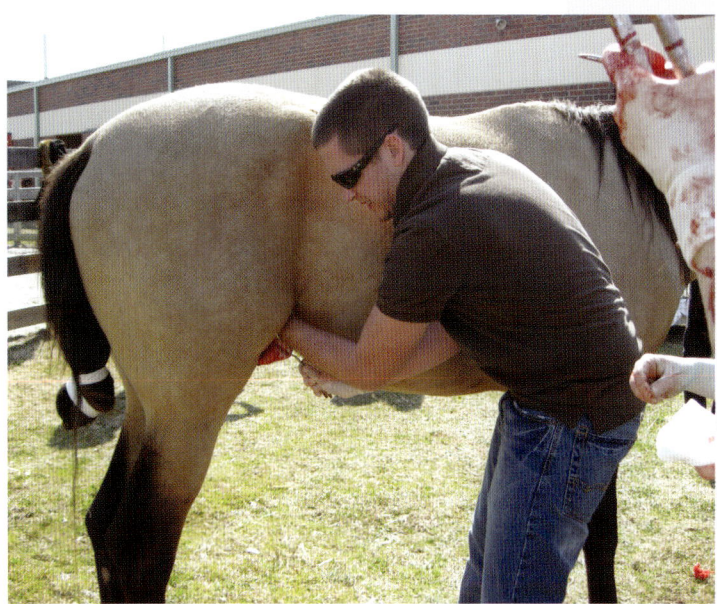

6.2 *Standing castration.*

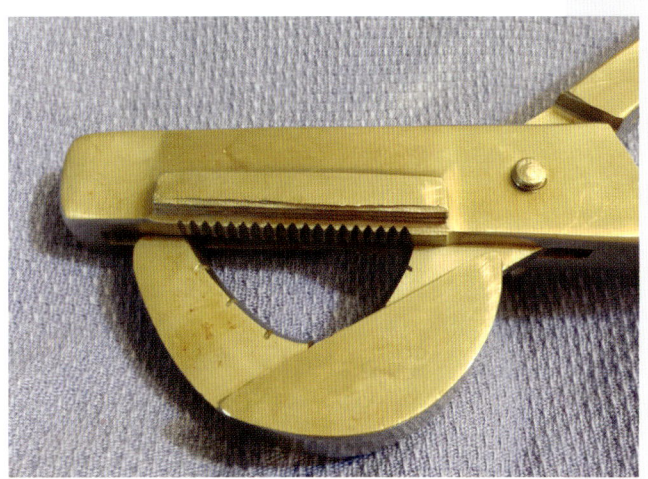

6.3 *One type of emasculators used for castration of horses.*

heal from the inside to the outside.

Your colt should stay in a stall or small pen overnight. After that time, he will need daily exercise to make sure there is no continued bleeding. Exercise increases the movement of body fluid, thus decreasing the swelling that often occurs after castration. Swelling is usually greatest at the fourth or fifth day post-operatively.

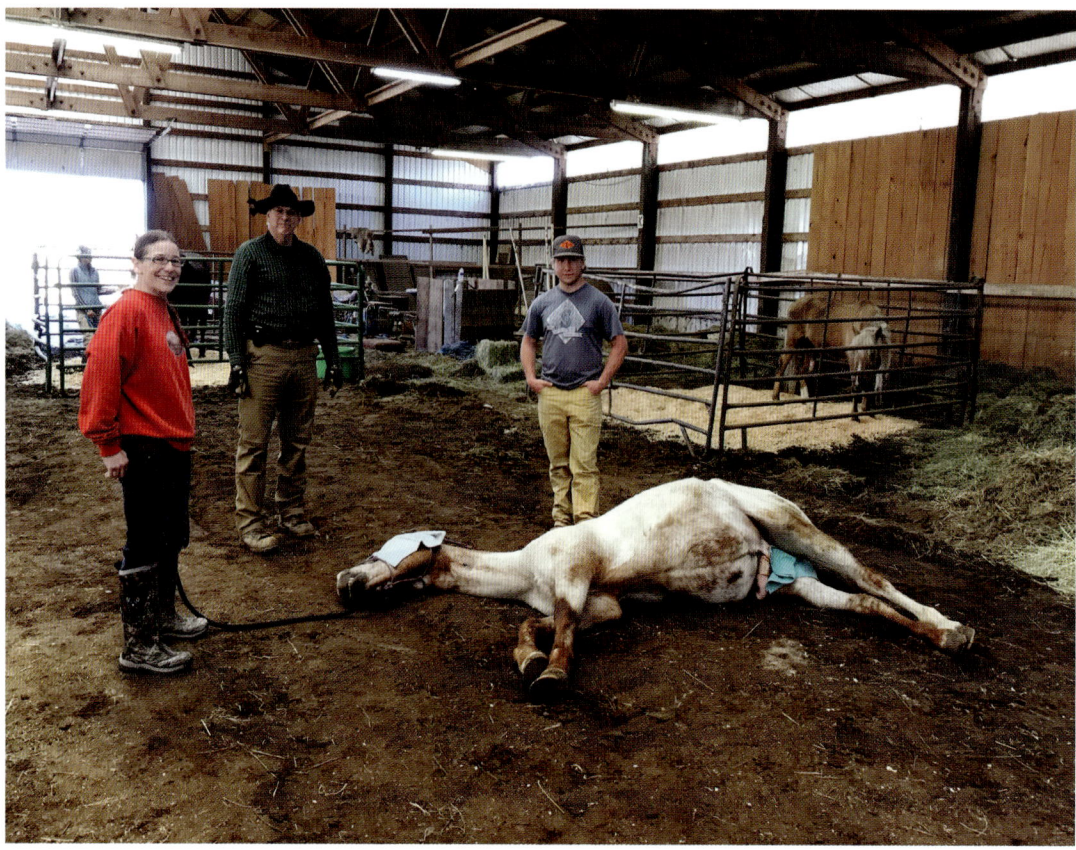

6.4 *Volunteers helping the castrated horse from fig. 6.1 (see p. 86) to recover.*

The drainage and swelling will continue for about two weeks as the surgical site heals. Historically, horse people used to cold-hose the area to help reduce swelling. This is no longer recommended, as research has shown that it predisposes the horse to infection.

Long-Term Expectations

Behaviorally, it takes about six weeks for all of the testosterone to be excreted by your horse's body. Testosterone is responsible for masculine behavior, so when it is absent, stallion-like behaviors diminish or disappear. Normal stallion behaviors include aggression, such as rearing or striking, lots of vocalization around mares, and the *flehmen* response—flipping the top lip up or wrinkling the nose to trap pheromones in a special nasal receptor (fig. 6.5). *Pheromones* are odorless, colorless biochemicals that are secreted by one animal and can affect the behavior of another.

Some geldings (20 to 30 percent) continue to exhibit stallion-like behavior, no matter the age at which they are castrated. This behavior is not due to hormonal influences, but is innate, psychic behavior.[83]

Because semen is stored in the internal accessory sex glands, it is possible for a gelded horse to inseminate a mare for up to four weeks after surgery. Mature recent geldings should be kept away from mares during this time to prevent accidental impregnations.

Castration Complications

Castration is the most common surgery performed by equine veterinarians, but any surgery can result in complications. About 10 percent of horses develop complications in addition to the expected swelling. Some of the complications with castration can be serious, so follow-up care is important.

Swelling: Nearly all new geldings will have some swelling. The larger the testes that were removed, the more the area seems to swell. Usually, the incision site is the only area that swells, but the swelling can extend into the prepuce (sheath), or to the hind legs. A typical swelling is the size of a grapefruit or a little larger, while extreme swelling is the size of a cantaloupe or watermelon, it affects the prepuce (sheath), and may inhibit the horse's movement. Some horses can be very sore from swelling and may show signs of colic or lameness.

What to Do About Swelling: Exercise! Although some pastured colts will move around enough to keep the tissue in the area well-drained, some simply stand around feeling sorry for themselves. Horses in stalls don't have the opportunity to self-exercise. At a minimum, I recommend 15 minutes of trotting, loping, or galloping twice daily as long as swelling is visible. Extreme swelling should be re-evaluated by a veterinarian.

Hemorrhage: Bleeding is going to occur in surgery, but it should be minimal. A slow drip of blood from incised skin and nearby tissues is expected for up to 24 hours. If you see a steady drip (more than one drop per second) or stream, your horse should be reassessed by your veterinarian.

What to Do About Bleeding: Keep the horse confined and as quiet as possible. Call your veterinarian immediately. Bleeding may occur after the horse stands up and his blood pressure increases. Having the horse confined in a small area for 24 hours after the procedure helps ensure that bleeding has stopped completely before starting his daily exercise program.

There are several ways your veterinarian may address the bleeding vessel. The blood vessel may be clamped temporarily, or the area may be packed with gauze. In extreme

6.5 The flehmen response, a normal behavior that is occasionally exhibited by any horse and frequently exhibited by breeding stallions.

cases, the horse may need to be anesthetized to find and stop the bleeding. Rarely, a horse may need a transfusion because of extreme blood loss.

Infection: This complication is not common. You may notice your gelding is extremely sore or has severe swelling. Infection will not be immediately apparent, but takes several days to develop post-operatively. It happens when the skin seals too soon. One study found serum amyloid A (a protein marker of inflammation) to be significantly lower when procaine penicillin was administered at the time of castration.

What to Do About Infection: Drainage of the area is key to preventing and treating infection. Call your veterinarian. Most likely, you will also need to increase your gelding's exercise. Although antibiotics can be useful, the surgical site may need to be opened to increase drainage. Rarely, the infection can ascend the remainder of the spermatic cord (*schirrous cord*) and invasive, difficult surgery will be necessary to remove the infected tissue.

Other Complications: Other complications are rare. A life-threatening one is *evisceration*, where abdominal organs protrude out of the surgical site. Trauma to the penis can occur intraoperatively. Infection within the abdominal cavity may occur as well. These complications require further, intensive medical intervention.

Cryptorchid Castration

The root medical meaning of *crypt* is hidden, and *orchid* is the root for testis. Cryptorchids are individuals in whom a testis fails to descend into the scrotum, and it remains "hidden" within the abdomen or inguinal canal. The medical term for the procedure to remove a hidden testis is a *cryptorchidectomy*. During normal development, the early testes must travel from high in the abdomen behind the kidney all the way to the scrotum. Other terms for a cryptorchid include *rig*, a *ridgling*, or a *high flanker*.

Prevalence of cryptorchidism in the general population is hard to define, but is probably less than 10 percent.[85, 86]

Why Cryptorchidism Happens: Genetics influence the development of cryptorchidism.[87] Some breeds are comparatively more predisposed to being cryptorchid, including Percherons, Saddlebreds, and Quarter Horses. In general, Thoroughbreds have the lowest prevalence of cryptorchidism, but some successful racing lines are known to have a higher incidence than the remainder of the breed.

Long Ears

Donkeys and mules have special needs for castration. With respect to anesthesia, some references indicate that increased dosages of anesthetic drugs are needed.[84] This is partially due to a species difference in metabolism. Also fearful, unhandled animals will need more sedation. Conversely, a desensitized and trusting animal will need less, even though he is a donkey.

Donkeys (and therefore mules) have larger testes when compared to horses, making them prone to increased bleeding. Veterinarians suture the spermatic cord, rather than solely relying on the emasculators to stop the bleeding.

Cryptorchidism renders a stallion less fertile and is considered a defect. Some breed associations do not allow registry of affected individuals. Every cryptorchid horse should be castrated because of the potential heritability of the problem. In dogs and humans, it is known that a retained testis is more likely to develop a tumor, but this is not well documented in horses.[88]

Horses are unique: the gonads of the fetus produce hormones that are important for signaling the maintenance of pregnancy. Because of this activity, the testes are relatively large at birth, but decrease in size after birth. Contrary to horse person lore, the location of the gonad at birth doesn't change over the horse's lifespan. A retained testis will not descend or "drop" later, no matter how long you wait. Some *high flankers* have a testis outside the abdomen, but not all the way to the scrotum. This inguinally located testis may be easier to identify after puberty when the testes enlarge to adult size.

Why Cryptorchids Often Need Help: A cryptorchid horse is more likely to find himself in need of a home. There are two reasons: behavior and expense. Any stallion can be aggressive and difficult to handle, and some horsemen believe cryptorchids are even worse than normal stallions.[89]

It is more expensive to castrate a cryptorchid horse than a normal horse. A cryptorchid castration is more involved: There are a variety of anomalous testicular locations, and there are multiple surgical approaches to castrate cryptorchid horses. Anesthesia time is longer, and the procedure should be done in a clean hospital operating room, rather than in the field. If the abdomen of the horse has to be opened to find the undescended

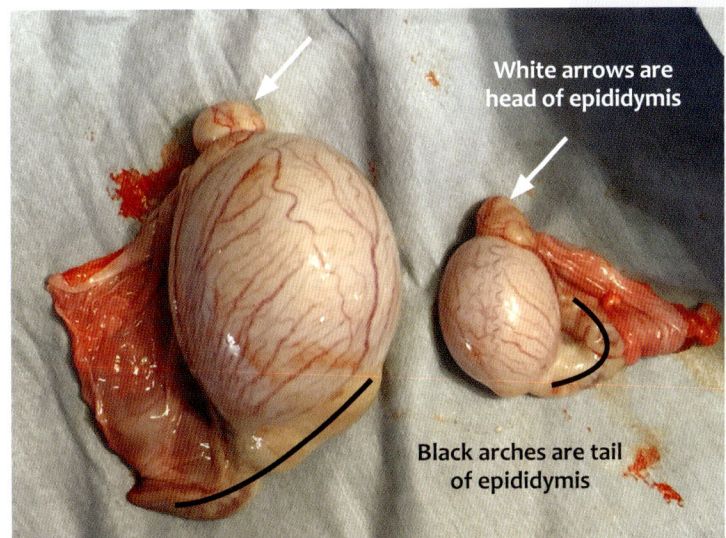

6.6 *The "retained" testis of a cryptorchid horse (on the right) is much smaller than the normal one.*

testis, the expense can go higher (fig. 6.6).

It is important for you to be able to identify cryptorchid individuals and understand the increased cost you will incur caring for them. They can be great geldings, and many are worth the investment, but the expense often means their former owners weren't able to afford the surgical procedure they needed, and that is the reason they are "unwanted."

The Proud-Cut Myth

A horse can be termed *proud-cut* for several reasons.[90] The most general sense of the term applies strictly to behavior: He appears to be gelding but exhibits stallion-like behaviors. The first reason is that he continues to have normal (but undesirable) masculine behavior after castration. It is rare for continued masculine behavior to occur because he was improperly castrated and testicular tissue remains. Sometimes the term *proud-cut* is used to imply that a surgical error occurred. In olden times, this was blamed on a portion of the *epididymis* (a portion of the sperm duct) remaining in the horse and continuing to produce testosterone and influence behavior. This belief is the myth! The epididymis, located adjacent to the testis, functions only as a storage site for sperm and does not produce testosterone.

Improper castration of cryptorchids can happen when only the descended testis is removed. Veterinarians considered this unethical. It can happen if a lay-person removes only the visible testis. This event occurred in the bygone era before good

The Proud-Cut Lottery

The heated conversation between husband and wife was in full swing when I opened the barn door. They were in disagreement about whether the mare in question was fat or whether her bursting belly contained a baby.

I took one look at the mare and informed the couple that their horse was most definitely pregnant. The wife nodded smugly. I confirmed the pregnancy with a transcutaneous ultrasound (a sonogram), pressing the probe to the mare's skin over her abdomen and showing them the baby's ribs and heartbeat.

The husband's horse, Rocky, was a gorgeous sorrel frame overo "gelding" he had purchased when the horse was about 20 months old (just before puberty) about 14 months prior. After puberty occurred, a testicle became visible near Rocky's scrotum. He had been an improperly castrated *high-flanker*. As soon as the couple noticed the testicle and Rocky's change in behavior, they removed him from contact with their mare. They were in legal discussion with Rocky's former owner, a rancher who had performed the castration himself, regarding being sold a one-testicle stallion rather than a complete gelding.

They thought the pretty, dun-colored mare, Rhonda, would not have conceived so quickly; after all, Rocky had just been a baby. The mare, however, had noticed Rocky's fertility before they had, and conceived a foal. Here we were, with the mare due in the next week or two. These were fairly experienced horse people, and they knew the mare had not received all the care she needed. They were worried. And, although they knew horses well, they had never birthed a foal. Luckily, Rhonda's body condition was appropriate, not too thin. The alfalfa hay commonly fed in the area was safe for pregnant mares.

We separated Rhonda from the rest of the group, and gave her private access to a large, sheltered stall and a clean pen. We updated all of her vaccines. We talked about all of the things that mares show when they are getting ready to foal: a fuller udder, sometimes dripping milk or *waxing*, relaxation of the vulva as well as the croup muscles and ligaments, and early stages of birth looking like colic. We talked about watching for the foal's head and both front feet being visible in a normal birth.

In lottery-like luck, everything went smoothly, and a beautiful dun frame overo colt was born one week later. We were all relieved. He was gorgeous and a rare color that many breeders and horse people desire and try unsuccessfully to get. This colt was not the first, nor the last, baby horse to be born with a "gelding" as a sire.

anesthesia was available: Inability to anesthetize the horse negated the surgeon's ability to effectively remove the undescended, hidden testis.

Hormone testing can determine if testosterone-producing tissue is present or not. It is important to screen the hormones of a suspected improperly castrated horse before he undergoes a major anesthetic episode and invasive surgical procedure.

PARAPHIMOSIS

Debilitated male horses can have an additional problem. They can become so weak, their muscles can no longer keep their penis retracted into the sheath. This problem is called *paraphimosis*. In cold climates, they may be subjected to frostbite, so it is important to keep the horse warm until his muscle function returns. There are ways to bandage or support the dangling organ with a sling while the horse gains weight and strength.

It is also possible for nerves to sustain permanent damage. If paraphimosis becomes permanent, the penis may have to be partially or fully amputated. This procedure can be done with the horse sedated and the nerves numb. Horses have a high quality of life after healing. If left untreated, the dangling penis can become injured or infected, resulting in systemic illness.

PREGNANCY EVALUATION IN MARES AND FILLIES

The natural cycle of the mare is a single ovulation every 21 days throughout the spring, summer, and early fall. A mare does not cycle when there is not enough daylight, so there is a period of quiescence called *anestrus* during the winter months. There is variation in mares' cycles, which is influenced by latitude or geographic location as well as the individual (presumably due to genetic variation).

A mare's early signs of pregnancy are subtle because as a prey animal, she defends herself by running. The fetal foal increases in size during the final trimester, but the pregnancy still sometimes goes unnoticed by caretakers until the last minute. Worse yet, if the pregnancy is not identified, it may become apparent only when a problem occurs or the mare aborts the foal. It can be shocking to see an emaciated mare that is still maintaining a pregnancy—just because she is very thin when you acquire her doesn't rule out pregnancy (fig. 6.7).

The sooner a pregnancy is identified, the sooner appropriate and special health care can commence. The point of helping horses is to provide adequate healthcare and emotional well-being for them. Ensuring you know a mare's reproductive status is critical for providing this care. If it seems I am over-emphasizing this point, it is because of the number of surprise foals I have seen.

Every mare or filly acquired should have a pregnancy check at the time of her intake examination. Palpation of the uterus per rectum is satisfactory for determining if the mare is pregnant in mid to late gestation. In late pregnancy, the ultrasound probe may be used transcutaneously (across the belly) rather than per rectum to evaluate the foal from a different perspective.

Ultrasound of the uterus per rectum is necessary in early stages of pregnancy, and an embryo cannot be detected prior to about two weeks. It is possible mating was not observed, especially if a mare went

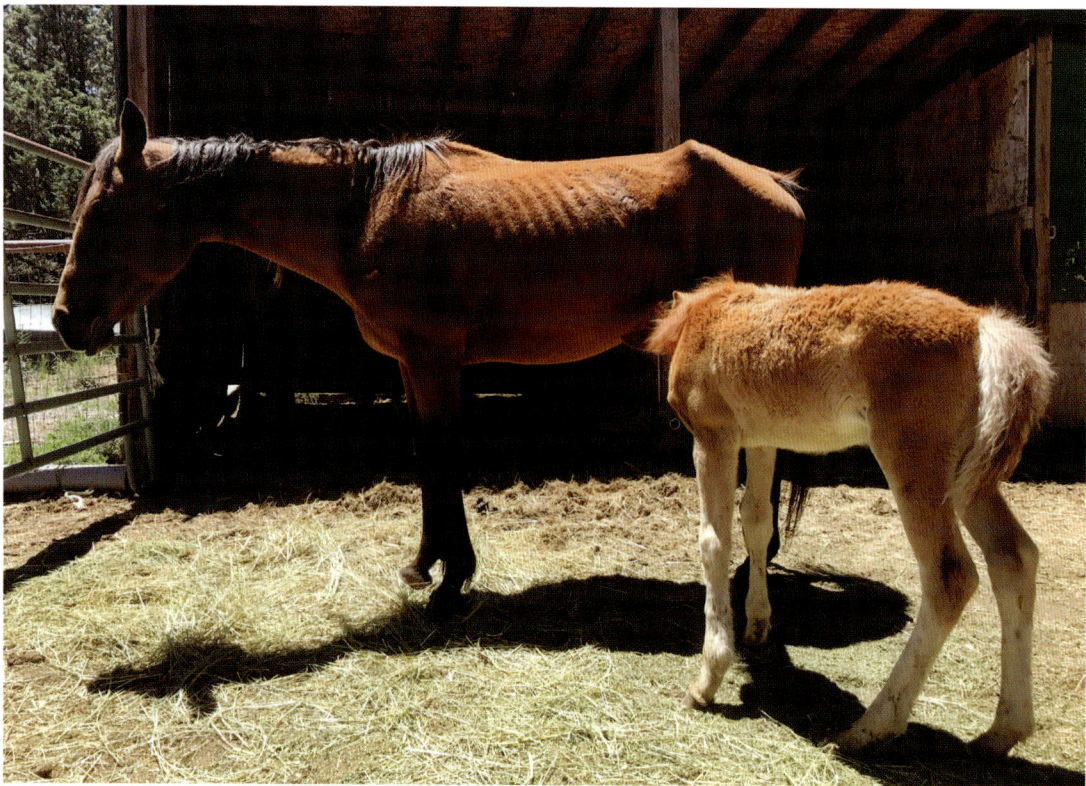

6.7 *Even a very thin mare can be pregnant, so all rescued mares should be evaluated for this condition.*

through a sales auction or was with a mixed herd. If a mare's history is unknown, the ultrasound should be repeated in two to four weeks to ensure a very early pregnancy is not missed.

Serum testing of hormones is available but is most useful in horses where an approximate breeding date is known. These tests can also be used in some instances, such as Miniature Horses, where standard pregnancy testing techniques cannot be used. Ultrasound is more commonly used, because it is less expensive.

Pregnant Mare Nutrition

Caloric Needs Increase: Because the equine fetus is small in early gestation, a mare does not have increased requirements for energy until late in gestation. In a thin rescue mare, her nutrition requirements will be based off her own nutritional needs first.

In the average 1,000-pound mare, the fetal foal gains almost a pound a day during the last three months of gestation—up to 80 percent of fetal growth occurs during this time. This is the time that your mare's nutritional requirements will change and be the most critical. In addition to needing more calories, she will need additional protein, vitamins, and minerals (especially calcium and phosphorus). Choose high-quality hay, and feeds that are labeled for pregnant mares.

Fescue: Fescue grass and hay should be eliminated from a pregnant mare's diet, especially in the last 60 days of gestation. Fescue

Two for One

The twenty-five eager veterinary students gathered for rounds in the veterinary teaching hospital. As we stopped at a patient's stall, the assigned student presented the medical case. Our patient, Sweetie, was an average horse: chestnut with a little bit of white, 15 hands, medium build, middle-aged, a quiet demeanor. Nothing special. She had unfortunately sustained a bad laceration on one of her front legs. Her owners loved her, although she was their first horse and they had little experience. When she sustained the wound, they were willing and able to have it treated.

The student explained about the anesthesia and surgical procedure that Sweetie had undergone earlier in the day to repair the wound, and relayed information about overnight treatments to the night-duty staff and veterinary students. One of the skilled veterinary technicians asked when Sweetie was due to foal. The student looked puzzled. The other students were quiet as the attending veterinarian told us that the mare was not pregnant. The technician and I looked at each other in surprise—we had both foaled out a number of mares for clients, as well as our own. The mare clearly had a very large abdomen.

I asked, "When did the owners acquire her?"

"They rescued her back in October, and she was thin at that time," explained the student. "The owners have been working on her gaining weight."

"She doesn't have any udder development," the attending veterinarian argued with me, "so she can't be pregnant."

I posed another question: "Has she been eating fescue?"

This type of grass was common in the area. Fescue can interfere with gestational hormone signaling, resulting in lack of udder development, reduced or absent milk production, prolonged pregnancy, and problems during the birth process. Nobody knew what type of grass or hay she had been eating at home.

I placed the ultrasound probe against Sweetie's belly. Sure enough, there were legs, and ribs, and a heartbeat! This mare had been through general anesthesia while late-term pregnant. The owners had no idea. It turned out that the mare had, in fact, been eating fescue, which had halted her milk production.

Sweetie was discharged from the hospital with medication to help counteract the toxin from the fescue, strict feeding guidelines, information about the birthing process, and an appointment for the next week with the reproduction specialists to more closely determine an expected due date. That appointment turned out to be unnecessary because her owners called early the very next morning—she had foaled at home. A beautiful, perfect foal! But no milk yet from the mare. The owners brought the mare and foal to the hospital for further treatment. A dedicated team looked after Sweetie and her colt for another week. Sweetie finally came into milk, and the colt thrived.

A mare with a surprise pregnancy is common in rescue situations, even when the mare is thin. The mare had not been expensive, but when Sweetie's people rescued her, they were 100 percent committed. This case resulted in a good outcome because her owners and the veterinary team worked closely to ensure she had everything she needed to restore full health of the mare and the foal that resulted from a high-risk pregnancy.

originated in North Africa and Eurasia, and a variety of species have naturalized throughout the world. It is common in the Northeast, Midwest, Central, and Southern regions of the United States because it grows best in humid areas. Tall fescue (Kentucky-31) is hardy and the most common. Fescue grows in bunches, it is smooth on the bottom of the blades but has ribs on the upper side. It is a flat-blade, cold-season grass with its fastest period of growth during the spring. When baled, it rolls up as it dries, making the blade stems look like a coarse hay. In mature grass, the small seeds develop in bunches at the stalk. To be honest, many grasses look similar. It is difficult to identify fescue.

The grass itself does not cause problems during gestation; the danger is in *Epichloë coenophiala*, a fungus that lives in between the plant's cells (often referred to as an *endophyte*). In the syndrome known as *fescue toxicosis* the endophyte produces hormone-mimicking substances that interrupt gestational signaling in horses. This results in a variety of problems including lack of milk production, problems during birth, decreased foal growth rate, and death of the mare and/or foal. A drug, *domperidone*, is available and is used to counteract the effects of fescue toxicosis.

Endophyte-free varieties of fescue grass are available. If you find out your mare is pregnant, it is critical to work closely with your hay and feed suppliers. Pure alfalfa, timothy, and orchard grasses are easiest to differentiate from fescue and are widely available, so sticking with those options for feed is best.

Vaccines for Pregnant Mares

Equine Herpesvirus: Mares need additional vaccinations during gestation. EHV-1 is also known as *rhinopneumonitis*; it is airborne, and usually causes respiratory signs similar to the common cold. It can also cause abortion (fetal death) in mares. Every pregnant mare should be vaccinated against EHV-1 in the fifth, seventh, and ninth month of gestation.

Quarantine protocols are designed to prevent the spread of EHV. This is especially important to protect pregnant mares—it prevents EHV spreading from new horses to pregnant mares in your herd. It also keeps a newly rescued pregnant mare from contracting any illness that may weaken her immune system and increase her susceptibility to EHV-induced abortion.

Other Vaccines: The interface between the uterus and the placenta allows oxygen and nutrients to pass to the developing baby, but prevents intermingling of blood. The barrier is variable among species; in most species it allows some antibodies of the immune system to pass from the dam to the fetus.

Horses have the most impermeable uterine-placental barrier, and antibodies protecting the mare from disease do not cross during gestation. A foal is born without antibodies, a critical part of long-term immune function. When the foal suckles *colostrum* (the first milk), antibodies are transferred from the dam to her offspring. Boosting all of the mare's vaccines four to six weeks prior to the expected foaling date increases the concentration of antibodies in colostrum and optimizes foal health.

The life cycle of some intestinal parasites includes the ability to be passed through the mother's milk to her foal. Mares should be dewormed two to four weeks prior to delivery to prevent this occurrence.

For a neglected mare whose date of exposure to a stallion is unknown, the timing of all these requirements can be difficult to achieve. However, the sooner the pregnancy is identified, the more closely the mare can be monitored. An assessment of her gestational development time frame can be estimated at the examination so that you will be able to provide your mare with everything she needs.

SPAYING MARES

In the United States when we refer to spaying a dog, we mean removal of both ovaries and the uterus. In mares, it is difficult to remove the uterus due to horses' large body size. Therefore, a spayed mare has only had her ovaries removed.

One medical reason to spay a mare is because she has developed an ovarian tumor.[91] Tumors originate from hormone-producing cells of the ovary. Tumors can produce either estrogens or testosterone. Therefore, a mare may have bad behavior that lands her in a rescue situation. An affected mare may either act as if she is in heat all of the time due to elevated estrogens, or she may instead act like a stallion—including increased testosterone-induced aggression or mounting other mares when they are in heat. A few weeks after the abnormal hormone-producing tumor is removed, she will return to normal behavior. Tumors can also cause episodes of colic.

If you suspect an ovarian tumor, a reproductive ultrasound will be used as the first screening test. These tumors may also be identified when your veterinarian evaluates a mare on intake. The ultrasound will reveal an abnormally enlarged ovary, with the opposite ovary being small and dormant because the hyperactive function of the enlarged, abnormal ovary causes the normal one to shut down. These examination findings can be confirmed with a blood test of hormone levels.

Although many horse people use a spay to calm particularly moody mares, evidence is that the opposite effect happens. A mare will show signs of heat based on lack of progesterone—so when there is no hormone cycle, she will behave like she is in heat. A recent study showed that mares with their ovaries removed show signs of being in heat for more days per year than those with ovaries.[92]

A GOAL OF PREVENTING PREGNANCIES

Stallions or colts and mares come with a specific set of reproductive issues relevant to rescue horses. I have seen a number of surprise foals, and aside from the goal of providing the best possible care to the needy horses we help, it is important to also prevent unwanted and accidental pregnancies.

CHAPTER 7

Little Lives:
Rescuing Foals

Because mares are so often pregnant at the time they are rescued, it's important to be informed about the normal birth process and normal foals. We'll also discuss the additional health, socialization, and handling needs of orphan foals.

THE BIRTHING PROCESS

A mare's pregnancy lasts over 11 months: about 342 days on average. The range is quite broad, with anywhere between 330 to 365 days considered normal. This can vary by about two weeks either shorter or longer.

It can be difficult to tell if a mare is pregnant by just looking at her. The majority of fetal growth happens in the third trimester and if horse owners are unaware that the mare conceived, it is often during the last month when people notice.

Predicting Foaling Time

Observing a mare's labor is important so that if a problem occurs, early intervention can save her life.

Development of the udder can begin as many as eight weeks prior to delivery (*foaling*), and will develop earlier in mares that have had foals before. Waxing is the dripping

> **Long Ears**
>
> **M**uch of the expected gestation and reproductive cycle of donkeys is similar to horses. Jennies with donkey foals have a longer gestation, which lasts between 360 to 375 days. A mule foal carried by a mare will result in a gestational length that is in between—the pregnancy will last longer than the time the same mare would carry a horse foal. If a stallion is bred to a jenny, the resultant rare offspring is called a hinny.

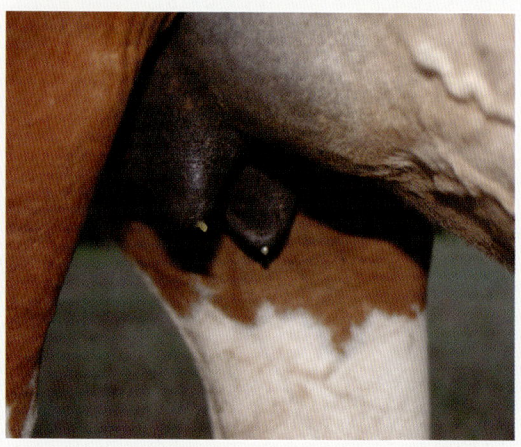

***7.1** This mare is very near foaling, with a full udder and dripping milk known as "waxing."*

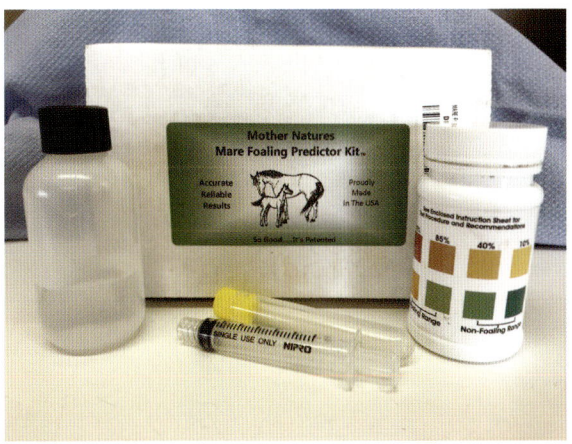

7.2 Using a commercial kit for testing a mare's milk properties—which change just before foaling—helps minimize sleepless nights waiting on foals to be born.

or leaking of milk and is often cited as the cardinal sign to watch before impending labor, but this can be variable (fig. 7.1). Intensity of signs shown by maiden or first-foal mares may be diminished by comparison.

Test kits are available that help predict when foaling will occur, and are particularly helpful if the breeding date is unknown (fig. 7.2). There are several competing brands, and they are based on the changes that occur in the mare's milk soon before she gives birth. Testing milk is 90 percent accurate within 72 hours of *parturition* (giving birth).[93, 94, 95]

As a prey species, horses have ways to avoid detection and possible predation. Mares show only a few subtle signs of readiness. A hormone called *relaxin* will peak soon before she foals. Relaxin causes the vulva to elongate, and the muscles and ligaments around the croup and tail head to soften. Many mares will develop a pointed appearance to the bottom of their belly within a few days prior to giving birth. In

Tragic Accident

Trisha called my office early one spring morning. She sounded terrified and heartbroken. She and her husband bred foundation Quarter Horses, and she explained her problem.

Early the previous spring, their stallion jumped a fence and was found in with one of his daughters, a small two-year-old filly named Blanca. Trisha and her family had hoped and prayed that she wasn't pregnant. Unfortunately, she was. The stallion was probably in with Blanca because she had gone into heat, incentivizing him to go over a fence when he had been previously content to stay within its boundaries.

Sadly, after they figured out that Blanca was pregnant, they didn't realize how close to foaling she was. They had not been watching her overnight.

Trisha had found Blanca down and suffering, and it looked like she had been struggling for hours. The filly had pushed so hard that the tissue surrounding her vulva and anus was torn, and her intestines were hanging out, frayed and dirty. The foal was still stuck in the birth canal and had been dead for so long it was beginning to rot. There was no option but to euthanize Blanca.

I sincerely wish that Trisha had called sooner. Most veterinarians are willing to advise and help. In horses, an early embryo can be eliminated using hormone injections and would have been less expensive than the emergency call, euthanasia, and burial costs. Even in late gestation, an elective terminal C-section could have saved Blanca. Close monitoring of the birth process and an emergency C-section might have saved her. I share this event in hopes you will be able to help your horses more than I was able to help Blanca.

nature, the mare will separate herself from the herd a few hours before foaling. Most horse people separate a mare that is close to foaling and give her a secure, oversized stall or paddock to herself.

The night she foals, the first stage of labor may appear as signs of colic. These signs can include pawing, rolling, repeatedly lying down and getting back up, flagging or swishing her tail, and flank-watching.

Foals are usually born between midnight and 4:00 a.m. with about 85 percent of foals born between 8:00 p.m. and 6:00 a.m. (fig. 7.3).[96] You are going to lose sleep monitoring your mare periodically through the night to be present for the foal's birth. This is one of the reasons why we try so hard to predict when she will foal—losing sleep for a few days is much better than losing sleep for a few weeks. Foaling attendants check mares hourly through the night, because if a mare is having problems, there is no time to lose. A foal can die in a short period of time, and the mare's life may be threatened as well.

Timing: Foaling Happens Quickly

Since everything happens so quickly in mares, it is a good idea to contact your veterinarian when you think your mare may be close. Work with her to make a concrete plan for help in case of an emergency.

The evening that you think your mare may foal, wrap her tail and clean her vulva and udder to minimize a foal's exposure to possible contamination.

From the time the water breaks to the

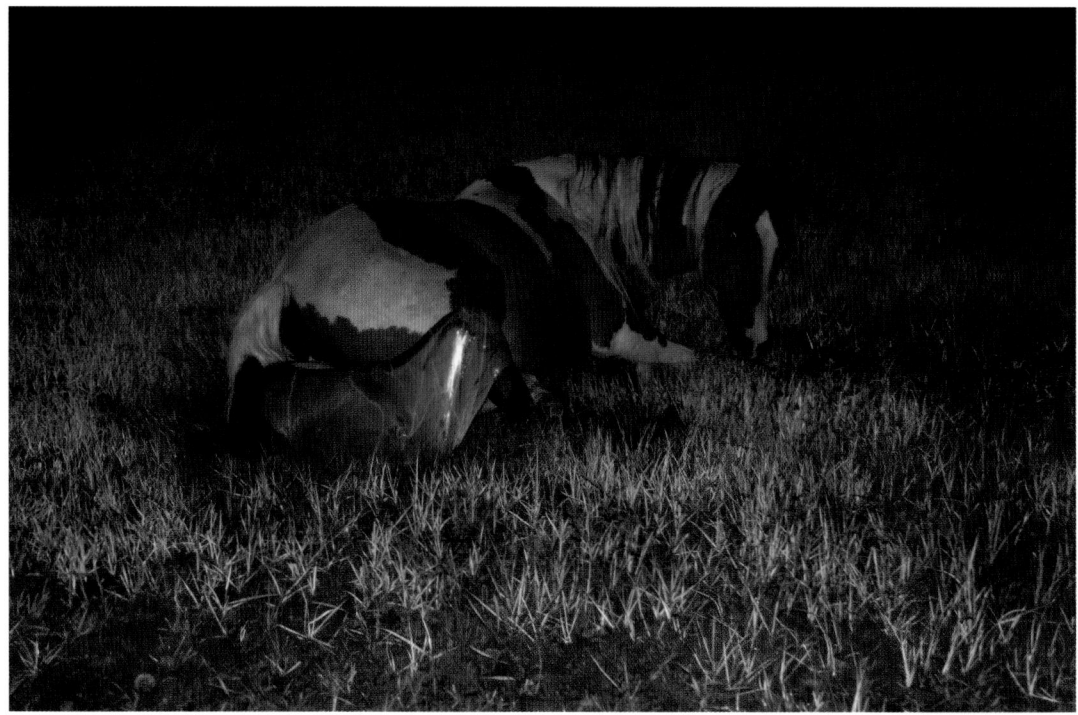

7.3 It is dark in this picture because foals are usually born during the night. Here it is just before dawn, and this mare (the same as in fig. 7.1—p. 98) is giving birth. The foal is all the way out but still has white fetal membranes over his body (note that his nose is clear).

time the foal is expelled should be 30 minutes or less. The mare will be down during the active birthing process of the foal, but she may stand up and lie back down several times prior to hard labor.

Foal Positioning Problems

For birth, the foal should be positioned like a diver, with both front limbs and the head extended. He must be viable and have normal structure to position himself. If you are observing the birth, you will first see a white bubble of fetal membrane tissue protruding from the vulva (fig. 7.4). Then you should see two feet, and shortly thereafter a nose above and 6 to 8 inches behind the tiny hooves. Hooves are covered in *eponychium*, a soft tissue present only during development that protects the interior of the placenta and uterus from damage from hooves (fig. 7.5).

Call a veterinarian immediately if you are observing the birth and do not see the two feet and head "diving" out, because this is an emergency. Improper position due to fetal foal abnormalities is a major cause of birthing problems in horses. You should also call for help if the mare has not made significant progress in a 15- to 20-minute time period. Horses are different from other farm species—a calf or a kid may be in the birth canal for several hours and still survive. This is not the case for a foal—he will perish quickly. Re-positioning a foal in the birth canal is tricky, and complications such as tearing the uterus can occur, so I don't recommend trying to do it yourself.

Red Bag

Another problem that happens during the birthing process is premature placental separation. This is termed *red bag* because

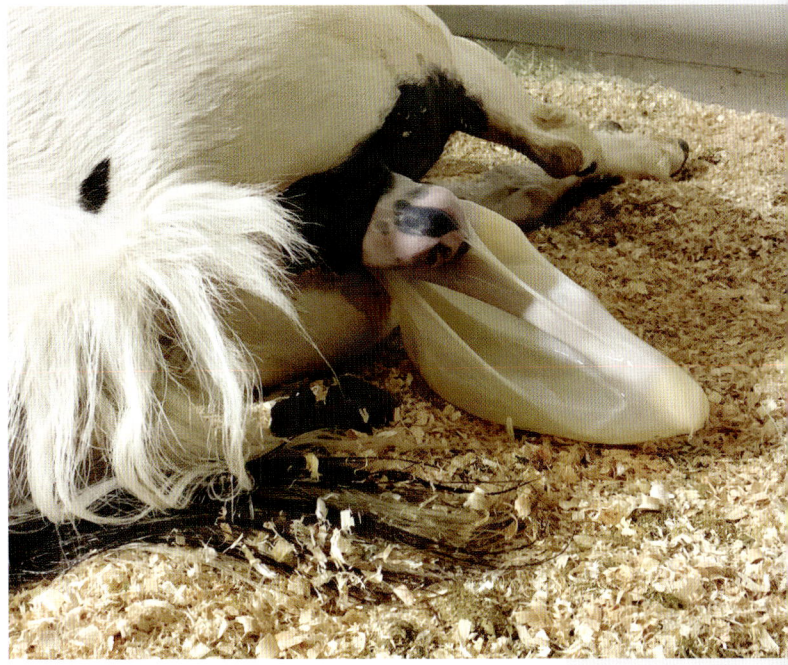

7.4 A normally positioned foal during the active, hard stage of labor, which takes less than 30 minutes for a normal horse birth. The forelimbs and head are extended and coming out first (the foal is positioned like a "diver"), which is normal. The white fetal membranes are still covering the foal, but will break shortly.

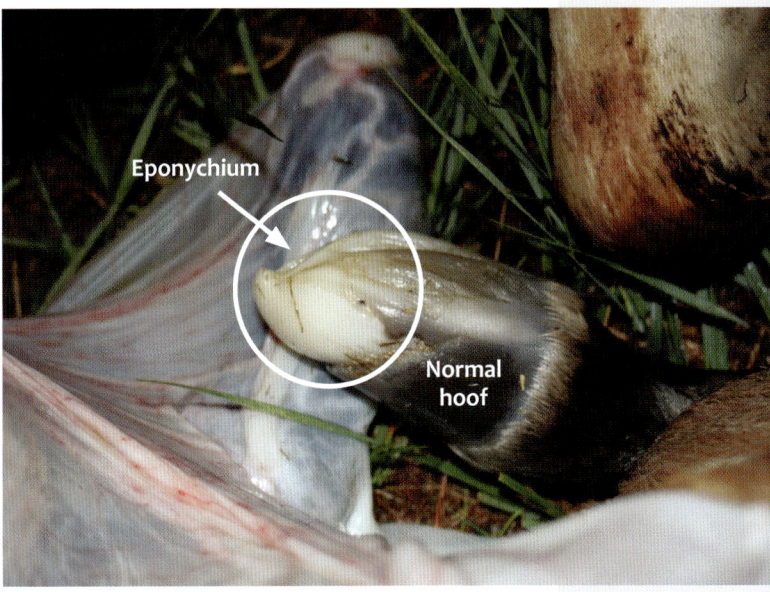

7.5 You can see the eponychium covering the foal's hooves to protect his dam's internal tissue during fetal development.

instead of observing the white bubble of the relatively tough fetal membrane, the entire lining of the placenta will appear with the foal. This lining is red and soft or velvety. In equines, the placenta must be intact to provide oxygen for the foal, and if it is prematurely separated from the uterus and expelled early, the foal will suffocate during the birth process. The abnormal red bag placenta must be opened immediately by cutting or tearing it, taking care to not cut the foal inside it. Opening it will ensure that the foal can start to breathe on his own. Fescue grass in the diet of the mare during late gestation can cause red bag, although other things such as inflammation or infection of the placenta can also result in this problem.

Normal After-Birth Sequence

After the foal is born, the placenta should pass within a few hours, and should be whole, with only one break where the foal came through. It should not be tattered or in multiple pieces (fig. 7.6). Your foal should stand within an hour. Before he stands, he will make many unsuccessful attempts. He should suckle within two hours. Shortly thereafter, he should defecate.

Suckling: Foals normally have a suckle reflex at birth, but they are uncoordinated. Initially, a foal may try to suckle his mother's elbows, shoulders, and hind legs. An experienced mare will guide her foal to the correct location. It will take him about an hour to figure it out, and the first time he latches on will be only for a second or two (fig. 7.7).

In the first week, he may suckle up to seven times an hour, less than 30 seconds each time. Under normal circumstances, very young foals often need multiple attempts to latch on, and will drink only a few sips at a time. As a foal's nervous system matures, he will latch on better, ingest more, and suckle less often.

A foal is born with a *naïve* immune system—it cannot yet recognize germs or pathogens. A foal must ingest and absorb antibody proteins (also known as *immunoglobulins*) via the *colostrum* during his first 24 hours of life. Colostrum is the first milk the mare produces, and it only lasts for a few days, gradually changing to regular milk. It is more yellow, thick, and sticky than the milk she will produce for the remainder of the lactation period. This ingestion of antibodies from colostrum is called *passive transfer*. The passively transferred antibodies will stay with a foal as his body encounters germs and begins to build its own bank of circulating immunoglobulin proteins.

7.6 A normal placenta. It should be passed within a few hours after birth. This often happens in conjunction with the foal suckling, which stimulates the release of oxytocin, a hormone that causes uterine contractions.

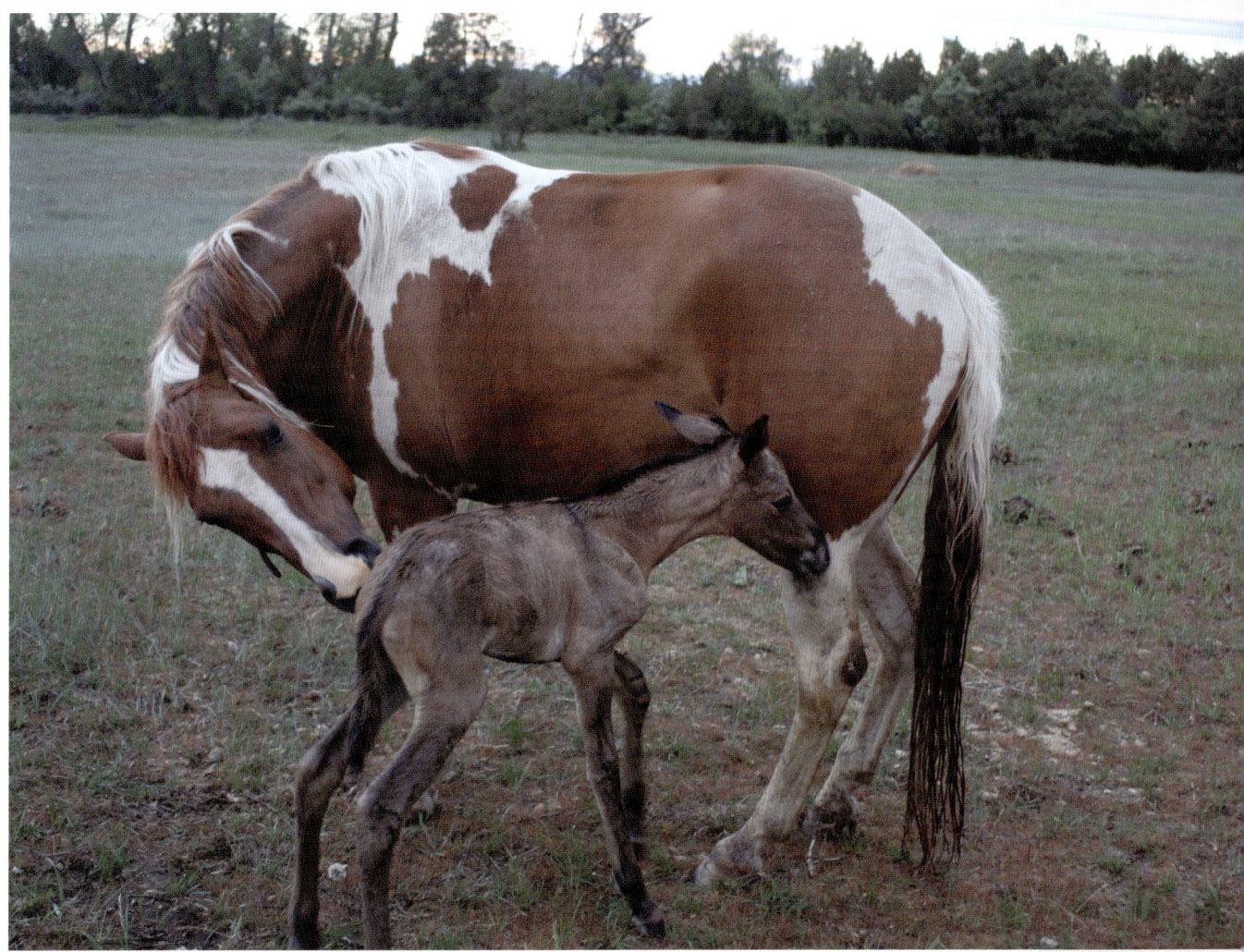

7.7 A newborn mule foal (the same foal and mare as fig. 7.3—p. 100) just learning to suckle. At first, a foal can't always find the right spot on the dam, but usually gets better at suckling pretty quickly.

Passage of Meconium: *Meconium* is the first feces that a foal expels, and it continues for up to 24 hours of age (fig. 7.8). The meconium appears as dark and tarry pellets. The first time a foal defecates should be within two hours of suckling. About 1 to 2 percent of foals are delayed and become constipated—they have a meconium impaction. A foal that has not passed feces in the first 12 hours of life is considered to have a meconium impaction. Foals that are born late and colts are somewhat more likely to develop this problem.[97]

A foal with meconium impaction will strain, sometimes producing small amounts of feces, and sometimes nothing at all. If left untreated, the signs will progress to colic, lethargy, and loss of appetite. Early treatment is an enema. Over the counter, phosphate (for example, Fleet®) enemas can be

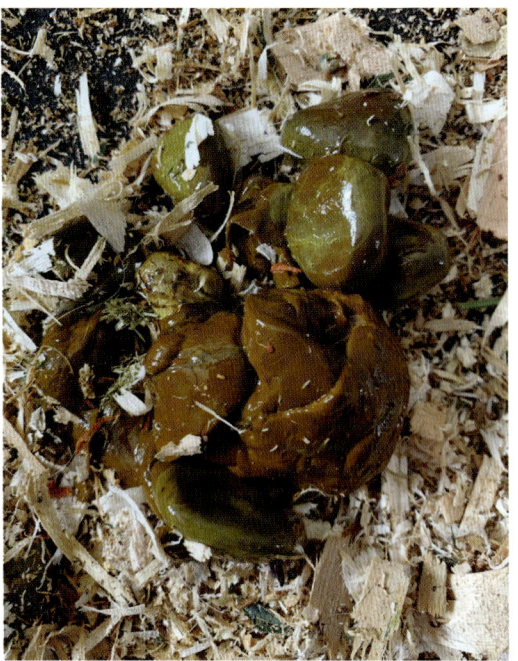

7.8 Normal "first poop" from a foal, known as the meconium. It is typically dark and sticky, as in the photo.

used but should not be repeated as toxicity can occur. Most veterinarians gently use warm, soapy water.

If the impaction progresses and enema treatment doesn't relieve the impaction, a foal may need repeated enemas along with intravenous fluids, pain management, and (rarely) surgery to solve the problem.

Normal Vital Parameters for Foals

- **Temperature:** 99 to 102.0 degrees Fahrenheit
- **Pulse/Heart Rate:** 80 to 100 beats per minute
- **Respiration:** 20 to 40 breaths per minute

FOAL EXAMINATION

The afternoon after he is born, your foal should be examined to ensure he is off to a good start. Your veterinarian will begin by assessing his vitals, which are different from those of an adult horse. Then, known locations of congenital problems unique to foals will be evaluated. Congenital means an individual is born with it, but does not necessarily mean there is a genetic cause—it can also be developmental. These potential problems include a cleft palate, a heart murmur, deviations of the bones or tendons, and umbilical abnormalities.

Temperature

A fever indicates inflammation or infection, the source of which may be identified during the remainder of the examination. Infection in foals commonly comes from the lungs, the umbilicus, and joints. Usually it takes a few days for infection to set in. Normal rectal temperature for foals is 99.5 to 102.0 degrees Fahrenheit.

Heart

Evaluating the quality of heart sounds is important, as well as heart rate. A *murmur* is a "whooshing" sound with each normal "thump-thump" beat and indicates abnormal blood flow. Murmurs can be present as the foal's body changes from specialized fetal circulation to normal circulation. The murmur should resolve within 72 hours, and your foal should be reevaluated to ensure that the murmur is not persistent and that the proper developmental change occurred. Heart rate for *neonatal* (just born) foals is 80 to 100 beats per minute—the normal rate decreases with age and size.

Respiration

When a foal has pneumonia, he will have a marked change in respiratory rate and effort. If abnormal respiratory noise is noted during an examination, further evaluation and treatment is warranted. Normal respiratory rate for foals is 20 to 40 breaths per minute. Like the heart rate, the normal rate decreases gradually as the foal matures.

Examination of the Limbs

Early identification and treatment of limb abnormalities is critical to a foal's athletic prospects and future soundness. Young foals may have tendon contracture or tendon laxity. In mild cases, each of these problems may be treated with exercise restriction and both typically improve over about two weeks.

Contracted Tendons: The tight, contracted foal buckles at his joints, usually his knees and/or fetlocks. He may walk on his tippy toes with the heels barely touching or not touching the ground. The extensor tendon on the front of the limb will appear tight and prominent (figs. 7.9 A & B). In an extreme case, the foal will be unable to extend his joints. He may not be able to stand or, instead, he may knuckle over and walk on the end of his flexed fetlocks with his feet dragging behind the bent joint. Consequently, his skin is quickly rubbed raw, even to the extent that bone is exposed.

Administration of *oxytetracycline* (an antibiotic) helps relax the contracture, but the scientific explanation for the mechanism of action is poorly understood.[98] Bandaging and splinting foal limbs relaxes the tendons and joints, but some cases require surgery. If the foal is unable to stand, he will not be able to suckle and get the colostrum

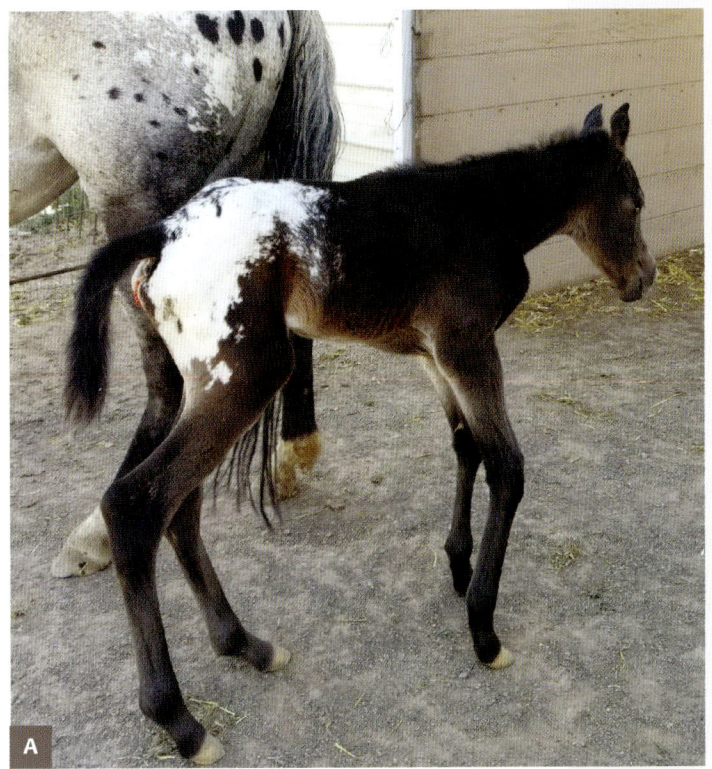

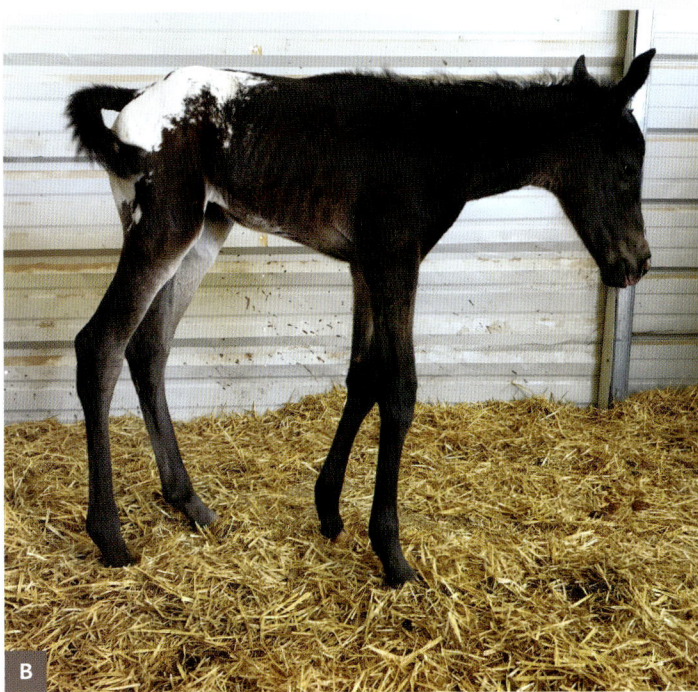

7.9 A & B A 12-hour old foal with mildly contracted tendons (A), and the same foal 24 hours later, after medical treatment.

he needs, leading to a downward spiral of severe health problems.

Tendon Laxity: On the other end of the spectrum, tendon, ligament, and joint laxity manifests with dropped or hyper-extended fetlocks, and the toes may not touch the ground (figs. 7.10 A & B). In severe cases, the back of the fetlock joints may touch the ground as the foal walks. Topical medical treatment and protection of skin is necessary. Glue-on baby shoes will help with proper foot placement.

Foals with laxity get stronger, and the problem resolves with time. Because splints and bandages are used to relax tight tendons, applying supports to a foal with laxity will worsen the situation.

Joint Infection: The spread of systemic bacterial infection will cause the joints of a foal to become infected. Early identification and treatment of this problem is the key for successful resolution of the infection and restoration of normal joint function. Sepsis will happen in foals that do not get enough colostrum.

A foal's infected joints may be treated directly by flushing them out and instilling antibiotics directly into the affected joints. Since these foals are sick, evaluation and treatment of immune deficiencies is necessary for recovery, and antibiotics will be administered systemically.

Growth Abnormalities: Monitor your foal's growth, especially his legs and orthopedic development. As he ages, growth abnormalities result in crooked legs or conformational defects—medically known as *angular*

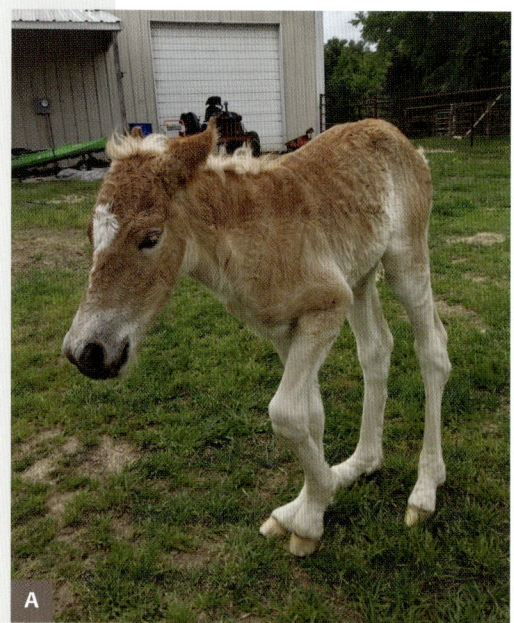
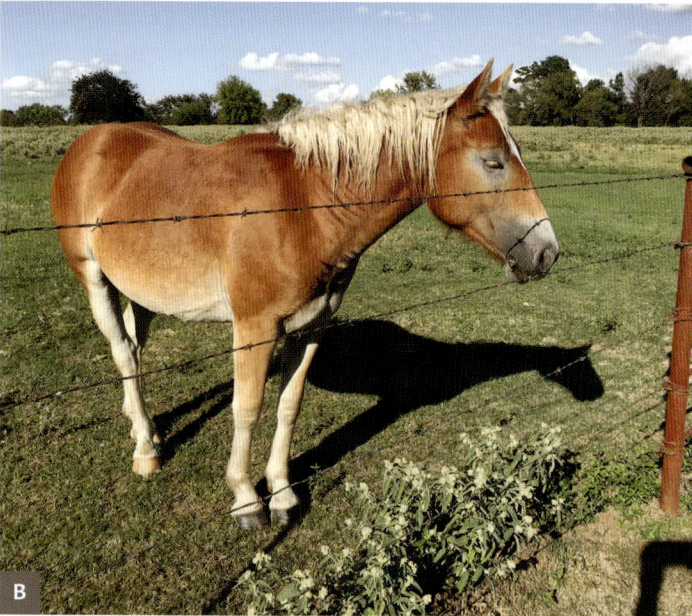

7.10 A & B A newborn foal with tendon laxity (A). She's otherwise normal (her head looks large because of the camera angle). After 2 to 14 days of rest or exercise restriction, these foals strengthen and become normal, as you can see in the photo of the same foal as a two-year-old (B).

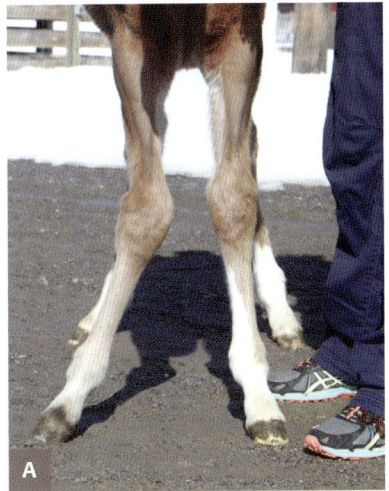 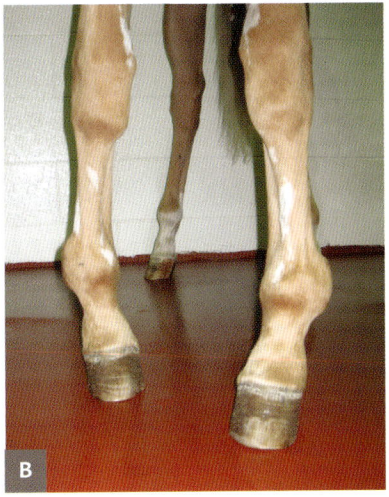 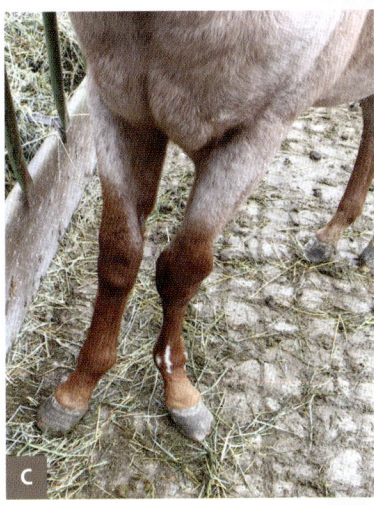

7.11 A–C *A foal with moderate right-sided carpal valgus (crooked knee), the most common limb abnormality, is shown in photo A. There are a variety of treatment options, and if treated, foals with this problem can be corrected (generally the prognosis is fair to good). A young horse with a severe fetlock varus (crooked ankle) growth abnormality is shown in photo B. She also had flexural deformities (severely contracted tendons) in all four limbs, although her hind limbs were worse than her forelimbs. Treatments were unsuccessful, and left scarring (white hairs). This filly was in excruciating pain and was euthanized. In photo C you see another young horse with a severe growth abnormality. This picture was taken at an auction yard. She has carpal valgus, fetlock valgus, as well as her left forelimb being rotated out. At her age, the growth plates have closed, and she has a poor prognosis.*

limb deformities. Depending on the foal's age, some can be corrected (figs. 7.11 A–C). Knees and fetlocks are common locations of angular deformity.

Conservative medical treatment of angular limb deformities consists of frequent corrective hoof trimming and rest. Surgical correction curtails abnormal growth, ensuring that your foal will develop proper conformation and maximize his athletic abilities.

Occasionally, foals will be born with immature bones in their knees and hocks. Their legs appear similar to those with laxity or angular limb deformities. X-rays are used to identify the partially formed bones, and the foal must be supported for a short period of time while the small, complicated bones of his legs mature (fig. 7.12).

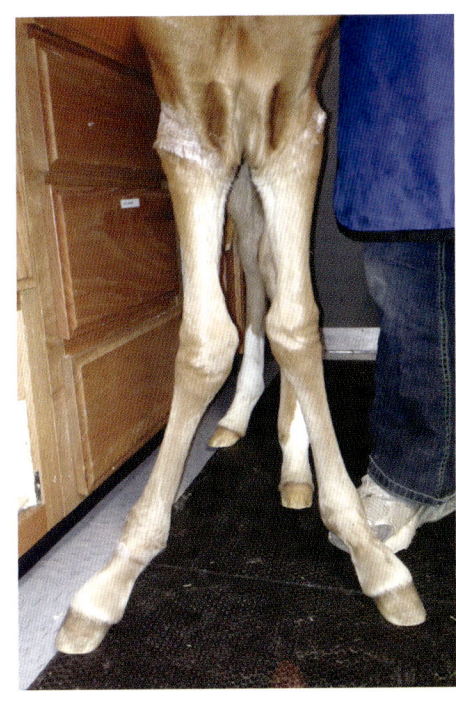

7.12 *An immature foal. Note the similarity in appearance to the foal in fig. 7.11 A (above). The only way to know when the bones of the carpus (knee) are not fully developed is by doing X-rays (radiographs).*

Part I: Caring for Horses in Need—107

In addition to evaluation of immunity, important areas on foals that should be evaluated are the umbilicus, ribs, and palate.

Evaluation of Passive Transfer of Immunity: Without absorption of critical antibodies via colostrum ingestion, a foal's immune system will not be able to function. Foals with failure of passive transfer have an immune system that cannot defend them, and may die if left untreated.

At 12 to 24 hours of age, all foals should be tested to ensure that passive transfer of immunity from dam to foal has been successful. To this end, your veterinarian should always test the amount of immunoglobulin class G (IgG). The cost is much less than treating a sick foal, which can be in the thousands (fig. 7.13).[98]

If early test results reveal failure of passive transfer of immunity, the problem

> ### Other Abnormalities That Warrant Veterinary Care
>
> As he grows, your foal must be re-examined if he shows any of the following signs:
>
> - Depression or lethargy
> - Decrease in appetite
> - Fever
> - Difficulty breathing
> - Milk coming from the nostrils when drinking
> - Coughing
> - Nasal discharge
> - Abnormal color of the gums: yellow, or either too pale or too dark
> - Straining to urinate or defecate.

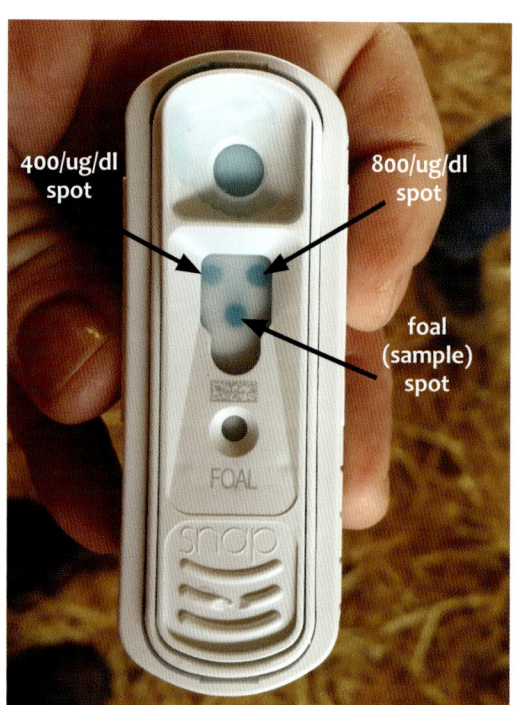

can be rectified. Equine veterinarians keep frozen plasma stocked throughout the foaling season, which has an ultra-high content of immunoglobulins. A plasma transfusion puts antibodies straight into the foal's circulation. His immune system will then be fully functional.[99]

7.13 Blood test results of a foal showing normal transfer of passive immunity by ingestion of immunoglobulins via colostrum ingestion. The dot on the left is the 400 μg/dL calibrator spot, the dot on the right is the 800 μg/dL calibrator spot and the dot on the bottom is the foal's test dot. Since the test dot is darker than both calibrator spots, we know the foal has >800 μg/dl of IgG. The test runs in just 10 minutes and tells us that immunity is adequate.

Umbilicus: The umbilicus is the site of attachment of the umbilical cord. In people, we call this our belly button.

The body wall should close around the umbilicus, with only a tiny divot at the point where the umbilical stump is. Sometimes the umbilicus doesn't close all the way, which results in a *hernia* (fig. 7.14). Although a hernia can exist for years with no problems, intestine can become entrapped in it, resulting in a serious, life-threatening emergency. Therefore, a foal's hernia should be surgically repaired at four to six weeks of age. Very young foals do not metabolize anesthetic drugs well, so waiting a few weeks until their physiology is more mature is advisable. The larger the animal, the more difficult it is to have a successful surgical repair on the first attempt, so you don't want to wait too long.

The umbilicus can also be infected, which is often related to failure of passive transfer of immunity. Long-term use of antibiotics may be successful in resolving the problem, but sometimes surgical removal of infected tissue is necessary.[100]

Finally, the umbilicus can have a *patent urachus*. The urachus is the normal fetal connection between his urinary bladder and the umbilical cord. It's the route that toxins use to leave the fetal body. It should close when the foal is born and the umbilical cord is broken. But occasionally it remains *patent*, or open. The patent urachus results in the umbilicus dripping urine. This opening may be closed by chemical cautery or by surgical correction.

Ribs: Foals on intensively managed broodmare farms are often born with an attendant observing them and assisting in

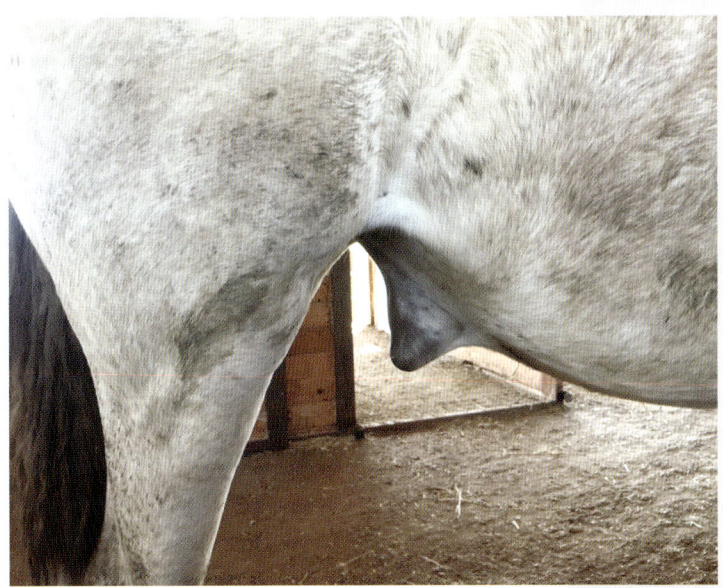

7.14 A filly with an umbilical hernia. She will need it surgically repaired.

delivery. This management practice must be used with caution, as improper pulling commonly results in rib fractures. A difficult birth or hard labor (even though it may appear otherwise normal) can also result in fractured ribs. During the special foal examination, each and every rib should be palpated to ensure all are intact.

Palate: The horse's palate is unique from other species in that a cleft palate will be at the back of the mouth, rather than visible from the front. It is difficult to view this area, and palpation of the roof of the mouth is the best way to identify this abnormality. A cleft palate will cause milk to drip from the foal's nostrils as he drinks. Because the mouth and the respiratory tract have an abnormal connection, aspiration of milk results in pneumonia. These foals need intensive management to survive, and surgery is required to correct the problem.

NORMAL FOAL BEHAVIOR

Observing your foal's behavioral habits will give insight about his health status. You can tell if your foal is having difficulty urinating or defecating if he is *flagging* his tail—that is, raising it and moving it as he strains (fig. 7.15).

A normal foal that is getting enough milk will go through a cycle of eating and playing, then sleeping. A foal should be suckling at least three to five times per hour during his first week of life. When a foal has had enough to eat, he will lie down and sleep comfortably. If a foal is constantly standing and seeking the udder, or is not seen taking a large number of naps during the day, he is probably not getting enough nutrition. There are a few reasons that a foal may not be getting enough to eat. A mare's milk production could be inadequate. Infection of the udder (*mastitis*) could be present, which will make the milk unhealthy or decrease its volume. Some mares behaviorally may not tolerate the foal suckling—known as rejection. Finally, the foal should be checked to make sure he is able to latch on and suckle successfully.

Conversely, if your foal seems to sleep all the time, is weak, or is having trouble standing or moving, he should be checked for underlying problems.

If you see your foal eating manure, don't worry, this is normal foal behavior. Scientists haven't fully elucidated why foals do this. The most plausible explanation is that he is populating his intestines with bacteria that will become part of the fermentation that horses depend on for forage digestion.

THE ORPHAN FOAL

When everything goes well, the hope and joy experienced with new foals is wonderful. Nature can be cruel, though. An orphan is a foal whose dam has either died or is unable to take care of her foal for another reason. This can happen at any time, from during the birthing process through several months of age. Foals are normally weaned between four and six months of age, so a foal would not be considered an orphan if his dam was lost at that age. Your foal should be examined immediately upon being orphaned or arriving at your farm.

Horse rescues may be involved with orphan foals due to involvement with nurse mare farms (see below). The constant care

---

Long Ears

Because they are a hybrid of two species, mules have an additional risk of an immune disease called *Neonatal Isoerythrolysis* (NI). NI is when the antibodies the foal absorbs from his dam attack and destroy his own red blood cells, causing severe anemia. His gum color may be pale or yellow, and he may be weak, prompting you to call your veterinarian. Although NI occurs in 1 to 2 percent of horse foals, it may occur in as many as 10 percent of mule foals.

NI is treated by preventing further ingestion of colostrum, instead relying on a plasma transfusion for immunity and milk replacer for nutrition. Severely affected foals need a blood transfusion to correct the anemia, and restore a healthy number of red blood cells. After several days (well past the time of colostrum absorption), the foal can safely suckle from his dam.[101]

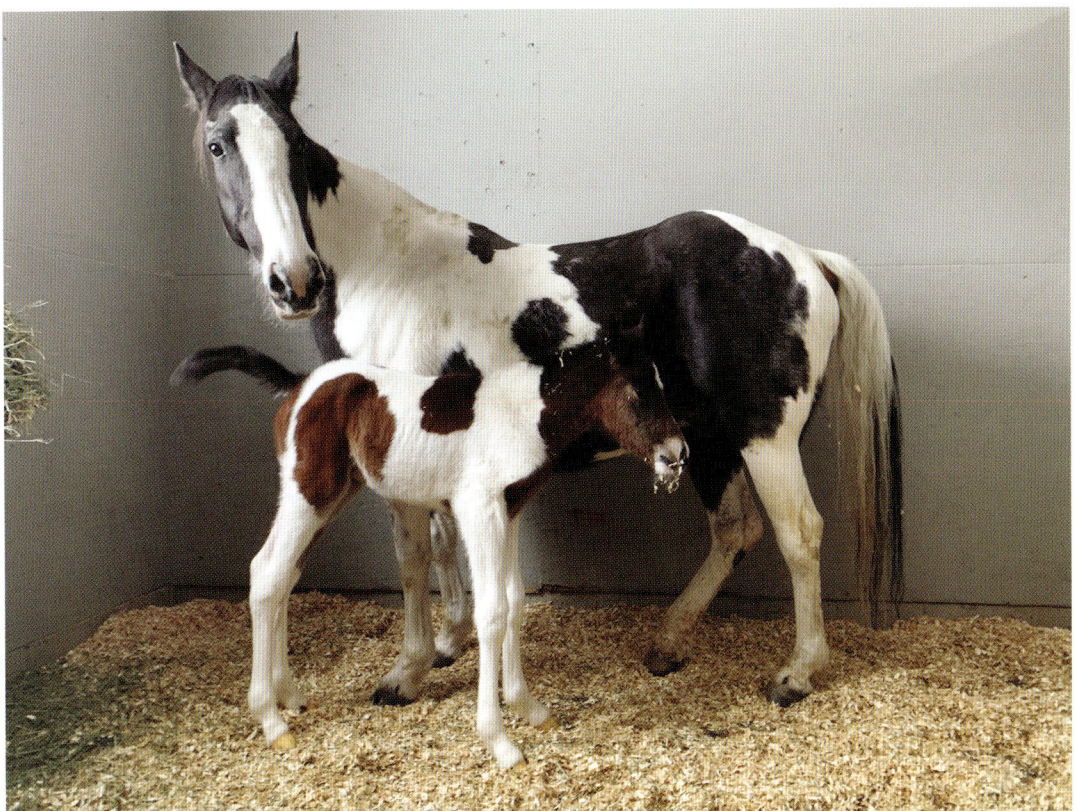

7.15 *A foal flags his tail as he attempts to defecate. Repeated flagging or straining indicates a problem to be evaluated by a veterinarian.*

needed by an orphan foal is exhausting. An orphan foal may be relinquished to a rescue group because of the original owner being unable to cope with the really hard work required.

Orphan foals also have a reputation for being skinny and slower growing than peers that suckle from their natural dam. But modern nutritional options are far superior to historical ones—we can do a much better job feeding these babies than was possible 30 or 40 years ago. Also, the quality of medical care available for sick and orphan foals has improved substantially in the last few decades. With commitment, your orphan can be as healthy and strong as any other foal in the pasture.

Feeding Orphan Foals[102, 103, 104]

Alternatives to Colostrum: Birth to 24 Hours:
When a foal has been orphaned at birth, the first thing to do is to make sure he gets colostrum or another immune system boost. Foals need at least four pints of colostrum. Large breeding farms may bank colostrum and freeze it. About eight to ten ounces can be saved from a mare, one time, after her foal has suckled. This small volume is filtered, pooled with colostrum from other mares, and stored frozen. Banked equine colostrum is commercially available, but you would have to pre-purchase it and keep it on hand—time is critical for establishing a healthy immune system.

> ### Nurse Mare Non-Match
>
> One spring, I helped Laura with a foal that was orphaned at seven days old. Laura's mare had a terrible colic, and died within about an hour of showing the first signs of pain. The mare was lying on the ground, struggling to breathe and the foal was standing nearby, occasionally nudging her. It was tragic watching the foal—she knew the instant her mother took her last breath, and began running circles around her dam and whinnying at the top of her lungs in distress.
>
> Laura immediately began working to find nutrition and companionship for her foal. She talked to Barbara over the internet—Barbara had the closest potential nurse mare, about 250 miles away. At first, we were excited about the match. After further discussion, Barbara stated that her expectation was that the young foal should travel rather than her mare. Needless to say, Laura didn't think hauling her recently orphaned foal that distance was a good idea. A match was not made.
>
> Laura tried several companions: a small pony, a quiet gelding, and one of her mares who hadn't had a baby that year—all failed. Finally, a friend's mare, who had reared foals of her own in past years, matched.
>
> During the weeks of matchmaking, Laura also worked tirelessly round the clock to make sure her orphan foal was eating, pooping, and acting as normal as possible. She burned up her vacation time, restructured her paddock and stalls, and used all of her own energy reserves feeding the foal every two to three hours through the day and the night. I visited the farm several times in the first week, administering fluids and enemas and working with her to devise a setup that would help this foal get enough good nutrition and companionship to grow up healthy, both mentally and physically. Thanks to Laura's efforts, this orphan foal thrived.

Orally supplemented colostrum is useful if the foal is less than 24 hours old; after that time absorption is minimal. Farm suppliers carry powder, gel, or liquid synthesized immunoglobulins. For foals, these resources are suboptimal. When mare colostrum is unavailable or the foal is more than one day old, the standard of care is to administer an intravenous plasma transfusion.

Any orphan or sick foal whose IgG status is unclear should be immediately tested. Common pathogens that he should be able to easily fight off can become a major source of severe illness if he has failure of passive transfer. It is also possible for the foal to have his immunoglobulins depleted if he has had high exposure to many pathogens, as would happen if he were to travel through an auction house or be intermingled with sick horses.

Nutrition from Two Days to Two Weeks: Neonatal foals must derive 100 percent of their nutrition from milk. The most ideal situation is to find a nurse mare (a horse "wet nurse") that will serve as a surrogate mother. Social media has become an excellent way to match mares and foals together. Usually, the mare's own foal is weaned early or died of illness. Rarely, a tolerant mare will accept an orphan and nurse two foals, but it's difficult for her body to meet this high demand for milk. If this is your best option, you will need to feed the mare large quantities of hay and grain. You should also supplement the foals' ration so that they are able to derive nutrients from another source.

When nature's milk is not available, a milk replacer is used. There are several good brands, and the one selected should be labeled specifically for horses.

Land-O-Lakes® Mare's Match® is a good one available from many online and local retailers (fig. 7.16).¹⁰⁵

Milk replacer for other species is different in lactose and fat content, so foals can get severe diarrhea with those formulations. Sometimes a foal that has had real mare's milk may be less willing to consume the replacer.

Frequency of Feeding: A young foal needs to be offered milk a minimum of every two hours (every hour is more ideal for the first week). After two weeks of age, the feeding schedule can usually be reduced to every three to four hours. All foals should have constant access to water, even if they also have access to milk replacer.¹⁰⁶

Feeding Containers and Methods: Bottles designed for calves have nipples that flow too fast and result in aspiration of the milk into the lungs and subsequent pneumonia. The human baby bottle, or a sheep nipple, will work better. When the bottle is inverted, milk should not flow from it. If it does, it's too fast. To ease the burden of feeding, the bottle can be secured to a wall. Ideally, the nostrils should be below the ears when the foal is drinking to help prevent aspiration pneumonia.

The best way to prevent aspiration pneumonia is to teach your foal to drink milk from a bucket or pan (figs. 7.17 A & B). (Remember: Bottles are bad, buckets are better.) This can usually be achieved with some effort, and should be attempted as soon as possible. First, dip your clean finger in the bucket of milk and allow the foal to begin to suckle. Repeat the dipping and suckling, gradually moving your hand closer and closer, and finally in to the bucket. Although some foals catch on very quickly, it may take many tries and repeated attempts, but it is well worth the effort. Your "bucket baby" is much less likely to develop aspiration pneumonia than a "bottle baby."

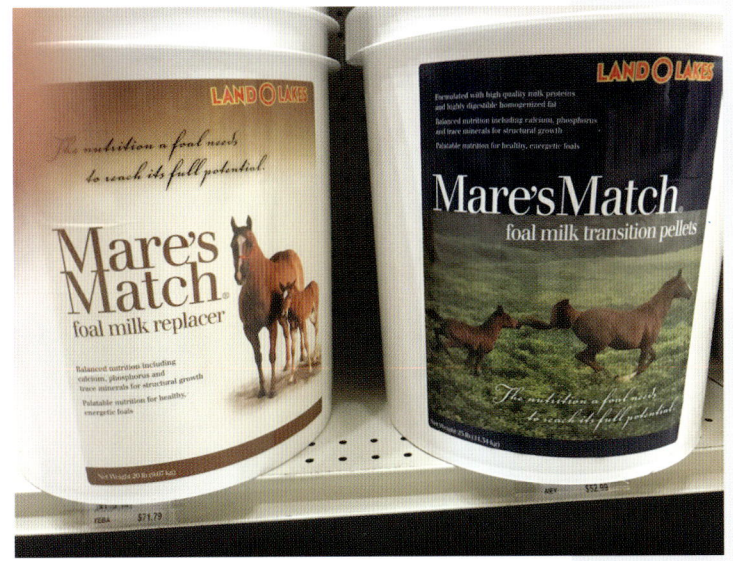

7.16 Commercial milk replacers are specifically available for foals.

A normal bucket baby can have milk available at all times. Depending on the climate, the bucket should be checked every four to eight hours to ensure that it is fresh and clean. If it has dead flies in it, has a foul or rancid odor, or appears to be separated, it should be changed.

Volume Your Foal Will Eat: You should expect your foal to drink about 10 percent of his body weight per day for the first few days. For example, a 90-pound foal will drink 9 pounds of milk, which is a bit more than a gallon. By two weeks of age, he will be drinking up to 25 percent of his body weight. A 120-pound, two-week-old foal will be drinking about 3½ gallons of milk each day.

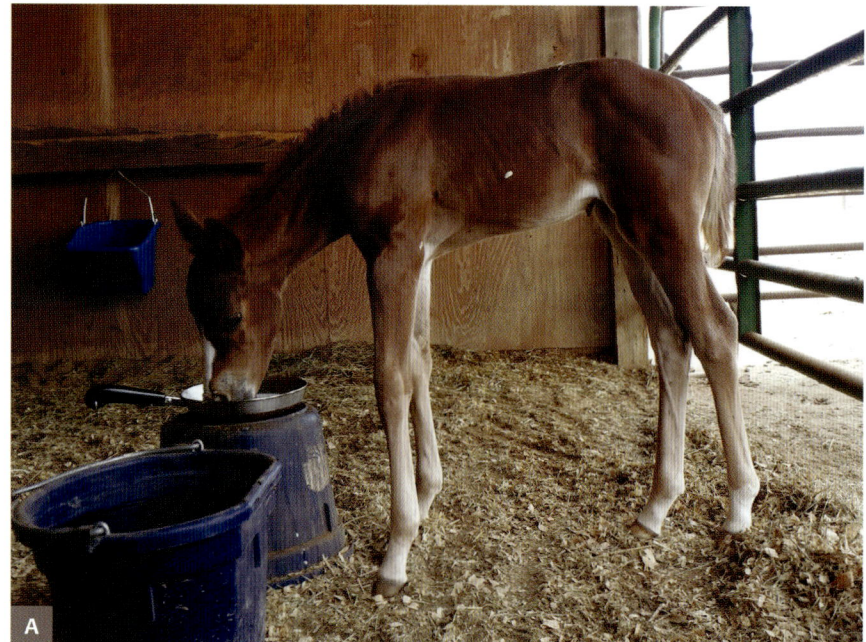

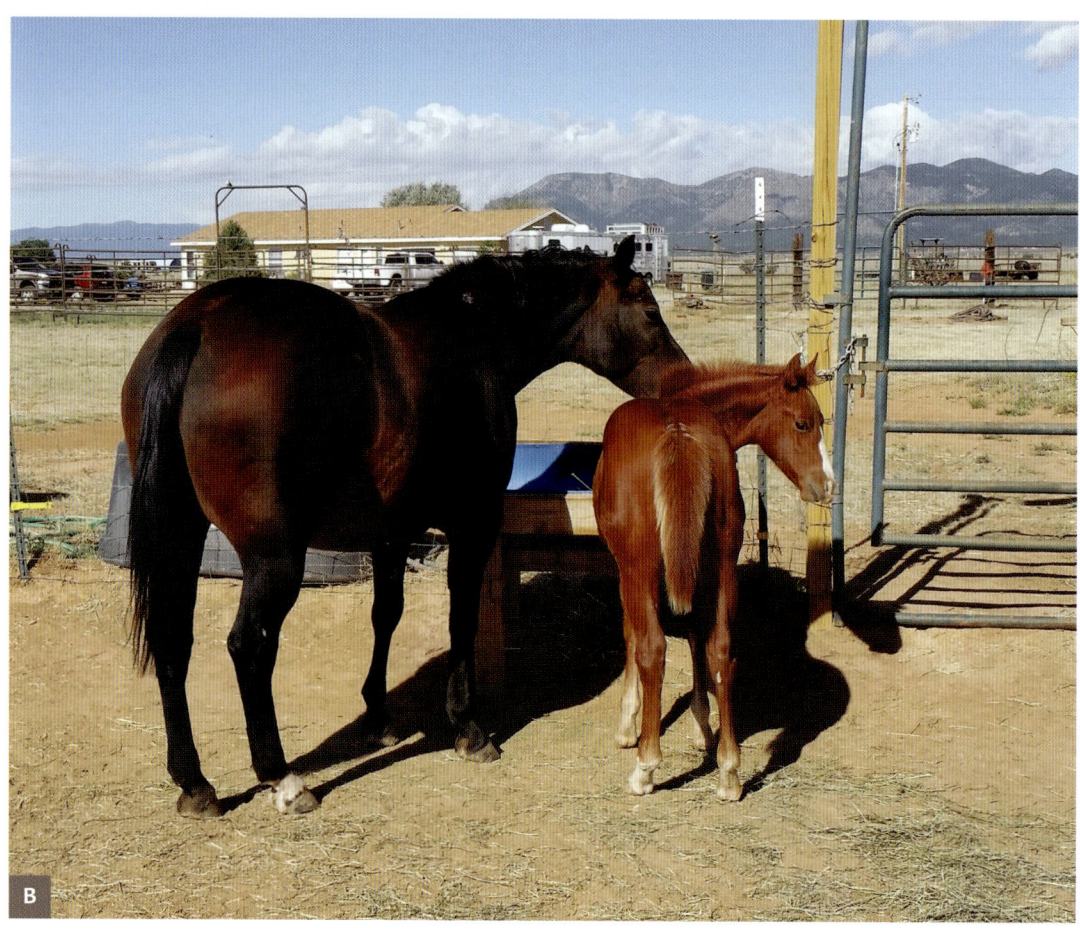

7.17 A & B A seven-day-old orphan foal learns to drink out of a pan on her first day without her mother (A), and the same foal at four months old with her adult companion mare (B).

If you note a decrease in what the foal has been consuming, that is a cause for concern. Contact your veterinarian and have your foal examined, especially if you note other concurrent abnormalities.

Feeding: Two Weeks to Two Months: As long as the colostrum and immunity are adequate, foals in this age group become easier to care for, bit by bit.

After about two weeks, milk replacer pellets can be added to your feeding routine. These are easier to manage than mixing and managing liquid milk replacer. Foal-Lac® pellets from Pet-Ag® are the original formulation, although other brands are available.[107]

As always, any changes you make in food for horses should be gradual. Offer a handful at a time and work up to 4 to 6 pounds per day over the course of two to three weeks. When your foal is eating this amount, the liquid milk can be discontinued, and the milk replacer pellets can be fed free-choice with continual access. The milk pellets should be fed until normal weaning time—usually about six months of age. One disadvantage is that the pellets have a decreased water content compared to liquid products. Monitor your foal closely because a decrease in water intake can lead to constipation.

Foals will start to play with plant roughage at around three or four weeks of age. Therefore, hay or pasture should be available starting at that age. When your foal is living with an adult horse, he will mimic that horse's behavior. The amount of hay and pasture he consumes increases until it becomes the staple of the foal's diet. The roughage selected should be the highest quality available; it should be green and leafy, no matter what type of hay or grass it is.

Event	Time Frame
Birthing process (parturition)	30 minutes
Standing	1 to 2 hours
Suckling	2 to 3 hours
Passing of meconium	30 minutes to 12 hours
Ingestion of colostrum	First suckle to 24 hours
Foal Exam and check IgG	12 to 24 hours, sooner if concerns or abnormalities noted
Dependent on milk for 100 percent of nutrition	Birth to 3 to 4 weeks
Starts eating some forage or adult food	3 to 4 weeks of age and beyond
Weaning	4 to 6 months

7.18 Timeline for Foals

Monitoring your foal's growth by height and weight is helpful to ensure he is meeting milestones. A "ribby" or thin foal is not getting enough nutrition. Overweight foals are prone to developmental orthopedic disease—cartilage or bones may not form properly. A foal should gain 2 to 3 pounds per day.[108]

Orphan Socialization

You have ensured that your foal is physically healthy and well-fed, so it's now time to critically evaluate socialization. Orphans have a reputation for growing up to be difficult to handle and disrespectful to their handlers.

Any foal can become spoiled or ill-mannered. It's not fair to the horse to allow him to develop behavior problems. A horse with bad behavior is more likely to find himself in need of a home or in an auction yard.

The less a human is associated with feeding, the less likely an orphan foal is to become disrespectful. Maintaining respect toward humans is another reason to transfer a foal to drinking milk from a bucket instead of a bottle.

The second critical aspect to prevent overly bold behavior is to allow a baby horse to learn how to behave based on interactions with adult horses. The most socially ideal scenario is to locate and match a nurse mare with your orphan foal.

At a minimum, orphan foals should live with another adult horse for socialization. The adult horse should be kind and steady, but no-nonsense. An experienced mare who has raised a foal but doesn't currently have one of her own may work, but a nice gelding can be fine as well (see fig. 7.17 B—p. 114). An unfriendly adult horse can severely injure a foal, so monitor the introduction and their early time together.

It is good for foals to have another youngster to cavort with. However, keeping orphaned foals in a group amongst themselves doesn't fully teach them how to behave within a herd as an adult horses should. Foals need to learn the body language and interactions of adult horses; the orphan needs to learn respect for others, and to know which signals mean to back off.

This doesn't mean that an orphan should be completely ignored by humans. Of course, like any other foal he should be trained to lead with a halter. He should also be taught to accept grooming and handling of feet. Training and handling of an orphan should closely match that of any foal you raise. People who have raised orphan foals will tell you that you must set boundaries in order to be safe, and that teaching *pressure-and-release* (see p. 120) is critical. These rules apply to orphans as well as normal foals.

HALTER TRAINING

Teaching a young horse to lead is the foundation of training for the rest of his life. Each horse has a unique personality and response to training, so your approach should change depending on the individual. Work with kindness and diligence, avoiding rapid movements that confuse or scare your foal.

When to Begin

During the first few days of life, working with your foal to ensure he is not afraid of being touched, brushed, or petted is plenty of handling. Two or three minutes once a day is enough time to achieve this, especially when his dam is gentle. In fact, brushing and petting your mare is one way you can help your foal to not be afraid.[111] A foal likes

> **Too Close for Comfort**
>
> I was once asked to evaluate a mare with a cut over her knee. I always listen to the heart as part of the physical examination, and when I did so she tried to kick me. When I touched the shoulder of her injured front leg, she tried to strike me. And, when I injected her for sedation, she tried to bite me. Later, I spoke with another veterinarian that had previously worked with her, and it turned out that the mare had been an orphan. She had not been taught respect for the people around her.

to be scratched, especially in areas that his mother would caress him, like the withers and the rump. He will also enjoy having his neck scratched.

After your foal is stable and strong—somewhere between 48 hours and one week—you should begin halter training. Waiting any longer results in a more difficult job as he gets stronger—the sooner he learns to accept the halter, the easier it will be for both you and him. Waiting too long also increases the likelihood of getting into a fight with the horse, resulting in possible injury to you or him. Foals are born about 10 percent of the mare's weight—somewhere around 100 pounds, and weaned at six months of age, weighing 500 to 600 pounds.

Putting on the Halter

You will need two people: one person will hold your foal, and the other will carefully put the halter on his head. The person holding the foal will lightly and gently hug or cradle him, with one hand supporting his

Nurse Mare Farms

There are farms that lease or sell nurse mares to look after orphans. However, the nurse mare's own foal is weaned early, thus becoming an orphan. This technique is occasionally used for large breeding farms of valuable show or race horses.

Many nurse mare farms are located in central Kentucky, where the Thoroughbred, Saddlebred, and Standardbred breeding industries are enormous. The Humane Society of Kentucky estimates there to be a few hundred nurse mares used each year.

Critics claim that the use of nurse mares is widespread, but this has not been my experience. During my training, I spent eight to twelve weeks at the peak of spring breeding and foaling season in Kentucky. As a veterinarian who dealt with sick and hospitalized horses, I probably saw nurse mares used less than half a dozen times a year. Carleigh Fedorka, the author of the equestrian blog *A Yankee in Paris*, wrote that she has assisted upward of 500 foaling mares in a year, and a nurse mare was needed to raise the foal only roughly 0.05 percent of the time—less than one per year.[109]

There are dedicated groups that care for and adopt out the orphans created from the use of nurse mares. Aside from the Humane Society of Kentucky's adoption program, Last Chance Corral is a rescue group that focuses on this special population of rescue horses. In 2016, high-profile horse trainer Stacy Westfall adopted two foals from Last Chance Corral, which only adopts orphan pairs. Their goal is for the foals to develop socially. By adopting pairs, they ensure that the foals have at least one equine companion.

JNP Horses in Hugo, Oklahoma, uses their own stallions to breed back their mares before leasing them out. All offspring are registered Quarter Horses. JNP Horses' hope is that their strategy allows some traceability of the offspring as well as helping them to be valuable horses. Their Facebook page is Equine Orphans: Past and Present.[110]

If a nurse-mare's foal is born in the fall, it will be fully developed and ready for weaning when spring foaling season arrives. Breeders can use this strategy for creating healthy foals while at the same time providing income from the mare in two ways (her own foal and her "rental" use).

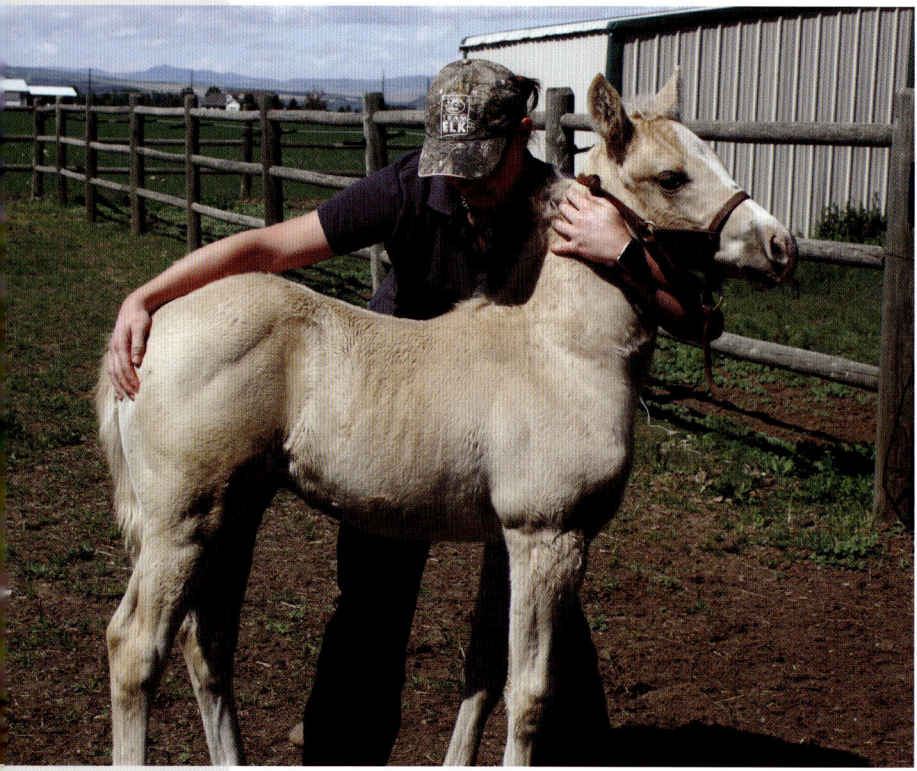

7.19 Here you see how you can "cradle" a foal to restrict his movement.

rump or holding his tail, and the other arm positioned under his throatlatch or neck (fig. 7.19). You want to cradle the foal and restrict his movement, but if you hold too strongly, he may "melt" and sink down to his knees or fold his hind legs up. It is prudent to allow the mare to continue to touch her foal. If you are between her and her offspring, that will be more distressing for her and possibly dangerous for you.

When the foal is safely restrained, the second person on your team can carefully and slowly place the halter on the foal's head and adjust it. Make sure that it is a good fit—too loose a halter may slip off his baby head and become a dangerous noose. Too tight a halter is uncomfortable and won't release pressure properly, making it more difficult for your foal to learn. You should be able to easily slip a couple fingers between your foal's face and the halter at all points of contact.

Many people allow foals to wear a halter for several weeks, until they are gentle and easy to handle. Because the halter can get caught on a horse's foot or on fencing or other objects, I recommend one that will break. This can be a leather halter or a nylon one with a breakaway function. Another addition to this is a *catch rope*, which is a small, short lead rope. A catch rope should be short enough that it will not get stepped on, and should not have a loop that might entangle your foal's leg.

Learning to Lead

Three main techniques or stages are used for foal training: 1) Allowing the foal to follow the mare, 2) using a "butt rope" to guide the foal, and 3) pressure-and-release. Whichever method or combination of techniques you use, limit yourself to only 10 to 15 minutes of total handling time. Although there is no current research, it is not recommended to work suckling foals in a round pen as trainers often do with adults. Hard exercise in this manner may exceed physiologic concussive forces on their developing joints, causing damage. Instead, stick with soft, slow work habituating your foal to being handled and led, but not allowing him to become pushy or disrespectful.

Following the Mare: It is easiest to start by allowing your foal to follow the mare, which requires a team of two people. The first person walks the mare, and the second person allows the foal to follow, but restricts his movement somewhat with the halter and lead rope. The foal won't be allowed to run circles around the mare. The idea is that you are guiding your foal, not getting into a tug-of-war with him. Usually foals will get the idea and walk along quietly after a half-dozen sessions or less. This isn't quite halter trained, but when you see that your foal accepts the restraint of the halter and the presence of a human, you can move on to the next step.

Butt Rope: Some foals are better at following their dam than others. A "butt rope" can be used to encourage forward movement (figs. 7.20 A–C). For the rope, use soft cotton to prevent a rope burn. The butt rope for a foal begins near the withers, goes around the back of the gaskin, just below where your foal's butt curves in and above the hocks, and then back around the other side near the withers. The long, loose end of a good lead rope attached to the halter works well. You want to keep slack between the halter and the withers. It takes a bit of manipulation to achieve this. Once you have the rope positioned, you will be able to

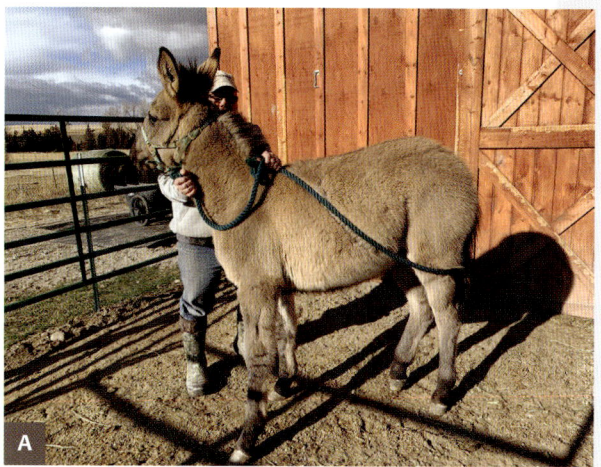

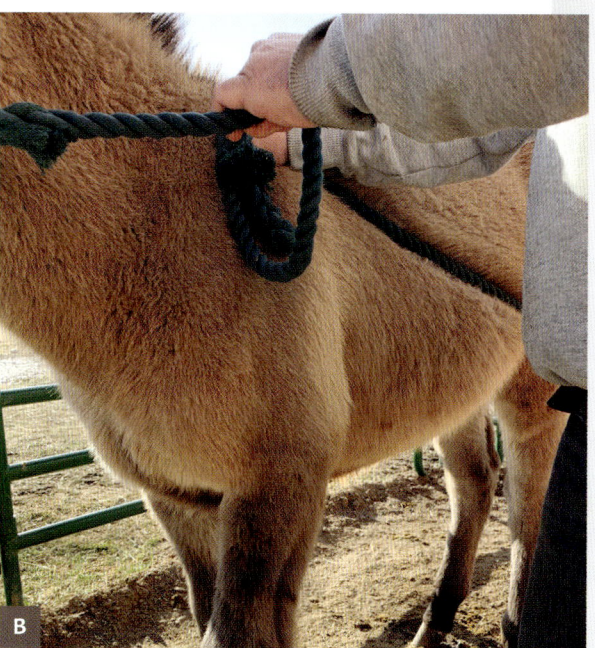

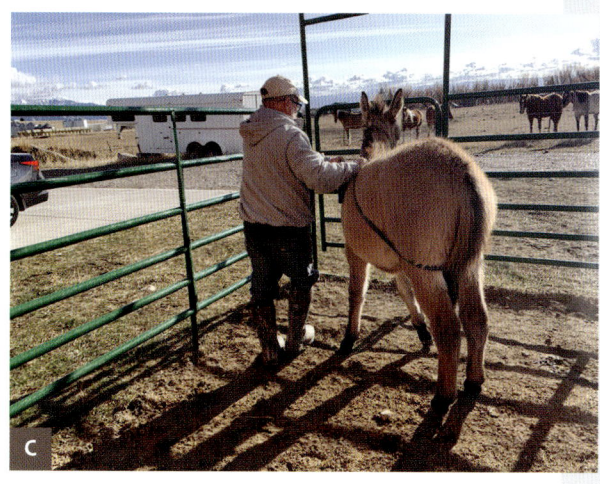

7.20 A–C The "butt rope" for a foal begins near the withers, goes around the back of the gaskin, just below where your foal's butt curves in and above the hocks, and then back around the other side near the withers (A). You want to keep slack between the halter and the withers (B). Positioned in this way, the rope allows you to apply pressure to your foal's rump until he moves forward (C).

apply pressure to your foal's rump until he moves forward, irrespective of pressure on his halter.

Pressure-and-Release: The final step after your foal has learned to accept the halter, and to move with you is to refine his training using *pressure-and-release.* This involves asking the foal to move his feet by applying a small amount of pressure to the halter when you pull on the lead rope. It's important to immediately release the pressure once he has moved. It works best to try to apply this pressure from side to side, especially in the beginning. He only needs to move one step in order for you to release the pressure. Once he has learned to consistently move one foot in response to pressure, you will then be able to ask for two steps. Although the building blocks are gradual, you will be well on your way to an excellent training foundation when the first step is achieved. Be patient and kind, but firm. Firm doesn't mean strong, it simply means that you wait on the foal to figure out what you want, and insist that you aren't releasing the pressure until his foot moves.

Pressure-and-release is tricky: too much pressure can cause the foal to resist, run backward, and flip over dangerously. Falling in this way can result in injury to the head, neck, or legs, including brain damage, blindness, or broken bones. With practice, achieving the pressure-and-release technique gives your foal a jump start on understanding how to respond to your cues. Riding uses pressure-and-release in some fashion, so by learning this early, he will learn how to figure out what you want him to do for many tasks later in life.

PICKING UP FEET

Being able to handle a horse's legs and feet is critical for long-term care and maintenance, including hoof trimming. At a very young age, it is difficult for him to balance on three legs. Allowing him to lean on a wall or on his mother can be helpful. As with all

> ### Advice Taken
>
> Sherry wanted me to geld her yearling palomino Mustang colt, Logan, and my assistant who was scheduling the appointment asked if you could "work with the horse." What she really meant to ask was if it was possible to put a halter and lead rope on him… which was not possible. The owner's interpretation of "working with" was that she could now touch Logan on the shoulder. He was still suckling off his untouchable dam, Sunshine. Sherry was well-intentioned, but she had a rough year with her own health problems cropping up after she had adopted Sunshine, who then unexpectedly produced Logan.
>
> I gave Sherry the contact information of a kind, brave horse trainer who I thought could help her. To Sherry's credit, she called the trainer immediately. The mother-and-son pair was herded from their large pasture into a small pen, and from there into the trainer's trailer. The trainer was able to separate them and get a halter on Logan within a day, and one on Sunshine within a week.
>
> Fast-forward a year: Sunshine is now ridable, Logan is being started under saddle, and Sherry's health has improved. She spends time with her horses daily and has even incorporated them into her therapy work. I'm so proud of her being mentally and financially committed to getting the help she needed when she was overwhelmed.

training, the idea is to start slowly and work incrementally to the ultimate goal over many sessions. I also recommend having a second person present, holding your foal's halter and lead rope.

First, work on touching each of his legs all the way down without him objecting. Always start by touching his withers as this is the one place he is most likely to accept touch. You want to touch him firmly—not too soft, which tickles, and not too hard, which may push or move him. Scratch his withers for a moment, allowing him to enjoy being touched. Maintain the touch and run your hand down his front leg. Try to stop just as he gets uncomfortable, but before he moves, stomps, or kicks. Repeat this process over and over, making sure you touch all sides of each leg. You will not, nor should you try, to accomplish all of this in one session. It will take a week or more.

When he accepts touch on all parts of all his legs, you may begin to pick up each leg. At first, you pick up a leg two or three inches, and only for a second. As he gains strength, acceptance, and balance, you can pick up the leg higher and hold it for longer. Remember, the higher you hold it, the harder it is for him to balance. Pick his feet out. Mime farrier work by scratching and tapping or firmly patting his hoof. Pet and reward him often for good behavior. Never frighten him.

After you have worked with and prepared your foal, your farrier should be involved beginning at six to eight weeks of age. Of course, if there are growth abnormalities, farrier care may begin earlier. Have him or her work with you and your foal every four to six weeks for baby hoof trims. It is well worth the financial investment for both training and for proper growth.

OTHER TRAINING

It is a good idea to make sure you can touch your foal all over. Teach him to allow you to touch every bit of his chest and abdomen. You should be able to touch his ears, and handle his lips to look at his teeth and gums. He should let you lift and touch his tail. He should accept grooming with a variety of brushes.

Understand that foals explore the world around them by touching, sniffing, or putting objects in their mouth. Don't allow them to bite you, but do allow them to look around and investigate new objects safely, for example brushing and grooming supplies.

AIM FOR A HEALTHY, SOLID CITIZEN

Although I have discussed many problems here, the majority of births are uneventful and result in a healthy and vigorous foal. An examination ensures he is healthy. Should a problem be identified, early medical attention is critical to foal survival. All foals are hard work, and orphan foals are more work. Saving your orphan foal's life and watching him grow up to be a healthy and sound solid citizen is well worth the effort. Critical parts of achieving a well-trained horse include appropriate socialization, early halter training, and handling of legs and feet.

CHAPTER 8

Unable to Rise:
The Down Horse

A recumbent or *down* horse is one that is unable to get up on his own. Usually, the horse is suffering from an underlying medical condition that needs treatment. It's critical to pinpoint and treat the condition as well as helping the horse get up. The longer a horse is down, the less likely he is to recover. A trained professional should be called to evaluate the situation and assist you.

The exhaustion of not being able to save a horse after investing significant emotional and physical energy can feel overwhelming. Nowhere in rescue is this more true than working with a down horse. In this chapter I'll discuss medical treatments for the down horse, as well as methods for assisting him to rise (fig. 8.1).

SAFETY

Personnel safety is the most important consideration for the feasibility of rescuing a down horse. Injured people cannot help a horse. Don't work with your down horse while you are alone. Wait for help. You should call your veterinarian, but it is also useful if you can get three or four horse-savvy and strong friends or neighbors.

Stay away from the horse's legs—work around his spine or back. Wearing a helmet is advisable, especially if the horse is flailing

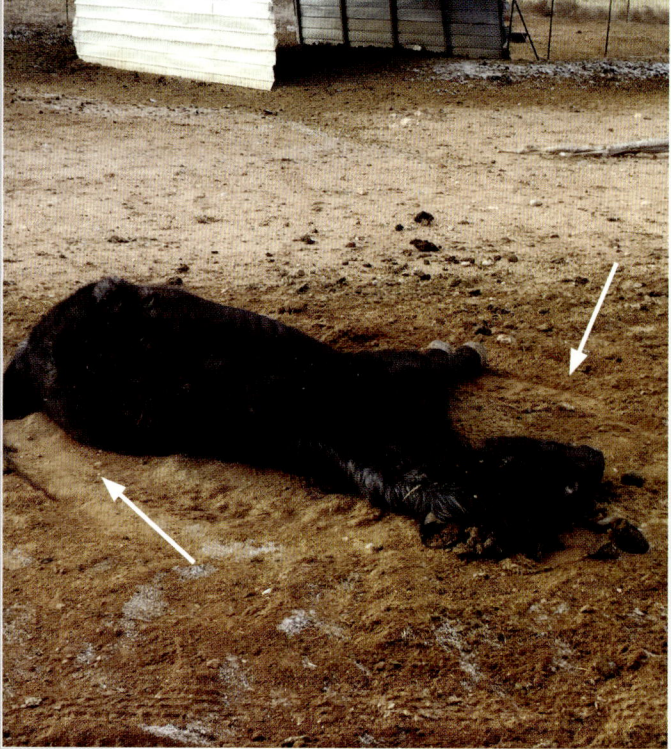

8.1 A "down" horse in poor conditions. He is thin and weak. Notice that he has made a gouge in the dirt near his forelimbs from repeated unsuccessful attempts to stand. (Note: His shelter is made of dangerous sharp metal.)

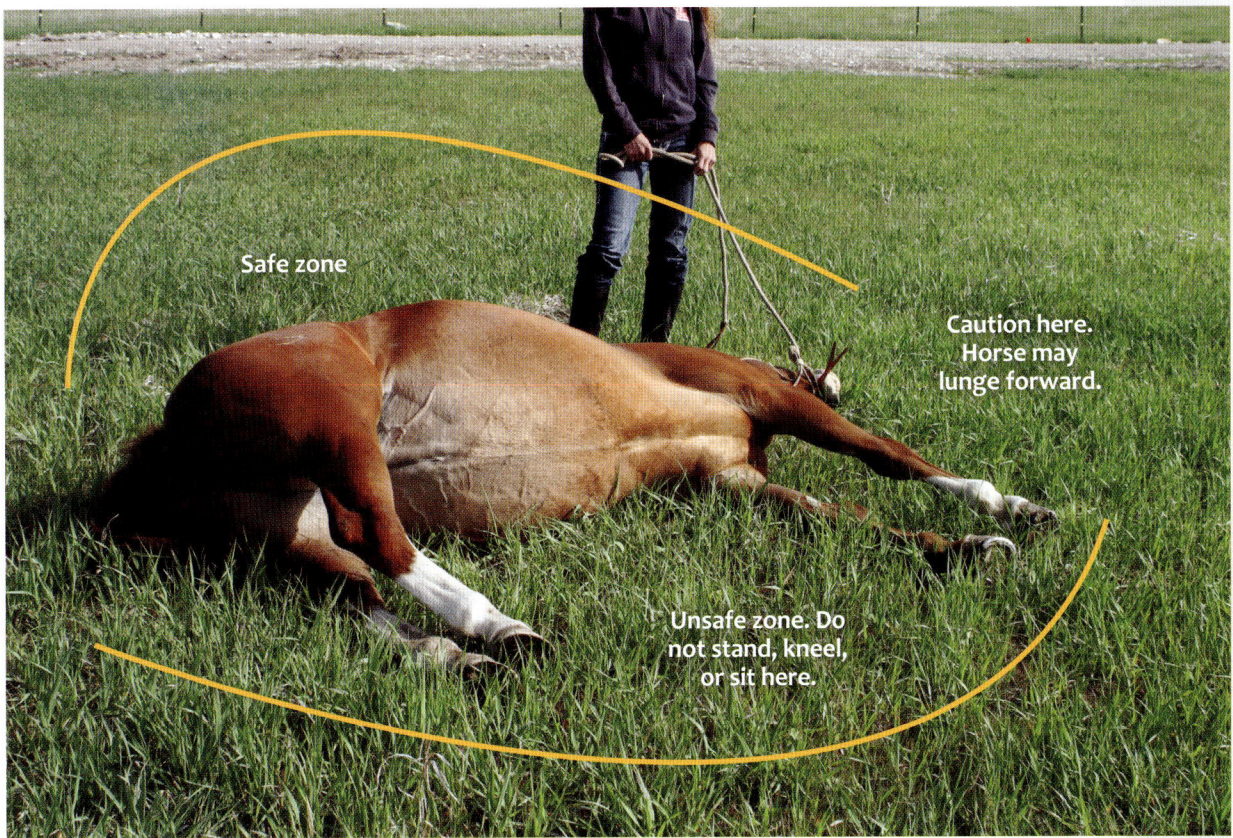

8.2 *This handler is in a safe location when standing near a down horse.*

or trying to roll. Never put your knees on the ground—you can squat, but you need to keep your feet under you so you can move quickly (fig. 8.2).

Putting yourself in harm's way could result in you being unable to care for this horse who depends on you. It may seem like the horse is a sweet, needy creature that would never hurt you. The reality is that from the horse's viewpoint he is in a life-or-death situation (which may actually be true), so he may panic and flail unexpectedly and dangerously. Protect yourself by adhering to safety precautions and never letting your guard down.

NORMAL SLEEPING PATTERNS

Before you can recognize "abnormal," you must know what "normal" is. Being down is different from sleeping. Horses can nap standing up, but they must lie down for deep sleep. They usually sleep between four and five hours total, but less than one hour will be in deep sleep. Deep sleep occurs between midnight and 4:00 a.m., but also there is a period in the mid to late morning where horses will nap in the warm sun.[112, 113] At least one herd member will remain awake and keep watch. Young horses sleep more often and for longer periods. When a sleeping horse gets up, he will shake himself off.

> ### Reasons Why a Horse Is Down[114]
>
> #### PAIN
>
> - Trauma: broken leg or pelvis
> - Muscle disease: tying up (myopathy), electrolyte deficiencies leading to muscle weakness
> - Colic
> - Laminitis or other hoof disease or damage
> - Generalized arthritis leading to lack of mobility
>
> #### NEUROLOGIC DISEASE
>
> - Botulism
> - Equine motor neuron disease (vitamin E/selenium deficiency)[115]
> - Equine protozoal myeloencephalitis (EPM)
> - Mosquito-borne viruses: West Nile Virus (WNV), Eastern or Western Equine Encephalitis (EEE/WEE)
> - Equine Herpesvirus (EHV)
> - Rabies
> - Toxins in feed or plants
>
> #### ENVIRONMENT
>
> - Being cast or malpositioned against a barrier
> - Slipping on bad footing
> - Obstacles in the way or a tight space
> - Natural disaster
>
> #### METABOLIC ILLNESS
>
> - Severe malnutrition and resultant weakness
> - Hypoglycemia (low blood sugar): can occur in sick foals or in refeeding syndrome

It is not normal for a horse to be recumbent for more than an hour at a time, or to stand up and immediately lie back down. It is not normal for a horse to struggle to get to his feet or to have marks in the ground around him where he has been moving his legs without getting up. It is not normal for a horse to collapse or to "dog sit" with his hips down and his shoulders up. It is not normal for a horse to get up and lie down repeatedly. These behaviors are signs of illness or colic.

REASONS FOR A HORSE TO BE DOWN

Most problems that cause a horse to be down fit into one of four main categories: pain, neurologic disease, environmental factors, or metabolic disease. Any problem can be complicated by obstacles, positioning, or natural disasters.

Any horse can slip and fall in bad footing, such as slick mud or ice. Occasionally, a normal horse becomes *cast* in his enclosure—he rolls to where his feet are up against a wall or trapped in a fence. He then cannot roll back over or get his legs back under himself to get up.

It is important to recognize that your horse could be down due to abdominal pain (colic) and not because he is physically unable to get up. Sometimes it is tricky to sort out exactly what the cause is, and there may be multiple factors that contribute to the situation—for example, he may be both arthritic and emaciated.

When a healthy horse is cast, he soon becomes an unhealthy horse. He cannot eat or drink, and his large body mass crushes his skin, muscles, and nerves. Horses that are

are down—particularly when in an awkward position—have a risk of contracting pneumonia. The longer he is down, the worse this can be.

Identifying Underlying Problems

First, it's a matter of determining if the horse is able to get up. Each instance and case is unique. Your veterinarian will assess the horse and do as much of a physical examination as possible. Circumstances and surrounding obstacles are limiting factors. Risking rescue for a horse who has a non-repairable broken leg or other medical malady with a poor prognosis is not advised. A malnourished horse who is down and unable to rise has a poor prognosis. In fact, trying to get him up may add to his anguish. In these cases, euthanasia may be the best option.

Your veterinarian is going to check the horse's vital signs. She will also determine if the horse's lungs are clear or if they sound diseased, and if the horse has a heart murmur or other signs of heart disease. A rectal temperature is needed. A horse who is down in cold weather can experience *hypothermia* (a dangerous drop in his core body temperature). If he has a fever, an infection that has affected the nervous system (for example, herpes virus) goes higher on our list of possible underlying causes. Your horse's gums should be evaluated to assess if he is dehydrated or has circulatory problems.

Since it is possible that your horse is colicking, discuss his recent eating habits, possible dietary changes, and defecation. Using a stethoscope to assess his gut sounds also clues your veterinarian in to gut health.

Your horse should be checked over for specific areas of pain or injuries and a determination made whether or not all four

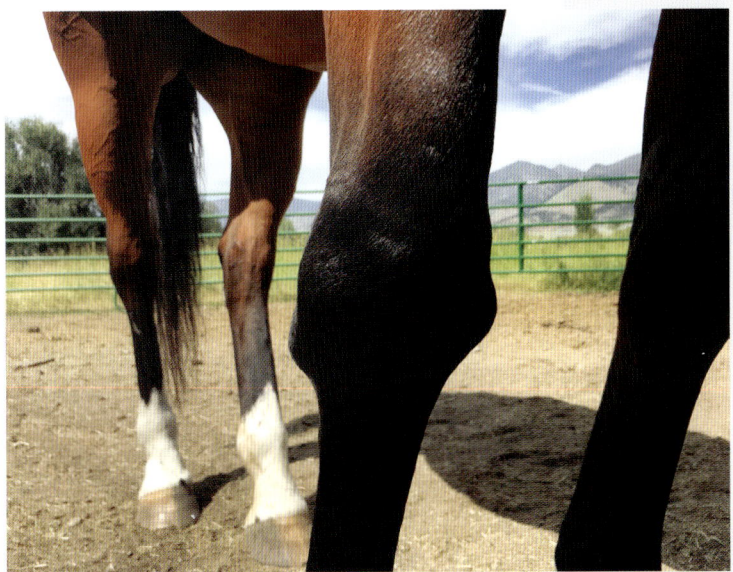

8.3 This horse has severe carpal (knee) arthritis. If he lies down with the affected knee on the ground, he could have difficulty getting back up.

legs can function (fig. 8.3). Look for cuts or abrasions on his legs, body, or face where the horse has injured himself in his repeated efforts to rise.

It is difficult to evaluate the horse's neurologic status while he is down. Indicators that a nervous system abnormality is present include a history of abnormal movement, especially if it has been worsening over time or the horse has taken a tumble, if your horse has twitches or tremors, *nystagmus* (rhythmically darting eyes), or asymmetrical muscle wasting. A specific, classic posture indicating the problem is within the spinal cord is dog-sitting, except his legs will be extended out from his body stiff in a pose known as *extensor rigidity*. If this pose is present, it doesn't matter how hard you try, he will not be able to rise or stand. It is rare for a horse who exhibits this pose to survive.

Your veterinarian may take the time to

run blood work before trying to get your horse up. The time it takes to check his blood work may be worth the investment, especially if the horse has been down for several hours. The laboratory panel will show any electrolyte imbalances that contribute to muscle weakness, which will need to be corrected before the horse can stand.

With intensive supportive care, a few horses will survive and recover after being down for several days. Since we cannot predict which ones these will be, all we can do is make our best effort to identify and treat what we can. As each hour and day ticks away, the likelihood of recovery progressively diminishes, and the enormous expense adds up.

Treating Underlying Problems

Regardless of cause, if you are going to save your horse, he needs first-aid care. You can provide this care while you are waiting for help to arrive, but only if you can do so safely.

The down horse may work himself into a lather or sweat trying to get up. When he stops trying and lies still, the sweat cools his body temperature, resulting in hypothermia. To warm him, dry off any wet hair, and then drape a blanket over him. Don't attach the blanket or leg straps to him as this will complicate his ability to get up.

If it is safe to do so, test your horse to see if he is willing and able to eat. If he has colic, his appetite may be decreased or absent. You may also want to offer him water if he has been down for more than an hour or two, especially in hot weather, because dehydration and electrolyte imbalances are likely. When the weather is cold or there is a possibility that your down horse has hypothermia, offer warm water.

If he is dehydrated, an intravenous catheter can be inserted into his jugular vein while he is down. This allows us access to administer medications or electrolyte-rich fluids. Fluids may include additives such as dextrose, B-vitamins, calcium, and potassium—nutrients and electrolytes that are critical to muscle function.

For arthritis or other pain, administration of bute or Banamine® will help. Hydrating the horse will ameliorate potential adverse effects of kidney damage that these medications can cause.

Some horses benefit from administration of a steroid, which reduces inflammation and triggers an adrenaline rush. This will amplify and direct his body's energy reserves to be useful, helping him have the ability to get up.

HOW TO GET THE "DOWN" HORSE UP[116, 117]

It's critical to set him up for success as failed attempts deplete his energy reserves, decreasing his chances of standing. We use all of our available resources, and give the horse any bit of help we can.

After providing medical treatment, we reposition and assist the horse to stand up. If it is safe, we put a flat halter with a lead rope on his head. A tail rope is also used for support. The knot used for this purpose is a quick-release modified sheet-bend knot (figs. 8.4 A–F). The halter and lead rope and tail rope guide the horse and provide support when he attempts to rise.

Dark-colored, soft fabric can be used to cover his head, protecting his eyes and avoiding injury. It may also help keep him calm.

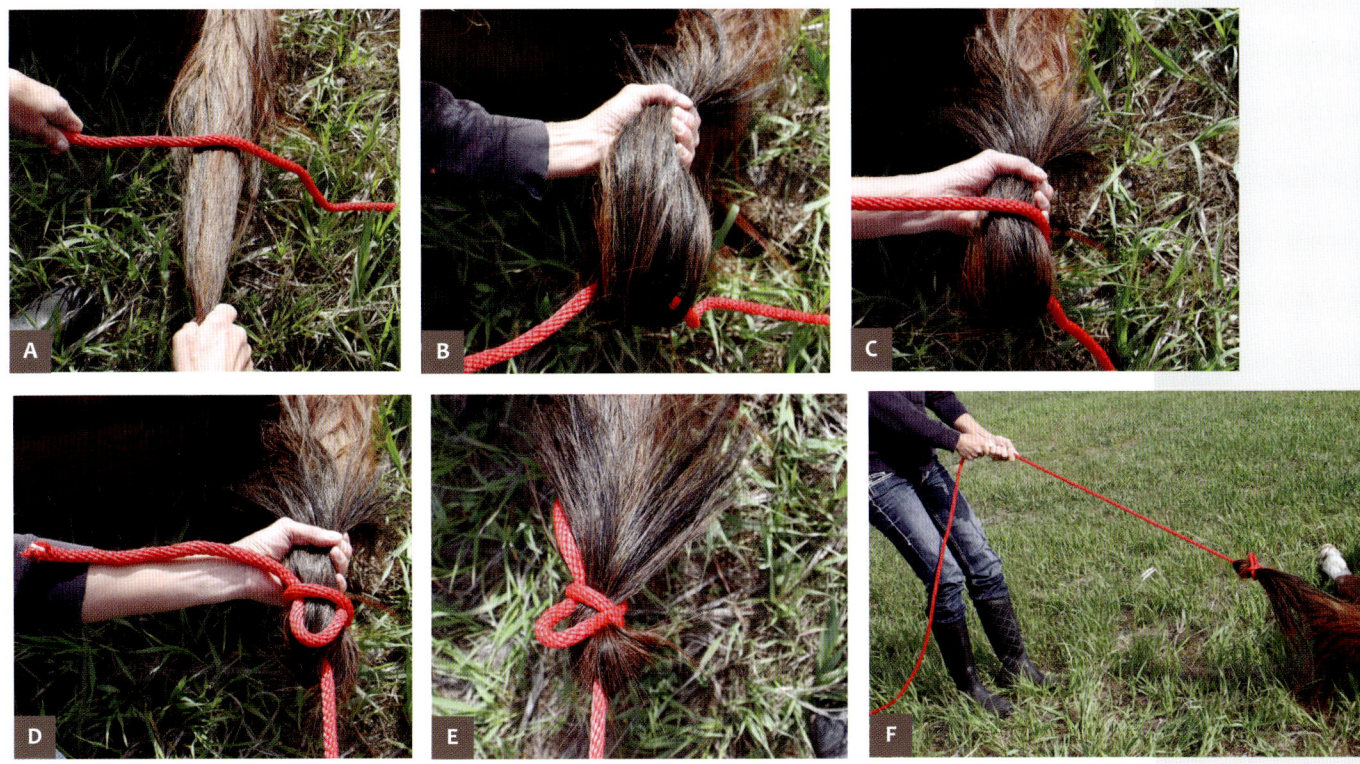

8.4 A–F Six steps to make a secure, quick-release, modified sheet-bend knot on a horse's tail to assist him to rise: Lay about a foot of rope over the horse's tail, which you will use to wrap around the tail and make the knot (A). Fold the tail over the rope (B). Bring the foot of rope underneath and all the way around the tail (C). Then bring the rope around the tail a second time and tuck the end of it underneath itself (D). Apply tension to secure the knot on itself (E). The tail can be pulled as a quick-release knot to undo it after the horse is standing. Tension can be applied to the horse's tail to help him to rise and keep him steady once he is up (F).

Identify and Remove Obstacles

For a horse who is down due to positioning and arthritis or weakness, we are going to reposition the horse before asking him to rise. His feet should be clear of debris, obstacles, walls, or fence. When the footing is unlevel, his limbs should be downhill from his body. To get up, your horse must be able to get his front feet forward, lift the front part of his body, and then lunge forward and straighten his hind legs. Clear the area to ensure there is ample room for lunging forward.

When there are obstacles in the way, move them. These may include fencing material such as boards or wire, round-bale feeders, buckets, pans, or troughs. Blankets attached to the horse should be removed. Anything that is in his path should be moved, both for the horse's success at standing and human safety.

Evaluate the surroundings: is there mud or ice preventing the horse from rising? If the footing is sticky or slick, use sand, gravel, or wood shavings to increase traction.

Rolling a Horse

We are going to roll or swing the horse so that his forelimbs are below or level to his chest. When feasible, rolling also gives the previously crushed muscles a chance to recuperate. Rolling can also be helpful for a horse who has a problem that reduces his orthopedic ability to function on one side, for example, a horse with severe arthritis of one knee. If your horse is cast, he must be rolled or moved away from the wall so that he has more room.

Your veterinarian may sedate your horse before rolling him to help prevent flailing. Wide webbing or soft cotton can be secured around the pasterns and fetlocks of the limbs on the ground side (one front and one hind). One person should guide and support his head. Others use the ropes on his legs to roll him from one side to the other (figs. 8.5 A & B).

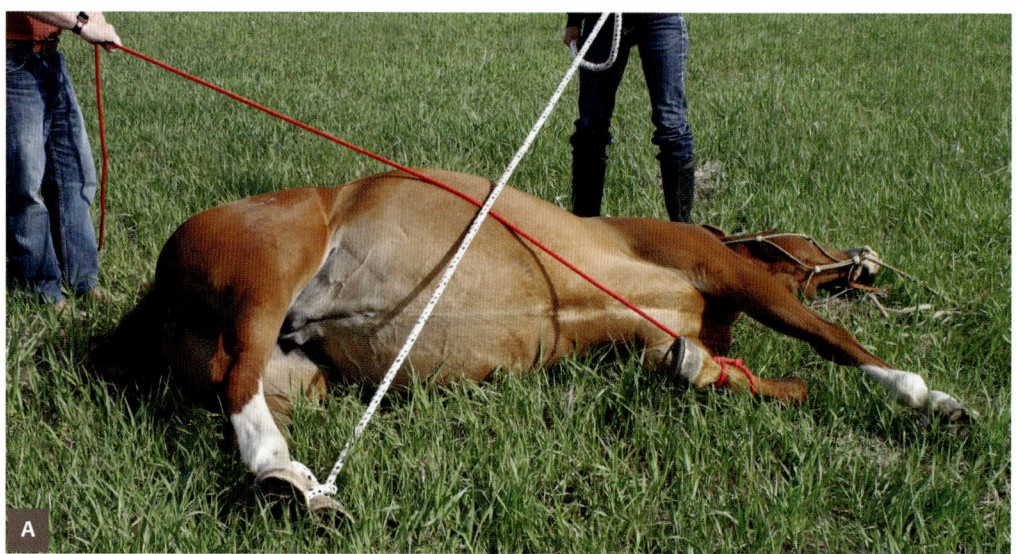

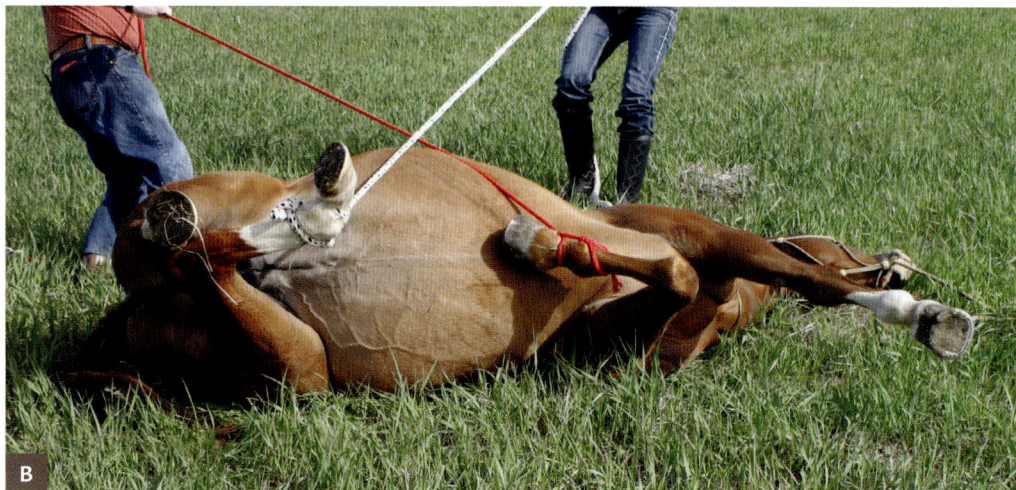

8.5 A & B Ropes can be placed around the fetlocks on the ground in order to turn a down horse (A). The horse can now be rolled over from a safe distance (B).

Sliding to Reposition

Two basic ways to reposition a recumbent horse without rolling him are the *forward assist* and the *sideways drag*. You need 4-inch nylon webbing that is 20 to 30 feet in length.

The simple forward assist is accomplished by passing one loop of wide webbing or thick cotton between the front legs and over his withers (figs. 8.6 A & B). The center of the webbing is at the withers, and the two tails of it will be between his forelimbs. You may use a painter's hook, boat hook, or other thin, stiff tool to pass webbing underneath the horse and manipulate its position. A tool will help you maintain space between you and the horse, keeping you safe. Then, with guidance on his head and tail, a horse can be pulled from a safe distance using the webbing.

A sideways drag is accomplished with two lengths of webbing or thick cotton. One will be placed around the horse's body at his withers, and the other will be around his flank (just forward of his pelvis). The center is at his body, and the strap tails over his back so that he can be pulled away from a safe distance (fig. 8.7). This is useful for getting him off bad footing or out of a depression or ditch.

Get Him Up (Prepare and Assist)

Believe it or not, the majority of the work to get the down horse up is done. Your preparation efforts should set him up for success on his first attempt.

He will still be guided with his halter and lead rope and tail rope as he stands and to help him support his weight. When I am leading a team, I put the person with the most equine experience and confidence on the lead rope. The tail rope will go to the

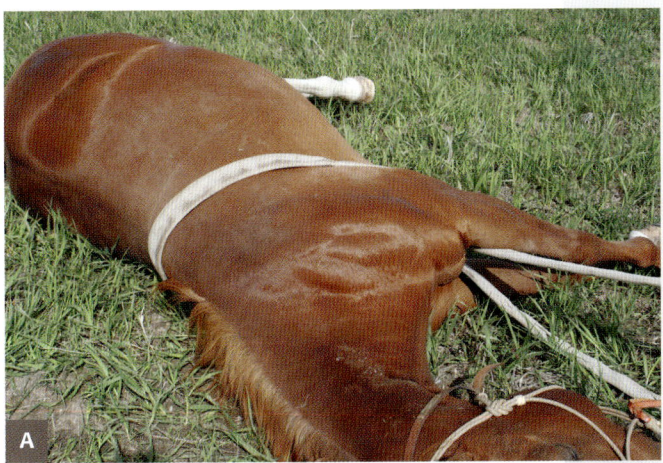
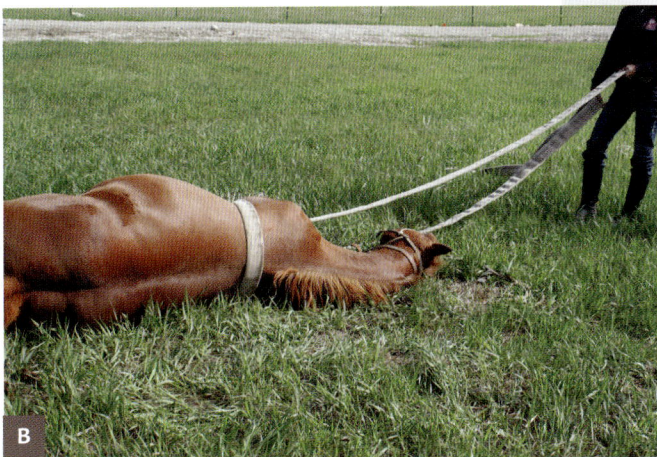

8.6 A & B *Two views of strap placement for a* forward assist, *which is a specific way of moving a down horse by pulling him forward after wide web straps are placed in the configuration shown here.*

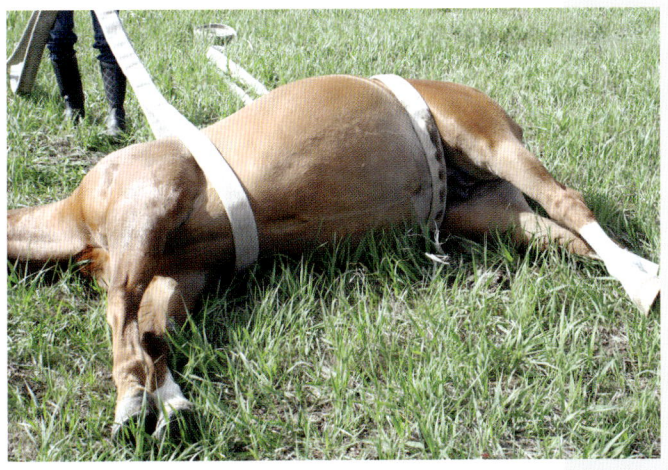

8.7 *Strap placement for sideways drag.*

Part I: Caring for Horses in Need—129

biggest, strongest person on our team. This person will help the horse lift the weight of the horse's hindquarters. When possible, the rope may go over a stall wall for additional leverage. Although the strong person may lift the tail from a close range, the rope allows them to steady the horse from a safer distance. The tail should not be pulled by equipment or tied to an immovable object.

Finally, after all this preparation, I ask the horse to get up. I will encourage him in a way that makes him *want* to stand. If he has made multiple attempts and failed, he may have given up. We want him to make one good, successful attempt and not deplete his energy reserve further. This may be the only way to save his life because a down horse cannot survive.

Once he is up, we support his head and tail until he seems more steady. I give him lots of petting, "good boys," and even a food reward.

If he is not able to stand using his own reserves, a team trained to use ropes, slings, and lifting equipment (such as a tractor bucket) may be needed to get him up (fig. 8.8).

LONG-TERM TREATMENT OF UNDERLYING PROBLEMS

If your horse was down because of colic, further assessment and treatment is needed.

The most common reason a geriatric horse is down is a combination of arthritis and weakness. The weakness may be due to either chronic disuse causing wasting of muscles because of the joint pain, or starvation. Your veterinarian may counsel you on ways to address these factors and help your horse long-term. We can drastically improve his quality of life by adding a pain management program to his regimen. If your horse has a low BCS, revise his nutrition plan with your veterinarian.

For a prey animal who defends himself by running, being down is terrifying. If a horse's arthritis is such that he has repeated episodes of being down, it is time to consider his well-being and say goodbye. Euthanizing him is kinder than repeatedly finding him down and afraid.

LONG-TERM DOWN HORSE

Unfortunately, for the horses that have diseases of the nervous system or have been down for more than 24 hours, the prognosis

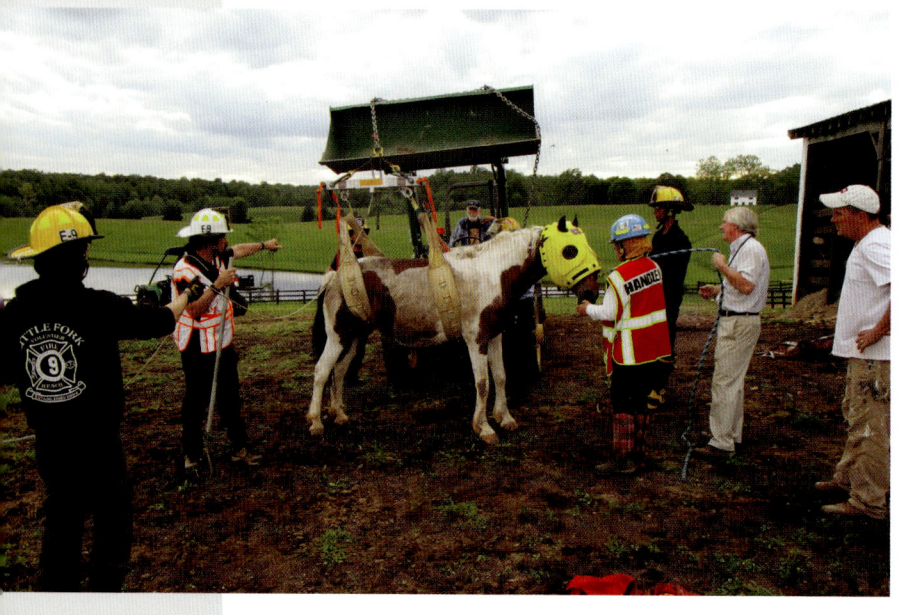

8.8 The Little Fork Volunteer Technical Large Animal Rescue Team in Culpeper County, Virginia, assists a horse to rise using a Becker sling.

is poor. It is rare for one to survive and be nursed back to health. It takes a very devoted and resourceful team. Round-the-clock care, very soft bedding, and a method of turning, assisting, and/or slinging the chronically down horse to support him at least part of the time is necessary. Some horses can get up but will only be able to stand for a few minutes at a time. There is hope for horses that gain strength and stand for a longer and longer period each day (figs. 8.9 A & B and 8.10 A & B).[118]

A down horse's personality is also a factor in his recovery. He has to be tractable

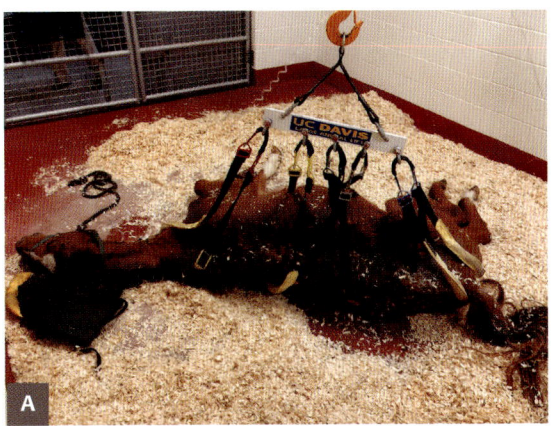
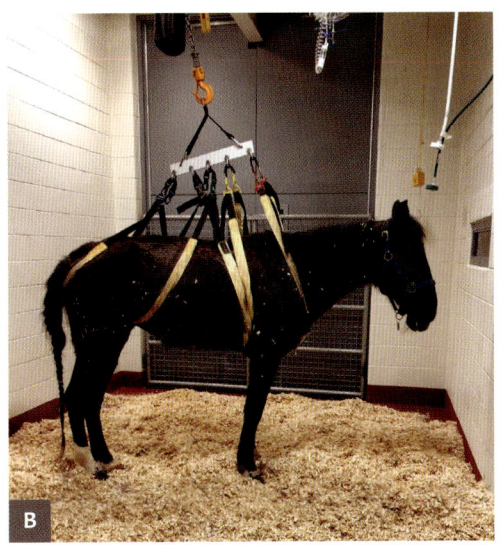

8.9 A & B Weak individuals may need sling support to stand. The longer a horse is down, the poorer his prognosis.

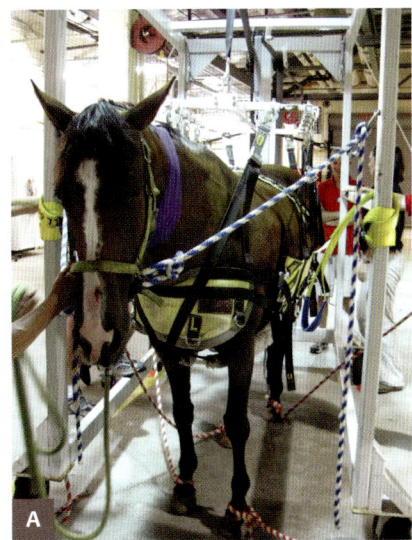
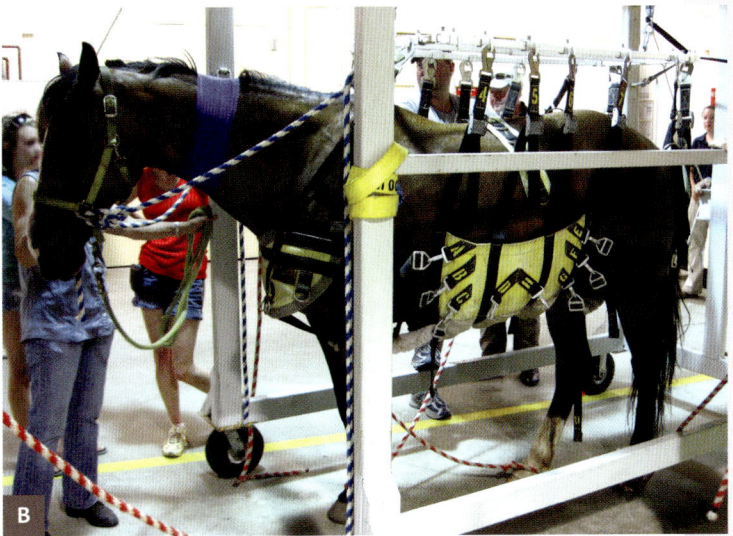

8.10 A & B A sling designed to assist a weak horse to walk. In this case, this horse is weak due to neurologic disease. The frontal view (A) shows the ropes attached to each leg to manually help the horse's step. The side view of the sling (B) shows the support on the horse's body and head. The wheels for movement of the sling frame are also visible.

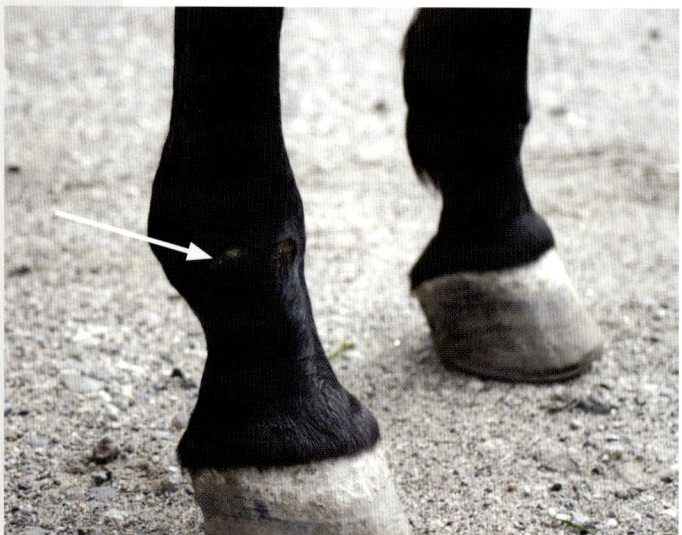

8.11 A "bedsore" skin abrasion on the front of a horse's fetlock. This is a common place for rubs to occur when a horse spends more time than normal lying down, especially on hard ground.

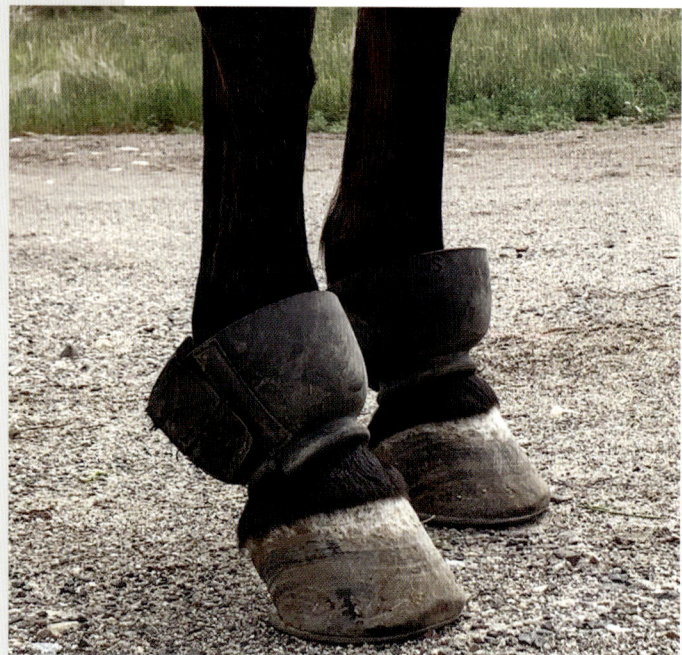

8.12 Bell boots can be used upside down to protect the fetlocks and facilitate healing.

and calm in order to allow people to handle him for nursing care. But he also has to be tenacious enough to have the will to live.

Bed Sores and Skin Injuries

Because horses are heavy, pressure sores on the skin develop rapidly. These *decubital ulcers* are more likely to occur in thin horses with a BCS of 3 or less. Lack of padding over bony prominences causes pressure points. Common locations are the point of the hip and the shoulder. Sores can also occur over the knees, hocks, or fetlocks, or on the horse's face (fig. 8.11).

Treating bed sores, especially on a down horse, is problematic. There is often a frustrating cycle of scab development and reopening of the wound. Treatment and prevention both rely on deep, soft bedding and rolling, repositioning, or lifting the horse periodically. It is recommended to do so every four hours. You should also keep flies off the wounds. There are a number of protective leg wraps and boots that are commercially available, and these will help protect and pad the sore areas of the legs (fig. 8.12). It is much more difficult to cover the hips and shoulders. A sticky bandage (Elastikon®) over a non-stick material with some gauze for cushioning may help. Salves and ointments should be used with caution. The best ointment for this purpose is SSD (silver sulfadiazine, an ointment used to treat burns in human patients), but triple antibiotic can help. Any other ointment (for example, nitrofurazone, scarlet oil, or corona) damages fragile tissue, delays healing, and should not be used.

Horses that have flailed around trying to get up may injure themselves and have abrasions or skin rubs as well. If this is your horse's first episode of being down, and you were able to get him up within twelve hours or less, these areas usually heal with no trouble.

If your horse is down because of colic and has rolled so violently that he has skin lesions, it is a bad episode and most likely he will need surgery to resolve the colic. These abrasions usually are on the face or head, especially around the horse's eyes. Without surgical treatment of the colic, the prognosis is poor to grave.

Use of Slings

There are several commercial slings available, and a homemade sling may occasionally be effective. Use of these is not without risk—pressure sores and compression of internal organs are problematic side-effects of sling use. A horse's legs are designed to support his immense weight. Weight is a problem for trying to support him via anything else.

The UC Davis Anderson sling attempts to work around these problems by supporting the horse from many different points, thus reducing the concentration of pressure at each point (see figs. 8.9 A & B—p. 131). The Anderson sling uses the legs as the main way to support the horse so that his abdomen and chest are not compressed.

The horse must tolerate the sling. Some horses panic when the sling is on them and they are lifted.

Another factor to consider is that with each passing day, the odds that your down horse will recover become slimmer. Knowing when to say goodbye after time, energy, money, and effort have been invested is tough. When the horse is not treatable in the field and must be hospitalized in a sling, the cost is often prohibitive for continuing treatment.

THE QUALITY OF LIFE QUESTION

The majority of horses that are down suffer from arthritis and some other factor, such as weakness due to malnutrition or environmental obstacles, contributing to their inability to rise. If a horse is only down for a short period, we can usually help him up, but should consider if the horse should be euthanized before he gets stuck down again. Treating your horse's arthritis pain and addressing malnutrition are the main ways to improve his quality of life.

Horses who are down because of severe colic or neurologic diseases have a poor prognosis. For horses with metabolic dysfunction due to starvation, it is possible to nurse them to health, but the time, energy, and money expended may be unreasonable or impossible. Even with extreme expenditures some will not survive.

CHAPTER 9

Urgent Rescue:
Working in Disasters

This chapter discusses a different type of horse rescue: those that are urgent or related to natural disasters. A disaster rescue may bring to light abuse and neglect that was previously undetected. Rescue facilities and shelters will have a population influx when a natural disaster strikes. Rescue leadership may serve as a community coordinator, using their network of established volunteers and foster homes to help horses displaced by disaster.

I'll first talk about disaster preparedness for you and your personal horses then address some guidelines for working in natural disasters and accidents. Next, I'll discuss basic first aid, and finally, I will outline specific medical problems from different types of disasters.

DISASTER PREPAREDNESS

Learn About Your Locale
Evaluate disasters your community has experienced in the past. Look at your terrain and determine what type of disaster is most likely. Consider where, specifically, your horse is housed. He could be at the base of a forest, near a river, or on the plains, rendering him susceptible to fire, flood, or tornadoes. If you live near railroad tracks or industry, hazmat exposure may be a real threat.

Find your local community emergency response team (CERT). Contact may be available through your local extension office. There is a CERT in every state. Learn what they recommend—they know local disasters best. Although many evacuation guidelines are general, it does you no good to prepare for a volcano if you live in Kansas. Training and credentialing workshops are available nationwide for individuals interested in learning to be a team member of a certified rescue effort.[119]

Plan Ahead
The severity and number of weather-related disasters is on the rise.[120] According to a Federal Emergency Management Agency (FEMA) survey, fewer than 40 percent of people have an emergency plan.[121] After careful consideration of the possible disasters that may strike in your area, organize yourself and prepare. Your horses are your responsibility, and good preparation will keep you ready in case you are displaced for any reason.

Prepare Your Plan: You need to have an evacuation plan in place, and everyone in your household or rescue group should know about it in advance.[122] It's a good idea to share your personal evacuation plans with neighbors, pet-sitters, and friends or family helping you. Your plan will also help them with *their* plan. Post evacuation plans in your tack room or barn, and keep a copy in your trailer as well.

For larger rescues or ranches, evacuating dozens of horses may not be practical or possible. Consider *shelter in place* options, whereby disaster risks are mitigated through land management and plans for emergency care at home.

Gather any items you may need such as halters, lead ropes, medications, and feed for your horses. Have a plan for leaving in five minutes, five hours, or five days.

Learn about your local authorities: Who is in charge if your horse is separated from you and you are trying to find him? Know what animal shelters may be available in your area. Your local animal control, emergency management team, or agricultural extension agent office are resources that can help you with this information, as well as local disaster response plans prepared by governmental agencies or organizations.

Location: Your evacuation location should be well beyond the geographic area that would be affected by your possible local disaster. For example, if you live in forested mountain terrain, plan to house your horses in the valley so they will be far away from fire danger.

You may have a friend in mind who can house your horses in the event of an emergency. Make sure far in advance that the friend is willing and able to do so. It is important that your friend be close enough that you can get to her in a few hours' time but far enough away she will not be experiencing the same disaster. Stay flexible and plan for a secondary shelter. Your primary plan may become inaccessible because of closed roads or other unforeseen circumstances. Once each destination is established, identify your route and alternative routes.

Prepare for Transport

Evacuate your horses early, well before requirements. You might be able to leave your house with your dog and cat at the drop of a hat, but coordinating the effort to move horses is more time-consuming.

For a variety of reasons, I advocate that every horse owner have a functional truck and horse trailer. It doesn't have to be brand new or fancy, just safe and in good working order. Otherwise, you could be at the mercy of other people during an emergency.

If you don't own a trailer, make sure you have at least two people you can contact to ship your horse in an emergency. If there is any question that evacuation may be necessary, get your horses moved as soon as possible. Plan extra time so your shipper can take care of your horses as well as her own.

Disaster preparedness is a motivator for trailer training, so school your horse and have him ready. The more stressed and fearful your horse is, the harder it will be to load him in the trailer, so train him to be confident in a variety of circumstances. Load him in the rain. Load him in the dark. Load him in the wind. Load him in the snow. Load him in the sun. Load him into a different trailer. You may not be there for your horse. Enlist the help of friends and family members for further training—just because your Mustang has learned to trust you and will go where you ask,

Make Your Go Bucket

- Your riding helmet.

- A halter and lead rope for each animal.

- Identification to attach to your animals (for example, ankle or fetlock bands, clip-on or braid-in tags).

- Emergency contact information for yourself, a backup person, your veterinarian and farrier, and documents showing animal identification and proof of ownership. You may also include a treatment authorization document with specific instructions about your horse.

- Any medications or special needs information for each animal—at least three days' worth.

- First-aid kit: bandage material (such as Vetrap™, gauze, and padding), a cleanser that can be used in eyes or wounds, a thermometer, and an anti-inflammatory medication such as bute or Banamine®.

- Some people advocate having feed ready to go—if you prepare this too far in advance, grain may spoil. If your trailer has a storage compartment for hay, it is a good idea to keep a supply at the ready. It can be occasionally rotated out when you change batches of hay.

- Bonus tools: flashlight, wire cutters, hoof pick, duct tape, and scissors.

- A premade kit can be purchased at lsart.org/ralphs-responders.pml that includes a useful visual guide for maneuvering stuck or down horses.[123]

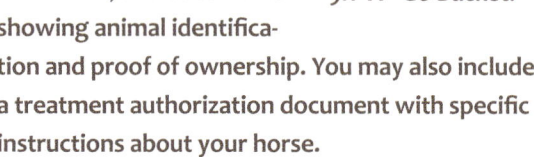

9.1 A "Go Bucket."

doesn't mean he will do it for others. Prepare for any variation you can think of.

During one fire in New Mexico, a husband and wife farrier team repeatedly drove into the flames and returned with loads of horses. They had to encourage, use ropes, and cajole horses in with food. The longer it took to load one horse, the longer the next horse had to wait, and the higher the risk to these volunteers.

Rescuers learned with Hurricane Katrina that evacuation of animals is also critical for evacuation of people and families to safety. Sometimes, people only evacuated because of law enforcement. Don't be that person. Law enforcement and rescue resources are needed to help everyone, but we should all do our part to prepare, and not be a resource-sucking victim.

Identify Your Horse

It's best to have more than one type of identification on a horse. You may not be separated from him, but if you are, there is a better chance you will be reunited when he is wearing visible identification. Livestock markers can be used. These are basically large grease markers (the size of "sidewalk chalk") made for water-resistant marking on animals. A crude, but useful technique is to have your picture taken with your horse.

Permanent, traceable identification is a critical component of being reunited; I advocate microchips for horses for this purpose (see previous discussion on p. 18). Louisiana is the only state that requires permanent identification for a horse to get a Coggins Test, and microchips are the best available permanent identification because of ease and accuracy of use. This regulation resulted in identification of many horses that would otherwise not have been returned to their families after Hurricane Katrina.

Keep the following documents in a watertight bag to take with you when you evacuate: Coggins test, identification photographs, and any proof of ownership you have (such as a brand inspection document or a bill of sale).

Other information to include is pertinent medical history and behavior quirks (such as indicating that your horse will not stand tied, is high-strung, or is a stallion). It's also a good idea to have a document with emergency telephone numbers: your veterinarian, secondary emergency contacts should you not be available, your farrier, and the contact information for people at your evacuation location.

Sarah's Story

One year in New Mexico we had a wildfire at the base of a mountain range (fig. 9.2). Even though it was small and in a rural area, more than 600 people and their animals were displaced from their homes.

Sarah is a retired teacher and is a strong-willed, tough community leader. She treats every animal and human she encounters with kindness and respect. She has mules and volunteers with the Backcountry Horsemen of America (BCHA) to pack in tools and maintain trails in our National Forests.

Because she lives in this mountainous area prone to fire, Sarah's personal mission is to ensure that everyone understands fire safety and evacuation precautions. She is a leader in her county's CERT. Each year she presents information at the local BCHA and Donkey and Mule Association meetings where she shows her Go Bucket and discusses disaster preparedness.

Until the fire, Sarah had never used her Go Bucket. When the fire started nearby, Sarah took her animals to her prearranged evacuation location. She then proceeded to work with other CERT team members to set up emergency shelter at the

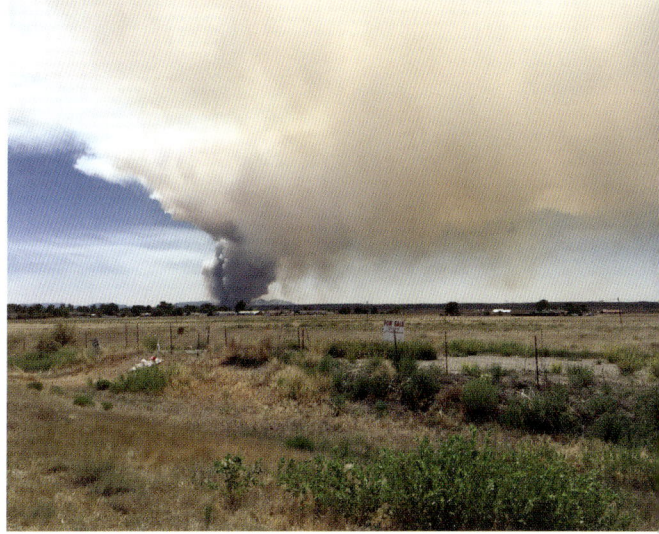

9.2 *The fire that displaced Sarah from her home.*

county fairgrounds. While organizing accommodations and caring for other people's animals, Sarah's house, equine shelters, and all vegetation on her forested property burned to the ground. Only a few metal panels were salvageable.

In what must have taken monumental emotional effort, Sarah continued to care for others as her home was destroyed. But because she was prepared, her life and the lives of her mules were spared.

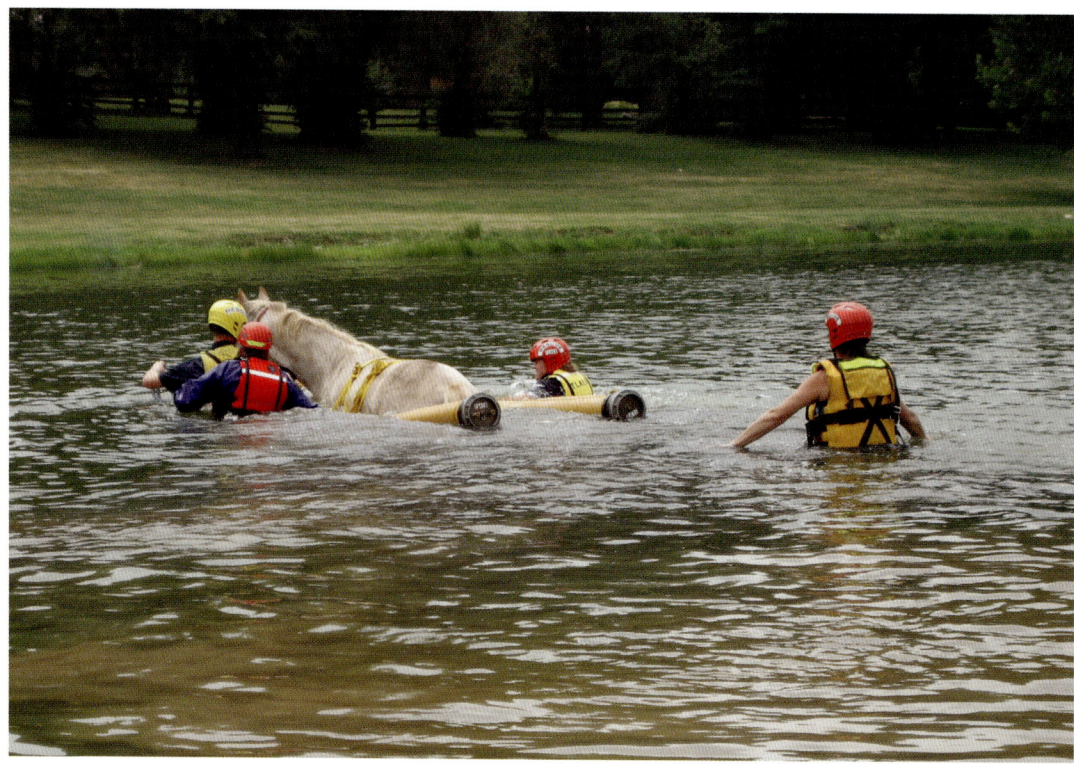

9.3 TLAER team members practice a water rescue. This trained horse is assisted with floats, and the humans are all wearing life jackets and safety helmets.

If you are working at a rescue providing shelter, identify horses as they arrive. During Hurricane Katrina, the rescue center run by Louisiana State University "took great measures to ensure every horse went back to its rightful owner." They marked each horse as he came in, and "the horses were photographed, microchips were scanned and logged into a system."[124]

GUIDELINES FOR WORKING IN NATURAL DISASTERS AND ACCIDENTS

Communication

Communication is essential for success in rescue. Ky Evan Mortenson asserts in *Horses of the Storm* (a book about rescuing horses during Hurricane Katrina), "Whether it was an actual rescue, volunteer coordination, or donated supplies being distributed through the appropriate channels, time and time again we learned nothing can take the place of clear communication and coordination."[125]

Emergency response teams include emergency rescue personnel, animal personnel, and community volunteers, and everyone must work within the incident command system. Being able to navigate this important communication network is critical for working to help animals during disasters and emergencies. Lone Ranger-type antics are likely to result in volunteers becoming victims. FEMA has free training courses for incident command at training.fema.gov.[126]

Incident command is designed to be

as small or as large as any event can be. It accounts for five main areas under the commander, as well as public relations as needed. The areas are operations, planning, logistics, intelligence or investigation, and administration with finance.

Identifying people and their responsibilities is important. During Hurricane Katrina, horses were identified as well. There were people that tried to falsely claim horses or harass volunteers, and proper use of identification markings or badges prevented this.

While you are caring for sheltered horses, keep written records on horse care. This is crucial for communication and looking out for their well-being. Records avoid problems like underfeeding, doubling up on medications, or losing track of a horse.

Technical Large Animal Emergency Rescue

TLAER is the acronym for Technical Large Animal Emergency Rescue, and refers to safely working within incident command to help horses in emergency situations such as trailer wrecks or traffic accidents, natural disasters, and barn fires. TLAER is self-described as "the practical considerations, behavioral understanding, specialty equipment, techniques, methodologies and tactics behind the safe extrication of a live large animal from entrapments… in local emergencies and disaster areas" (fig. 9.3).[127]

According to Dr. Rebecca Gimenez Husted, co-author of the TLAER textbook, "An unjustified difficult, dangerous or high-tech approach is sometimes employed by rescuers." Furthermore, "the excitement of rescues tends to break down the use of teamwork and common sense."[128]

Dr. Husted traverses the world educating potential members of a technical rescue team. I have had the fortunate opportunity to learn from TLAER in different terrain and geographic challenges (fig. 9.4). Look for training opportunities in your area (tlaer.org). Another group, the Equine Emergency Response Unit, puts on a variety of courses as well (eerular.org). Disaster apps are available from the Red Cross to download to your phone and include hurricane, earthquake, tornado, flood, pet first aid, and a general emergency app.

During an emergency, be aware of your surroundings—don't get between a horse and a wall or rock or other immovable structure. If the horse is down and can't get up, stay away from his legs and feet. Wear

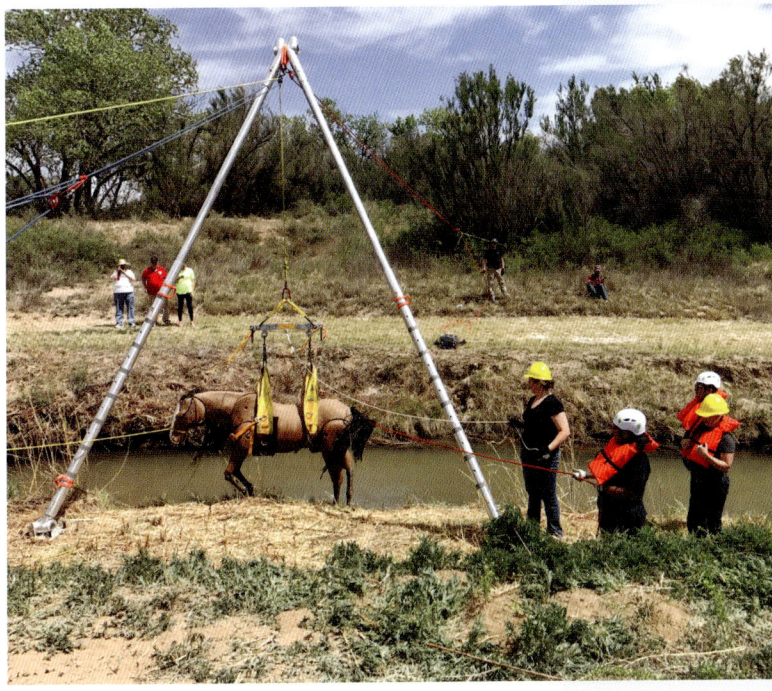

9.4 TLAER training where team members practice a water rescue with a mannequin. Notice the safe distance from the horse (a live horse could kick if personnel are too close), and the use of ropes to guide the horse's relative location in the sling and A-frame. Also, team members are wearing safety helmets and life jackets.

a helmet. Don't go onto ice with a horse, or enter a burning building. It's terrible for horses to die, but you want to preserve your life first and foremost.[129, 130]

As a volunteer in a coordinated effort, you may be asked to assist with basic or advanced tasks. Everyone on the team is needed and important. Volunteers that clean stalls and feed horses are critical, but not glamorous.

FIRST AID FOR HORSES

Horses can panic and be flighty. When injured, they may not allow safe handling of the affected area. No horse is worth getting hurt yourself, so don't take risks that compromise your own safety.

When a horse is injured or ill, evaluate his vital signs, and reevaluate them periodically (every 30 minutes or so). Trends away from normal are a bad sign.

Leg Wounds

Wounds occur most often on legs, so check all four of your horse's legs from hoof to body, on the outside, inside, front, and back of each leg. If you find a wound, and especially when it is bleeding, a bandage should be applied (see p. 82 for instruction). Clean the wound then apply the bandage material you have. It should be tight enough to stop the bleeding. If it bleeds through the bandage, simply apply another layer of bandaging on top. If you take the first bandage off, it will disrupt the clot that is forming underneath. Disturbing the clot can result in further extensive hemorrhage (figs. 9.5 A & B).

Next, make sure the horse can walk. When a limb is unstable, do your best to stabilize it with a splint made from a board or PVC pipe and bandage material. Most broken legs do not heal well, so euthanasia may be the best option.

Eyes

Although leg wounds account for the majority of injuries to horses, eye injuries also occur. You can tell if a horse can see out of his eye by checking his blink response. If he blinks while you pass your hand or finger near his eye, he likely can see. If there is damage to the eyeball itself, a non-stick pad and a bandage over the head can be applied to protect the eye from further damage. Elastikon® works best for this purpose as it is

---

Normal Vital Parameters for Horses

Temperature: 99 to 101.5 degrees Fahrenheit

Pulse/Heart Rate: 36 to 44 beats per minute

Respiration: 8 to 16 breaths per minute

Potential Response Team Members

- Firefighters
- Emergency Medical Technicians (EMTs)
- Police or sheriff's departments
- Veterinarians and veterinary technicians
- Animal control officers
- Community volunteers

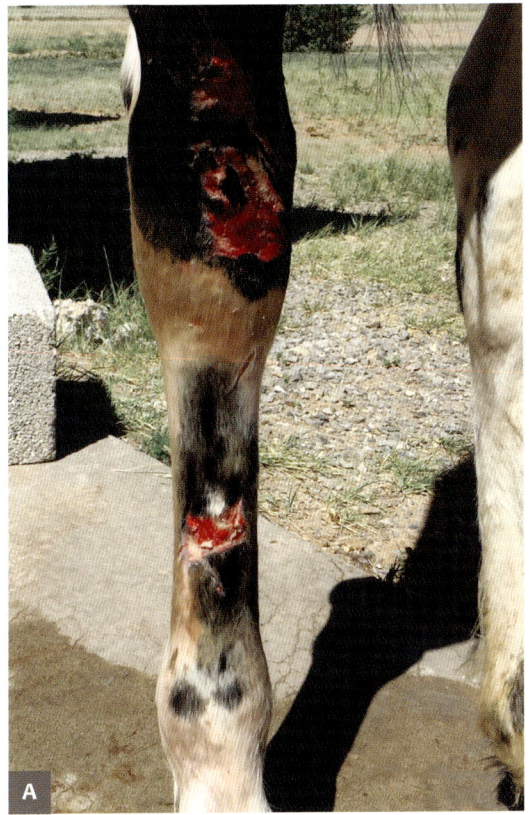 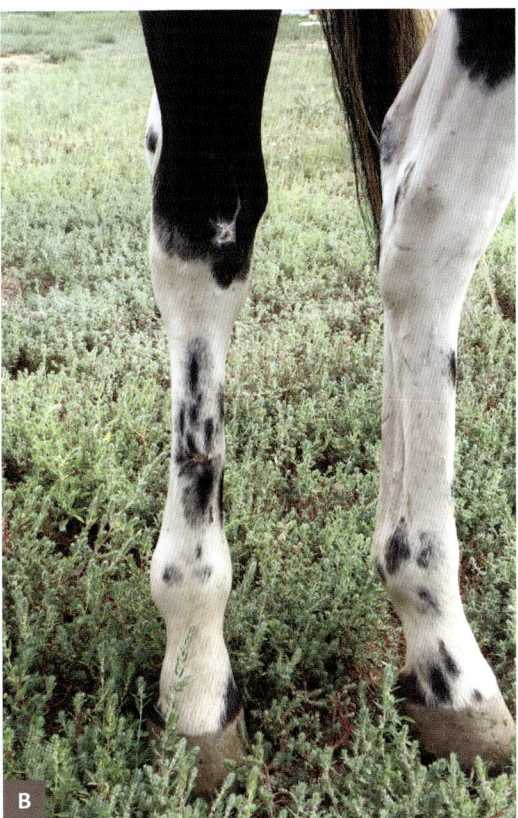

9.5 A & B This horse sustained leg wounds when he was being loaded in the trailer to be evacuated from a fire (A). Trailer training in a variety of circumstances will help mitigate anxiety and injury to horses. The same horse, with his leg wounds healed (B). He will always have a scar.

sticky and stays in place well. Make sure the other eye stays uncovered so that the horse can still see.

Wounds on the Body

Most wounds on the body heal well. First aid consists of stopping bleeding, then preventing contamination. You may administer pain medication (bute or Banamine®).

The deepest wounds may enter sterile body cavities, such as the chest and abdomen. When a wound enters the chest, cover it to ensure that dirt, debris, or contamination cannot enter. If the abdominal cavity has been compromised and intestines are open, the horse will not survive and should be euthanized at once.

After any wound has been attended to in the field, arrange for transport to a veterinary facility or shelter for further treatment and intensive care.

SPECIFIC DISASTERS AND THEIR EQUINE HEALTH CONSEQUENCES

In the United States, geography is varied. Possible disasters include earthquakes, wildfire, hurricanes, floods, oil spills, tornadoes, extreme heat, extreme cold, and (rarely) volcanoes. Barn fires also happen. Aside from specific problems that are caused directly by the disaster, post-disaster stress and colic is common as a result of changes in shelter, food, and water.

Fire

Any fire burning near horses is terrifying. Wildfires or structure (barn) fires can result in smoke inhalation. Horses are susceptible to burns of their skin as well as heat damage to hair, hooves, and eyes. Once the barrier function of a horse's skin is lost because of damage, he will be susceptible to serious injury and loss of body fluids and proteins. Initial damage may not be immediately apparent. Charred skin may slough days or weeks later.

It can take months for burns to heal, and extensive scarring will occur (fig. 9.6). Treatment is a matter of intensive care support (intravenous fluids, antibiotics, and meeting nutritional needs) as the horse recovers from smoke inhalation and caring for skin as it heals. Hospital expense can be exorbitant.[131, 132, 133, 134]

Floods

It is as the old saying, "Water, water everywhere, but not a drop to drink." Hurricane high tide salt water is not palatable or safe for horses to drink. Overflowing freshwater sources can be contaminated with toxins, chemicals, or debris.

During floods, horses will be loose as fencing and barriers are covered in water. They may travel for miles. Horses standing in or traveling through high water may become entangled in debris that is not visible from the surface. Prolonged immersion leads to skin infections of fungus, bacteria, or both.

The barrier function of the skin is lost over time as the skin degrades by soaking. Think of your raisin-like fingers after soaking in a hot bath for too long, but expand that over hours or days. Skin can degrade to such an extent that it sloughs.

After horses are rounded up and identified, attending to their injuries, dehydration, and medical needs is important. Centrally located shelters and communication are critical for returning horses to their homes.

High Winds

Hurricanes and tornadoes are high-wind situations that can cause collapse of shelters, or result in dangerous flying debris that injures animals. If your shelters are old or not sturdy, your horses may be safer outside. High winds can cause trees and utility poles to crash into horses' fields and shelters. When fences are damaged, horses can easily escape. Finally, horses may be struck by flying or unstable debris and injured.

As horses are located and their injuries are treated, shelters must be prepared for ensuing bandage changes and medical care, in addition to seeking out the owners of each animal.

Heat Waves

Horses are cold-adapted animals and do not cope well with excessive heat. They should have access to clean water and be provided with shelter that gives shade. Work with horses in the early morning hours when it is cool, not in the brutal heat. Horses can be hosed or sponged-off to help them stay cool.

Blizzards and Snow

Blizzards occur in northern states. Most states are prepared with snow plows, sand,

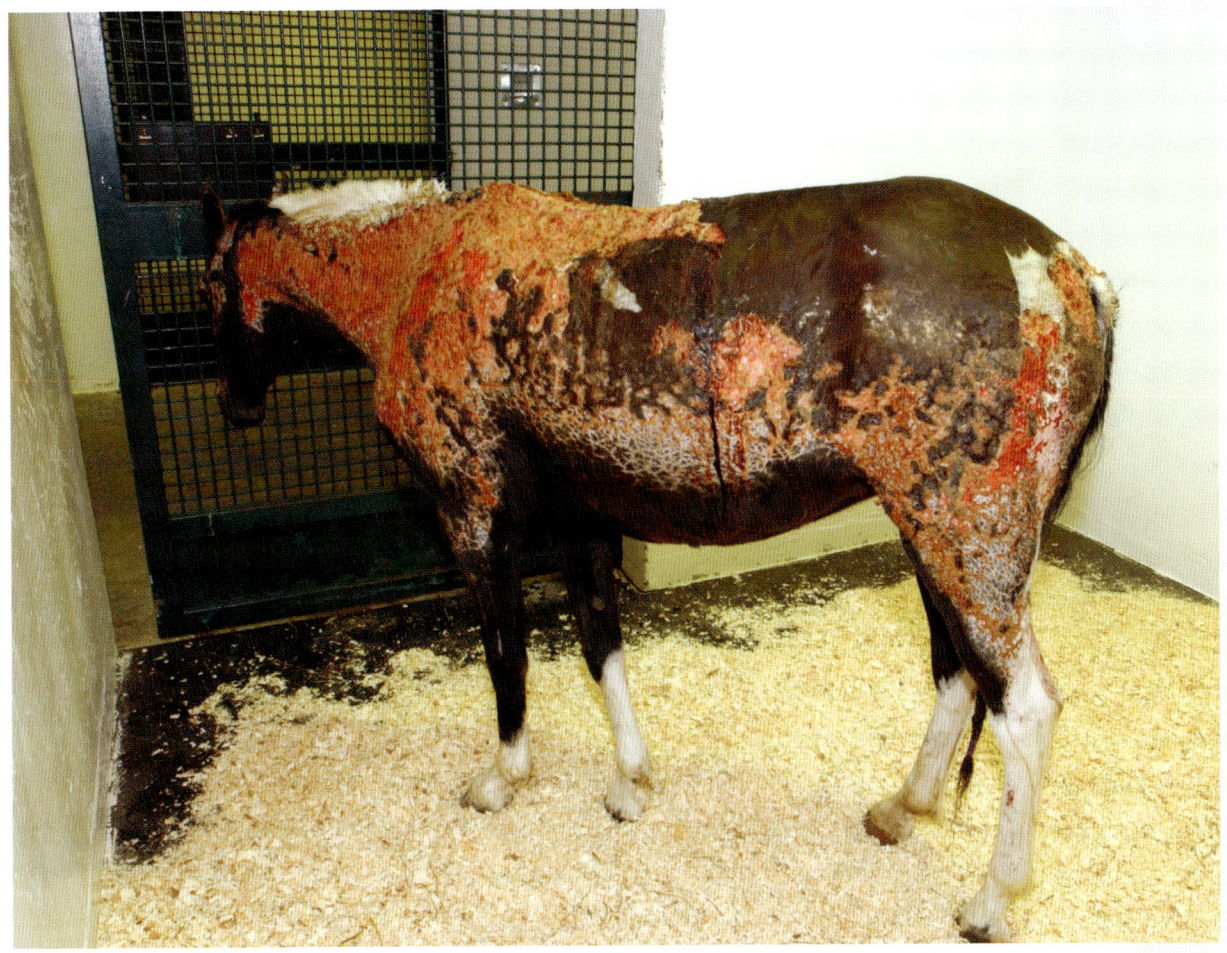

9.6 This horse has extensive burns from a structure fire but ultimately survived. Healing took months.

and other efforts to ameliorate poor road and weather conditions. However, rural areas (where most horses reside) are served last. Extreme cold can decrease accessibility to water because of the water itself freezing, or because weather conditions prevent animals from getting to it. Snow conditions can also make taking hay or forage to horses difficult. In states with minimal winter weather, a cold snap can be a disaster. Southern states don't have infrastructure for clearing snow, and many people may not have stock tank heaters, access to enough forage, or ability to get to their animals after the snow.

The first priority is to ensure animals have enough food and water. Watching the weather and planning ahead is important. Stock up on hay or other forage, and if you think you won't be able to get to your animals after the snow, put plenty out so they can have full access. As the forage is broken down by microbes in a horse's gut, heat is released, helping to keep him warm.

Even with no stock-tank heater, there are some ways to keep water thawed in milder unexpected cold. For example, half-fill clean milk jugs with water, seal the lid and put them in the tank. The movement they create as they float around will prevent freezing. Warm water can be periodically added to buckets and tanks, as long as they are accessible.

Falling Through Ice or into a Swimming Pool

Occasionally, a horse falls through ice or into a swimming pool. Because of the vertical walls of the swimming pool and the nature of ice, it's nearly impossible for the horse to get himself out. In these cases, a forward assist may help.

Horses that spend hours trying to swim to stay afloat or get out of the water are susceptible to hypothermia and will sustain muscular damage. As the muscles release toxic metabolic byproducts, the kidneys can be damaged.

Slow warming of the horse using dry air is important. Don't rub—this action dilates vessels, worsening tissue damage. Protecting the kidneys by having the horse in intensive hospital care with intravenous fluids and monitoring blood work will be necessary for recovery.

BE PREPARED

The primary goal of disaster preparedness is to first ensure you are not a victim. Next, you can be a volunteer who cooperates and works within the incident command system on a team. Everyone's role is important, but there is only one incident commander.

Specific disasters can lead to specific medical problems for horses. Enhance your first-aid skills for the most common and likely problems in your region. Disasters are not exclusive, so preparedness should be broad. Hurricanes bring flooding in conjunction with severe winds. Fires often occur after earthquakes, especially around structures where gas or propane lines have been disrupted. If you are prepared for evacuation from one disaster, you will also be ready for evacuation for a different reason.

CHAPTER 10

A Good Goodbye:
Euthanasia

Despite our best efforts, it is not possible to save every horse. Saying goodbye and ending a horse's life is sad, but it is better for him to be euthanized surrounded by caring people than it is for him to suffer. A horse could live under horrible conditions, suffering from malnutrition and dehydration. He could go through an auction house, be held in a feedlot for several months, take a really long and hard trailer ride, and end up in a foreign slaughterhouse. He may also have an incurable disease with a poor prognosis. By comparison, a humane and peaceful euthanasia is a good option. Although you will feel overwhelmed by heartache, you may take comfort in knowing that you truly are helping him.[135]

MAKING THE DECISION

When the time comes to make the decision, you need support from your family, friends, other people in your rescue network, or your veterinarian.[136]

If a horse is owned by a rescue group, board members or officials in the group should make the decision together. If you personally own the horse and your family members assist you financially or physically caring for him, it is also important to involve them in this decision. Getting a group of people or a family together in consensus on this judgment call is emotionally taxing and can worsen grief. In the case of rescues or group ownership, it is helpful to discuss health and euthanasia options in advance. Having an agreement and guidelines in place will ease confusion and reduce strife in situations where emotions run high.

When you are the sole caretaker for a horse, euthanasia and loss is a heavy burden to bear alone.[137] The decision to end a life is the most difficult responsibility a caretaker has. The AAEP has published *Euthanasia Guidelines*, which acknowledge the role of the equine veterinarian as an animal advocate. The *AAEP Guidelines* recommend that you and your veterinarian explore options and alternatives together before making the final decision. Each situation is unique, and your veterinarian will have valuable input.[138]

COMPASSIONATE GUIDELINES

The intent of the *AAEP Guidelines* is to help make a decision about euthanasia that is fair to the horse. It states that a horse should not have to:

- Endure continuous or unmanageable pain from a condition that is chronic and incurable.

- Endure a medical or surgical condition that has a hopeless chance of survival.

- Remain alive if he has an unmanageable medical condition that renders him a hazard to himself or his handlers.

- Receive continuous analgesic medication for the rest of his life.

- Endure a lifetime of continuous individual box stall confinement for prevention or relief of unmanageable pain or suffering.

A horse who is in continuous or unmanageable pain can have weight loss despite good dentition and appropriate feed offered. If his orthopedic pain is significant, he will lie down more than a normal horse, thus spending less time eating. You may not ever see him lying down, but he can develop rubs over his hips, hocks, or shoulders. He may also alter his posture in such a way that standing is no longer energy-efficient.

Pain in horses is expressed through subtle facial expressions: tight wrinkling may be observed around the lips, nostrils, and eyes.[139] He may hold his ears back, even at rest, and have strained chewing muscles. His attitude can be grouchy with ear-pinning and tail-swishing as a response to handling requests or minor movements. It is important to recognize these subtle indicators of pain.

A horse should be able to mentally "be a horse." When he is in a box stall, he cannot run from predators, nor can he socialize with others. Each horse is an individual, and some will tolerate stall rest better than others. A temporary period of stall rest for a recoverable injury is understandable, but a protracted and indefinite period of living in a stall is not fair to the horse. In older horses, with a gradual decline, the time point at which euthanasia is the best option is not always clear.

Statistics show that the leading cause of death in geriatric horses is old age followed by colic and cancer.[140] Some geriatric horses will have an event such as a terrible colic,[141] or an episode of choke. This event triggers an immediate and well-defined time point for euthanasia. Of the horses that succumb to old age, only 36 percent die on their own. The other 64 percent are humanely euthanized, and the most common reasons are weight loss and inability to ambulate. "Inability to ambulate" may mean anything from chronic, severe arthritis pain to a horse who is down and unable to rise.

Other Reasons for Euthanasia

There are situations where euthanasia is warranted for younger horses. This is heart-wrenching. The younger the horse, the more devastating it can feel to have to let go. Consider the *AAEP Guidelines* with respect to a young horse who needs continuous analgesics for relief of pain or would need to be in a stall for the remainder of his days. The lifespan of a horse ranges into the thirties, which is a long time to be in a stall.

Medical and surgical treatment with a hopeless prognosis is cruel. When a horse will not survive his condition, euthanasia is the only way to end suffering. An example of this is a horse with an inoperable broken leg.

Sometimes the time for euthanasia isn't as clear. What about the neurologically abnormal horse who cannot be safely ridden? Will he fall on a handler who is leading him? What about the moderate to severe colic where surgical intervention is not an option? How long do you wait for medical therapy to work? What about a sick orphan foal? How many other horses could be helped with the same dollars that are being poured into him? How likely (or unlikely) is he to recover?

These are intricate questions. There is no blanket answer for any given situation. The interplay of many factors will affect outcome.

Euthanasia decisions are challenging to discuss with your peers, your family, and your rescue group. I encourage everyone to have compassion for each other and to not judge harshly. Facts can be obscured by emotion, and passing judgement makes a painful choice more difficult.

EUTHANASIA PROCEDURE

Whether the horse is in the hospital or on the farm, your veterinarian will need a signed *Euthanasia Consent* document before proceeding (fig. 10.1). You or a representative from your group or family will need to be able to sign this legal document and portion of the medical record. You also need to decide if you want to be present for the euthanasia procedure. This is an individual choice, with no right or wrong answer.

There are several acceptable methods of euthanasia for horses. Both the AVMA and AAEP sanction these methods:

1. Intravenous IV administration of an overdose of barbiturates.

2. Gunshot to the brain.

10.1 A "Euthanasia Consent" form. This example is courtesy of Bluebonnet Equine Humane Society.

3. Penetrating captive bolt to the brain.

4. Intravenous administration of a solution of concentrated potassium chloride only if the horse is already unconscious (as for surgery).

5. Alternative methods may be necessary or acceptable in special circumstances.

Although methods one and two are fairly self-explanatory, the others need clarification. A penetrating captive bolt works similarly to a gunshot, but the device is reusable. It is a heavy bolt, contained

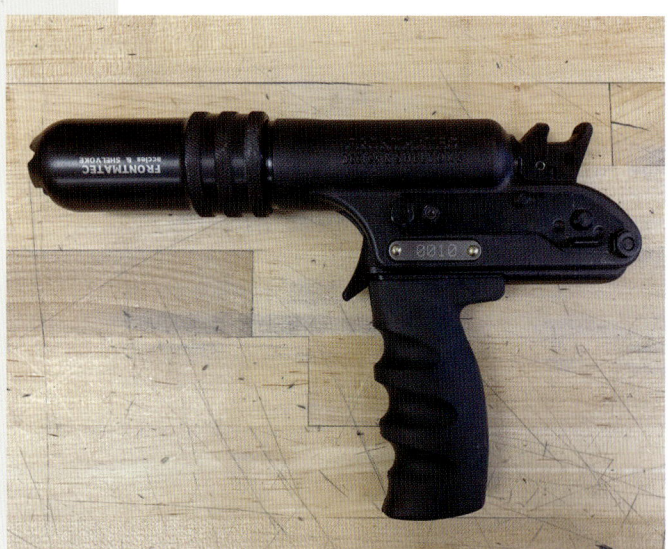

10.2 *A "Captive Bolt" is sometimes used for humane euthanasia of horses.*

within a column (akin to a miniature cannon) with a spring mechanism that is reusable. Newer designs may be shaped more like a pistol. Like a bullet, the bolt penetrates the animal's skull and brain, causing instant death (fig. 10.2). It is safer than a live firearm because there is no chance of over-penetration or ricochet.[142]

Intravenous potassium chloride is only used when the horse is anesthetized. For instance, during colic surgery, when evaluation of the abdominal organs determines that the horse's prognosis is grave. This is not an appropriate choice for an awake or conscious animal because it causes muscle contractions.

"Special circumstances" leaves an open area for a veterinarian to use her best judgment in the case of an emergency or traumatic situation. The veterinarian should keep the safety of handlers and the suffering of the horse in mind during these extenuating circumstances.

Some states license euthanasia technicians. These individuals are trained in the use of drugs and procedures relating specifically to humane euthanasia. They must meet legal requirements and adhere to guidelines mandated by the state. State laws may also allow animal shelter employees to euthanize unwanted animals. Finally, some states explicitly allow a law enforcement officer to use his or her gun for euthanasia of large animals in the case of emergency. State laws are variable, and it behooves you as a rescuer to know the laws in your state and ensure that they are followed.

Most Common Procedure

In practicality, barbiturate injection is the most widely used technique by veterinarians in the United States. Barbiturates are drugs that are used for general anesthesia. They cause depression of the central nervous system. In the case of euthanasia, a high overdose of an ultra-fast-acting barbiturate causes the body to shut down—the animal ceases breathing and the heart stops beating.

Many veterinarians will sedate the horse first, so that he is quite drowsy (but still standing) when the barbiturate is injected. Some veterinarians will also place a catheter in the horse's jugular vein for better assurance of accurate injection. A few veterinarians will anesthetize the horse prior to injecting the lethal dose.

Sloped ground or slippery footing can affect safety. The horse will usually fall downhill. Because of the variability of the situation and the safety factors, euthanasia procedure should be discussed with everyone present. The horse is a very large animal, and no one can completely control how he will move or react. The number one priority is human safety. Your veterinarian may want to go over safety precautions with you prior to proceeding.

With a handler still holding the horse's halter and lead rope, the barbiturate overdose is injected. Because of his high flight and prey drive, a horse will remain standing as long as he has any consciousness. Response to the barbiturate injection is variable. Movements the horse makes are unpredictable. His fall may be fast, slow, sudden, smooth, traumatic, or anything in between. Younger horses who are not systemically ill tend to have more movement. Horses that are flighty or have a lot of adrenaline due to an injury tend to exhibit more movement. If you are present when a horse is euthanized and you think the horse is coming toward you, move your feet and get out of the way!

After the horse goes down, he may still move or twitch unpredictably. It is unsafe to be near his feet, but it is fine to be by his withers, back, or the top of his head or neck. Know that he is unconscious *before* he goes down, and he is not aware of your presence at this time.

Confirming Death

We know that a horse has finally passed away when regular breathing stops. Your veterinarian will listen for a heartbeat, which should be gone. She may also check the *corneal eye reflex,* an indicator of central brain function. After all three of these indicators confirm the horse's death, the peripheral body reflexes of the diaphragm may cause several sudden and hard muscular contractions. This is the body's final reflexive effort to retain life, even though the horse is brain-dead and the heart is stopped. It doesn't always happen, but when it does, you may have to endure watching five or six of these contractions, which, in medicine, are termed *agonal breaths.* Because of the location of certain large nerves, the muscle contractions can also cause the head and neck to move. The agonal breaths seem traumatizing, but they usually occur after the corneal reflex has ceased, so there is no indication of consciousness.

Aftercare

You may want a keepsake to remember your horse. Along with framed photos,

Saying Goodbye to Buddy

The whole family was present to say goodbye to Buddy. He was a well-loved, special, geriatric gelding that had taught both daughters how to ride. The family prepared a grave so that he could be buried on their property. As is typical, we walked him near to the grave, and I sedated and then euthanized him.

Usually, when a grave has been prepared, a veterinarian will euthanize the horse nearby and then his remains can be moved over and into it. But Buddy fell over backward with his legs straight up in the air and his back deep in the grave. The wife and I both looked at each other in surprise! Then I noticed that her husband was trying to get in the hole to retrieve the halter and lead rope! I had to physically stop him. In his sadness, he wasn't thinking of his own safety, and he was willing to dangerously get in a deep hole with a 1,000-pound animal that was still reflexively twitching his legs.

many people keep portions of their horse's mane or tail, and it can be made into a bracelet or other jewelry. Others keep a shoe or a hoof-print impression in clay. A useful website, hoofbeats-in-heaven.com, is dedicated to horse loss support.

Aftercare of the horse's body is a challenge since horses are so large.[143] Burial on your own private land may be an option. Jurisdictions across the country have a variety of requirements for this, and some outlaw burial altogether. Private pet cremation services may be able to transport the body for cremation. In some areas, either government or private rural individuals will have a pasture burial option. In many states, a state-supported laboratory system will inspect the horse's body to determine the cause of death and subsequently dispose of his remains. This investigation is a *necropsy*, which is also known as a *post-mortem examination*. After necropsy, the horse's body is often cremated.

State laboratories are often associated with a university or a veterinary teaching hospital. Many states encourage and partially financially support a necropsy to determine the cause of death. For example, Kentucky has one of the most well-developed state laboratory systems for dealing with deceased horses. This is because the horse industry is such an important part of the state's financial health, and a disease outbreak could result in economic turmoil. Using necropsies as a surveillance tool prevents this occurrence.

Cost

The cost of euthanasia (the procedure and the farm call fee) is one reason why some horses continue to suffer in unsanitary and illegal conditions. If you wish to bury your horse at home, a backhoe will have to be hired. If a landfill accepts the body, there is a fee, and if somebody has to move the body for you, you will have to pay for that, too (an amount that will depend on the distance). Cremation is the most expensive option. Note that not all crematoriums are able to accommodate an entire horse.

TAKE HOME MESSAGE

The idea of rescuing or helping horses is to save them from a horrible and untimely death elsewhere. Some horses have diseases or problems that are life-threatening. Many geriatric horses have problems that are manageable for a very long time, but they will eventually need to be put down because of long-term suffering. You as a rescuer need to be prepared to make the difficult decision for a humane and peaceful death in the case of an emergency, for an incurable problem, or for an older horse.

PART II

Training Horses in Need

CHAPTER 11

Understanding Unique Training Considerations

In Part One, I covered a lot of medical information. The remainder of this book is devoted to training your rescue horse. Training guidelines take into consideration the unique medical needs as well as the mental needs specific to horses that have been neglected or abused.

Chapter 12 (p. 155) is critical for any horse person to read as it discusses equine sensory physiology and behavior. Further chapters cover training, from a foundation of trust, to haltering unhandled adult horses, training for medical care, and on to groundwork and riding. Not every training chapter will apply to every horse, nor will this book be able to cover all training topics in-depth. However, each gives you a foundation to target your horse's particular needs, while keeping in mind health conditions from which neglected or abused horses suffer.

When working with your horse, remember that a well-behaved horse is more likely to retain a good home. Outside of addressing his medical needs, training him is the most important action you can take to ensure he has a good home long-term. Even if you plan on keeping him forever, unforeseen circumstances can arise.

If you reach a point where you feel as though you are in over your head, or are not making progress in your training, seek help. It's a matter of good horsemanship as well as safety.

TRAINING APPROPRIATE BY BODY CONDITION SCORING (BCS)

It is important to consider your horse's Body Condition Score (BCS) before beginning any training with him. I've outlined important factors here; refer back to page 28 for BCS details.

BCS 1 to 2

Focus on providing medical care, water, and feed. Work on petting, brushing, and haltering. Make sure you can touch the horse's legs all over. He may not be able to balance if you pick up a foot. As he gains weight and strength, cautiously and gently teach him to pick up his feet, but don't hold them up for more than one or two seconds. No exercise or unnecessary movement. After refeeding, leaving the quarantine enclosure for a five- to ten-minute session of hand-grazing is a good way to spend time together.

BCS 3

Begin in-hand groundwork, staying low-key and slow during this time. No cantering, but you may begin one- to two-minute increments of trotting. Your goal during this time period is to help the horse build muscle while he is still gaining weight. Walking up hills and then coming down in a widely-arced "S" shape increases fitness. Walking the horse through arena work that includes ground poles, barrels, cones, or other obstacles requiring him to bend his body or pick up his feet is appropriate. This is a good time to practice walking in and out of enclosures or barns, trailers, and stocks (chutes or small metal stalls meant to contain horses and restrict their movement to facilitate examination or procedures—fig. 11.1 and see Entering and Being Restrained in Stocks, p. 202). Try to not stress the horse out, and don't work so hard that he breaks a sweat or burns excessive calories. Keep everything calm and quiet.

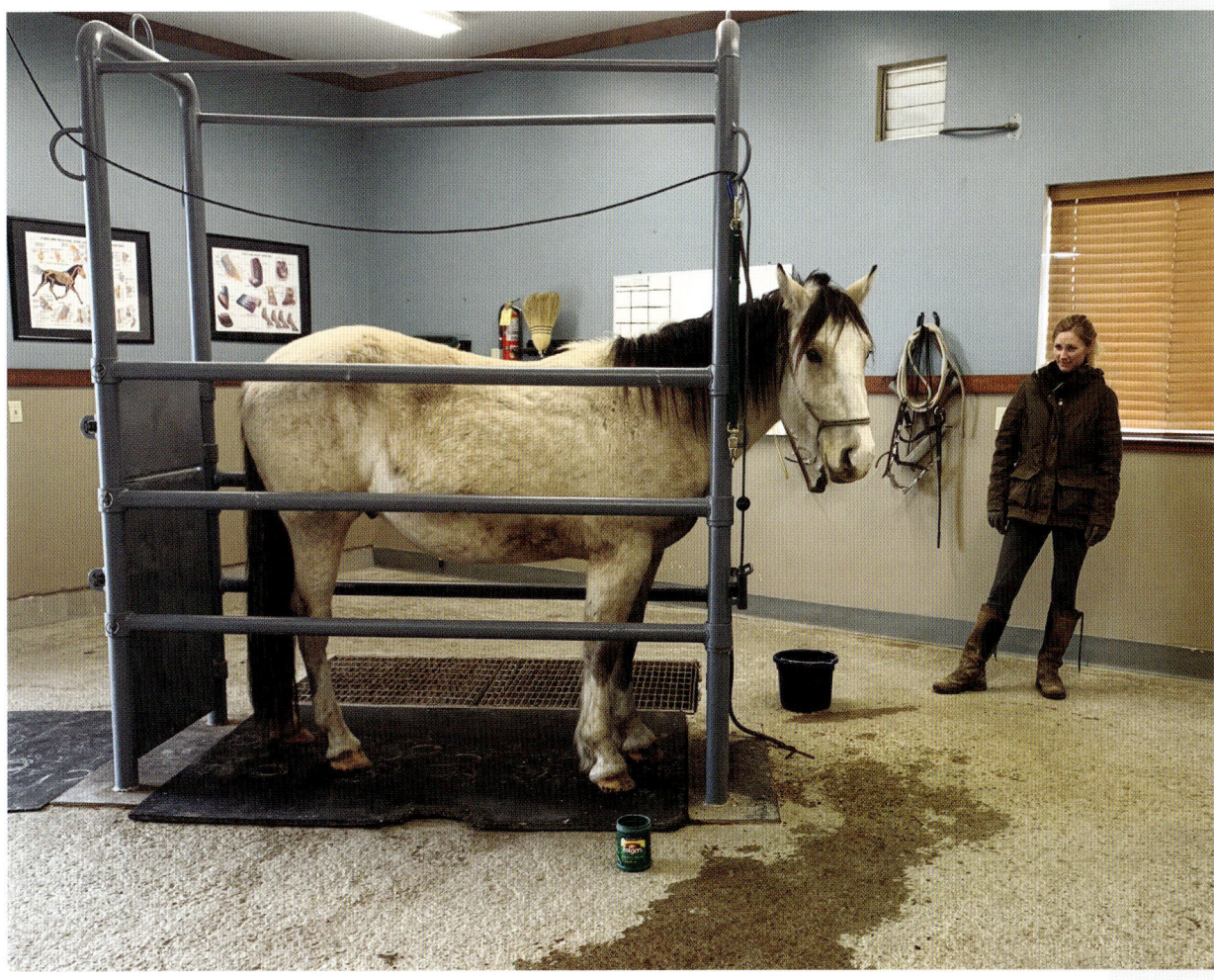

11.1 Stephanie has trained her horse to walk quietly and confidently into stocks. The buckets in this photo contained treats, which she correctly used for positive reinforcement during the training process.

BCS 4

Your horse should now be healthy enough to exercise more vigorously. Gradually work up to 10 or 15 minutes of in-hand trotting, and then start adding a few canter strides into your groundwork. Watch closely for any signs of pain or lameness. Get him to build more muscle. Work for correct, immediate responses, rather than the sluggish movements typical of a weak horse. Asking the horse to move around you in circles on a longe line (as in natural horsemanship or longeing) builds his strength and communication skills. You may tack him up and practice ground-driving as you prepare him for riding. Prepare him physically and mentally for a veterinary examination.

BCS 5 to 6

Your horse should be reevaluated for soundness by your veterinarian before riding him. If he has low-grade pain or subtle lameness, your training will be slow, and it isn't fair to him to ask him to work while in pain. Lameness is one of the most common problems in rescued horses. If he isn't sound, work with your veterinarian to formulate a plan. If he is deemed sound, riding can commence.

BCS 7 to 9

Have these horses been killed with kindness? Overweight rescue horses exist. For example, a client brought me three Miniature Horses to evaluate—all of which had a BCS of 9! Their former owner had passed away, and in the interim period, the minis were free-feeding off a round bale. Being too heavy carries significant health risks. Overweight horses are prone to painful arthritis due to overloading their joints, causing stress and inflammation. Laminitis or founder as a sequela of metabolic aberrations is a serious risk.

While these fat horses need exercise, you still should stick with an organized training plan. It is safer for you because you want to ensure that there aren't holes in his training. Incremental training will also protect the horse from injury. Start slow—rigorous in-hand walking for five minutes each day may be an increase for an unfit horse.

CHAPTER 12

How Horses Sense and Respond:
Sensory Physiology, Training Concepts, and Thought Processes (Fear)

This chapter introduces sensory physiology of horses, behavioral science, and training techniques. I have already alluded to ways horses respond in medical care and rescue situations. Now, I will discuss in more detail the reasons why horses behave in certain ways.

The most important training tip for you to take from this chapter is to stop, wait, and read your horse before reacting. Figure out your horse's thought process—it is key for developing trust in your relationship with him and progressing through training.

Although you train your horse every time you interact with him, you want to wait until health issues have been resolved before proceeding with structured or intensive training.

SENSORY PHYSIOLOGY

Equine Vision

Most of what science has elucidated about horses' perception of their environment has to do with vision. This is because humans rely heavily on vision and because vision is a testable sense. We can design experiments to help us understand what and how horses see.

When training a horse, it's important to understand that what he is seeing is different from what you are seeing. There are several features of your horse's eye that make his perception of the world dramatically different than that of predatory species like humans or dogs.

Field of View: A horse's eyes are set wide on his head, far in front of his body. He has a wide-angle view of the world—almost 360 degrees. He sees nearly the entire horizon without turning his head, but the majority of the world is seen with only one eye at a time (*monocular* vision). There is a small blind spot right behind him, which is why if you must approach a horse from behind, it is a good idea to talk to him so that he knows you are there (fig. 12.1).[144]

A horse cannot perceive distance within his monocular vision range. A lack of *depth perception* can be described as the world being a large painting with objects sliding around on it. In this type of vision, relative distance is impossible to know. One way for you to understand his vision is to cover one of your eyes for five or ten minutes and walk around. It's difficult to tell how objects are

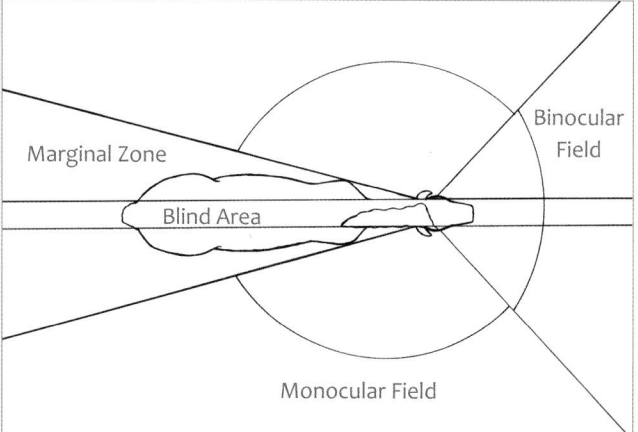

12.1 *The horse's field of view.*

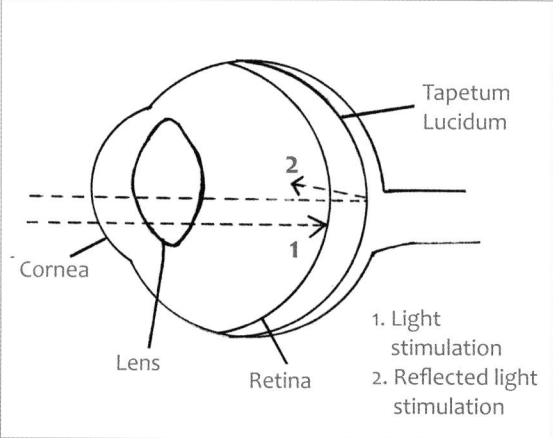

12.2 *The horse's eye, including the reflective* tapetum lucidum, *which allows light to stimulate the retina twice.*

spaced without the information from stereo (*binocular*) vision using both eyes.

Binocular vision and depth perception for horses is restricted to a small slice in front where the fields from each eye overlap.[145] Your horse's ability to bring an object into sharp focus is limited to close objects. This is why he lowers his head to inspect a nearby novel item. Conversely, he may raise his head to see something far away.

Color Perception: Based on the types of cells in the back of the eye, we know horses can see a narrow range of color that includes greens and blues, but not reds. The horse's view of the world is muted compared to the bright rainbow we perceive.

Light Perception: The horse's eye is the largest of any land mammal—even larger than an elephant's. It takes his eyes about seven times as long as our human eyes for his pupils to widen and constrict to adjust for changes in light, such as walking from the bright sunlight into a dark barn.

Slow adjustment is one reason why many horses hesitate when entering a dark area—a time when horses and people commonly miscommunicate. The horse may hesitate because he is momentarily blind. A handler might give the lead rope a tug, expecting the horse to follow him right into, as far as the horse can tell, the abyss. If you give him a few seconds for his eyes to adjust before pulling on the lead rope, he will then go forward more willingly. When light and footing change, your horse may need to put his head down to inspect it before moving forward.

When light enters the eye, it stimulates the cells of the retina in the back of the eye. The stimulated retinal cells send an electric signal up nerve cells to the brain. The horse's eye has a reflective surface beneath the light-sensing cells of the retina, called the *tapetum lucidum*. After the light passes through the retina, it hits the *tapetum* and is reflected back, stimulating the retinal cells a second time (fig. 12.2). Once the pupil has adjusted to the darkness, horses can see quite well in low light. The *tapetum* is the reason dogs, cats, and horses have superior

Blind Trust

Acuity of other senses helps horses compensate for vision deficits. I once did a pre-purchase examination on a cute, quiet, and compliant large pony named Merlin. A pre-purchase examination is a screening tool to help people interested in buying a horse make an informed decision—a veterinarian evaluates the whole horse for any problems. I was evaluating Merlin on behalf of a purchaser who lived far away.

Merlin was quietly standing tied when I arrived. He turned toward me when I approached and briefly touched his nose to my arm when I untied him. The first thing I noted was scarring of the cornea, iris, and some other major eye abnormalities. Right away, I tested this pony's vision. He had no menace response when I poked my finger toward his eye to see if he would blink. He didn't blink. He couldn't see my finger. I shined a light in each of his eyes, testing each of his pupil's response to light. His pupils did not constrict at all in response to the bright light.

We were in a large indoor arena. There were doors at the north and south ends, letting the sound of an occasional passing car through. There was another horse, with a rider, working in the northeast corner. We could hear that horse's footsteps and breath.

I set up a raised pole about 4 inches off the ground. I led Merlin over it, and he stumbled. I proceeded to do a number of figure eights and approached the pole from each direction, from a variety of distances and angles, both at the walk and the trot. He did not stumble over it a second time. I moved the pole. He lifted his feet up at the previous location of the pole. Then, he stumbled over it the first time at its new location. He didn't know where it was when I moved it. But then, presumably based on the sounds of the arena and his inner spatial orientation, he didn't stumble a second time. I turned him in a dozen tight circles, making both of us dizzy and trying to disorient him. Still, he knew exactly where that pole was. I repeated this exercise and with each repetition, he stumbled over the pole just once after I moved it.

I was impressed by Merlin's ability to compensate for his vision deficit and with his trust in humans. He never hesitated to be led by his halter and lead rope.

I called the purchaser, and explained what I was seeing. I wanted to know what she would be using him for. Would Merlin be used as an indoor riding pony? He might work well for that purpose—he was kind and gentle and he was orthopedically sound. He could navigate a limited world easily. No, she wanted him for a driving pony and expected him to go outside on trails in unknown areas. We felt that his blindness would render him unsuitable for her purpose.

Later that afternoon, I received an angry telephone call from the seller. He was horrified because I had told the purchaser that Merlin was blind—the seller flat-out did not believe me. We discussed my examination findings at length. He told me all about how Merlin loaded in trailers, was ridden, and interacted with his other horses. The seller did not believe or understand that the pony could be blind and maintain such an apparently normal life. How is it possible that a horse can assimilate so much spatial information with a complete lack of vision? Awareness of what and how your horse sees—and how acute his other senses are—is critical for successful training.

White-Associated Deafness

Animals with extra white patterns of their hair or fur may have congenital deafness (they are born without the ability to hear). Behind the eardrum, mammalian ears contain fluid, small stones, and specialized nerve cells with hair-like projections. When sound vibrates the eardrum, it causes the stones to move within the fluid, stimulating the nervous system's hair cells, and relaying the information to the brain.

Melanocytes (cells that contain and produce pigment) are necessary for inner-ear hair cells to survive. If an animal has a defect in melanocytes, it will not produce pigment, and will have lots of white, which can adversely affect the inner ear hair cells. Splash overo horses may be apron- or blaze-faced and have high white socks, with white sometimes extending to the horse's body or belly (fig. 12.3). One particular splash overo line has produced successful reining horses. Even though many have hearing, some horses with these markings are deaf, even when both of their parents had full hearing.

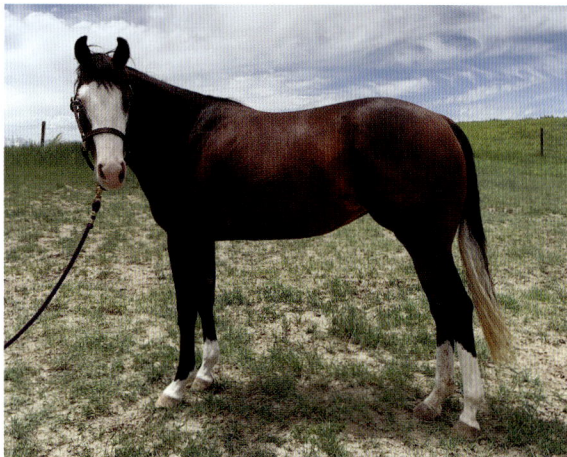

12.3 *A splash overo horse, with the characteristic blue eye, blaze face, and high white socks. At least five genes have been identified that result in this color pattern, and two can result in deafness.*

night vision compared to humans. Their eyes maximize use of minimal light.

A wide, horizontal pupil gives the horse a panoramic scene with only a small blind spot. But the scene is blurred, muted, and he cannot tell how near or far an object is until it is close in front of him. A horse easily senses motion, alerting him to possible predators even in low light. Your horse isn't sure what an object is until it is right up close. He has instincts born over millennia of being hunted, so his response to an unknown moving object tends to be to run first, and figure out what it is later.

Other Senses

Humans rely strongly on vision to help us understand the world we live in. Horses, on the other hand, use vision in balance with other senses. Hearing and smell play a role in how a horse responds to stimuli. Unfortunately, we don't know much about how the horse hears or smells. Information on tactile or touch sensation and taste is almost nonexistent.

Hearing: Horses can hear a wide range of pitches and tones. In fact, their hearing is almost as good as a dog's. High-pitched sounds are used by predators as a communication signal. Think of a pack of coyotes yipping and calling to each other compared to the low, soft nicker a mare will use for communicating with her nearby foal. For this reason, talking to horses in a low, calm tone is helpful and soothing, whereas high-pitched, sudden noises can unnerve them. Horses have 10 ear muscles (compared to humans' paltry three) that move each of their ears 180 degrees.[146, 147] Where their ears are pointing tells you what they are focused on. Ear movement also is how a horse can narrow down the location of a sound.

Sense of Smell: The horse's nose is large, with a vastly increased surface area compared to our tiny, insensitive "schnozzes." This surface area contains many odor-sensitive receptors. Horses can perceive odors from other animals, smoke, humans, and medications almost as well as dogs.[148]

Understanding His Senses

You can now understand why your horse behaves the way he does in certain training situations. Being aware will allow you to work with your horse more effectively.

A good example is figuring out how changes in weather influence your training session. Horses are nervous on a windy day, which creates training problems. Think about it: His sense of smell is distorted, the wind obscures noises, and everything is moving, so detection of a predator is difficult. No wonder your horse is fearful in the wind.

TRAINING PRINCIPLES

The behavior-shaping strategies discussed on the pages that follow are critical for training, but still do not explain the "magic" of horsemanship, nor fully acknowledge the special relationships that we see between horses and humans. Horses look out for us in more ways than we can imagine. Accidents and horses are always going to be part of the equestrian equation, but they seem to happen far less often than they would if the horses weren't looking out for us. There are lots of successful horse trainers, and they use a variety of techniques. Consistency, kindness, and lots of repetition are key for meeting any training goal. For their part, horses are usually kind, forgiving, and intelligent. They try hard to satisfy our requests and expectations.

Positive Reinforcement

Current behavioral science asserts that *positive reinforcement* is the most effective way to train a horse. Positive reinforcement rewards behavior; it encourages a response. For example, you ask the horse to go in his stall, and when he enters he finds his feeder has a scoop of grain in it. Rewards can also be in the form of your voice ("Good Boy!"), a treat, or petting and scratching him.

Conversely, early behavioral science in horses asserted that the basis for training horses should be negative reinforcement. These behavioral experiments demonstrated that horses did not respond to positive reinforcement. Newer research studies have proved that mantra to be false. Horse training is steeped in tradition, and some of the traditional methods disregard positive reinforcement, instead relying on either negative reinforcement or punishment.

Older behavioral science missed the mark because our relationship with horses has changed over the last few decades. At one time, horses were almost all working animals, but now they are primarily companions. How we interact with, and our expectations of, horses have changed. It's difficult to feed a horse treats while riding, so when behavior studies focused on a horse's performance under saddle, the conclusion was drawn that the best reward for a horse is to leave him alone.

Intrinsic Reward and Bribery

There are two extensions of positive reinforcement: *intrinsic reward* and *bribes*.

Clicker and Positive Reinforcement Training

Clicker training relies on positive reinforcement.[149] Positive reinforcers come in two varieties: primary and secondary. Primary reinforcers are those that are necessary for survival or innate to the animal: food, water, or pleasure. Secondary reinforcers are used to indicate to the animal that the primary reinforcer is on the way.

For example, in Pavlov's famous experiment,[150] a bell was rung and dogs were then fed. The food was the primary reinforcer. The dogs learned that the bell was associated with food. Soon, they drooled and salivated for the bell alone, even when no food was present. The bell became a secondary reinforcer.

In clicker training, the clicker is a secondary reinforcer to which an animal is conditioned. The noise the clicker makes is specific, unique, and clear. It also allows the trainer to be precise with timing. Almost all zoo animals in the United States are now trained with clicker or other secondary reinforcement training to stand for hoof trims, blood draws, or other veterinary care. Other secondary reinforcers can be a whistle or your voice, as examples.

We may inadvertently create secondary reinforcers. For example, when I feed my horses, they know the sound of the feed room door and that food is following shortly.

Intrinsic reward can occur for any behavior—whether desired or not. An example of intrinsic reward is when a horse breaks into the feed room and finds the grain bin. Now that he has learned how to open the feed room door to eat, he will seek to do so again and again, trying to get back in for a yummy feast.

Bribes are when food or other primary reinforcement rewards are given before desired behavior has occurred. A common example is using a bucket of grain to lead a horse into a trailer. Bribes can sometimes be useful to get the job done. For example, a handler can feed the horse carrots to distract him during injections. While bribes can help the horse to have a positive rather than a negative experience, they don't work for long-term training. Recognize when a bribe has been used, and work on training the horse for the desired behavior. In order to be useful for long-term training, the bribe must be transitioned to post-behavior positive reinforcement.

Traditionally, horse people are taught that horses become mouthy and demanding when they expect treats. If administered appropriately, this is a low risk for most horses. When offering a treat, if the horse is seeking too strongly for your comfort, close your fist around the treat and bump him on the nose. When he stands quietly, the treat can be offered. He should take the treat respectfully. You are shaping his expectations: He does well, he gets a treat. He does well, but becomes pushy or disrespectful, he loses his treat opportunity.

Some trainers assert that no horse should ever be fed a treat, reasoning that thus, no owner will ever allow a horse to get pushy. I have a little more faith in you than that. Positive reinforcement is a useful strategy for training. You be the judge of what your horse and you can handle. Remember that there are other methods to reward your horse such as petting or scratching, and using your voice positively.

Negative Reinforcement

Negative reinforcement is when a cue is given, the horse has a response, and the cue is then removed. It is also referred to as *reinforcement withdrawal*. Negative reinforcement is *not* the same as punishment. This can be confusing. You are taking away an uncomfortable cue or reinforcer.

An illustrative example is pushing your horse's hip over. You push, and the horse moves over. Therefore, you stop the cue. This can be a push with your leg while riding or a push with your palm while on the ground. The concept is the same.

Approach-and-Retreat

To appreciate the effectiveness of *approach-and-retreat* techniques, it is important to understand foot movement. To the horse, moving his feet—even if it is just a few inches—away from an object or person that he is uncomfortable with is successful in avoiding noxious contact.

The approach-and-retreat technique is used to desensitize a horse to objects. You want to push your horse slightly outside his comfort zone. Using this method, he should keep his feet still. You want to get close enough for him to pay attention then step back away or retreat. For example, for a horse who you are training to accept brushing, you may start by stepping into his pen, holding the brush. After he accepts this, he may demonstrate curiosity and investigate the brush. You can touch him on his withers while holding the brush in your other hand, and then retreat. You can then touch his withers first with your hand, then with the brush, and then retreat. Finally, you may begin in soft, slow strokes to brush him, stopping as he is tense, but before he moves his feet to escape. In this way, you can work up to brushing his entire body.

Approach-and-retreat in conjunction with positive reinforcement uses a horse's innate prey drive as well as his food drive. When properly applied together, they yield rapid training results with solid mastery.

Punishment

Punishment is administration of a painful or unpleasant stimulus after a horse has

> ### Click It or Ticket
>
> To illustrate the difference between negative reinforcement and punishment, my friend Jess helped me with an example.
>
> Jess is supposed to buckle up every time she drives her car. But sometimes she is in a hurry or has her hands full, and she forgets. When she gets in her car and starts driving, the car makes an annoying dinging sound. When she buckles up, it stops. This is an example of negative reinforcement. The mildly uncomfortable signal is removed when she does what she is supposed to.
>
> If Jess is busy, and perhaps also talking on the phone, she may ignore the dinging sound. When she drives past a police car, she is pulled over and gets a ticket for blatant disobedience of the "Buckle-Up" law. This ticket is punishment. It is unpleasant, and it occurs after undesired behavior.

demonstrated an unwanted behavior. Punishment is intended to discourage or eliminate an unwanted behavior. When used in an immediate way and without anger, punishment is not necessarily abuse. If it stops the unwanted behavior, it is considered a successful tool.

Behavioral science advocates punishment as a last resort, but we should acknowledge that horses use it with each other. When a lower-ranked gelding invades the lead mare's space, she will pin her ears to ask the lower-ranked horse to move. If that horse does not move away, she will then punish him with a bite or kick. Once he moves away, they will go back to living in peaceful harmony.

To have any effect, the key is that the punishment is meted out instantly and according to the level of infraction. Most people innately understand this with respect to horses as it wouldn't make sense for that lead mare to seek out that encroaching gelding later in the afternoon and bite or kick him for no apparent reason. Sometimes we forget, however, because we have memory and societal communication techniques that separate punishment from the infraction. For example, you may restrict your child's curfew if he arrives home late. Each night of restricted curfew, he remembers why. Your horse doesn't have the same communication skills to understand delayed punishment.

Many behavioral scientists and animal trainers advocate never punishing an animal. In some situations (zoos, for example, where there is a physical barrier between the trainer and the animal), this tactic works well. In order for this to work with horses, a trainer has to be exceptionally in tune to the horse's language in order to predict behaviors early enough to head them off, rather than reacting to them afterward. People enjoy horses' power and strength; conversely, their size and strength can hurt a human if misdirected. An example where punishment may be necessary is a horse who bites his handler. The handler may need to react with a swift, brief, physical retaliation.

There can be long-term negative consequences to punishment, such as the horse becoming fearful and head shy if he is hit on the head repeatedly. Each horse is an individual and what one horse needs or tolerates will not be the same as another. Under no circumstances should a horse be allowed to bite a handler, but there are many ways to strategically prevent and diminish biting behavior, of which punishment is an option.

Abuse: Discussion of negative training tools would be incomplete without a discussion of *abuse*. Abuse is overusing punishment or negative reinforcement to the point of injury. The injury may be intended or accidental. A spur rowel used to the point of bleeding is abuse, whereas properly applied it is a tool for precise communication. A whip may function as an extension of our arm for clarifying cues to the horse, but it can also be used excessively and without cause, causing a horse to be fearful. Abuse may be physical or mental, although mental abuse to horses is poorly documented.

THE FEARFUL HORSE AND RESCUE TRAINING

When it comes down to it, training a rescue horse is no different than training any horse: He thinks and acts like a horse. However, because of his history, some responses may

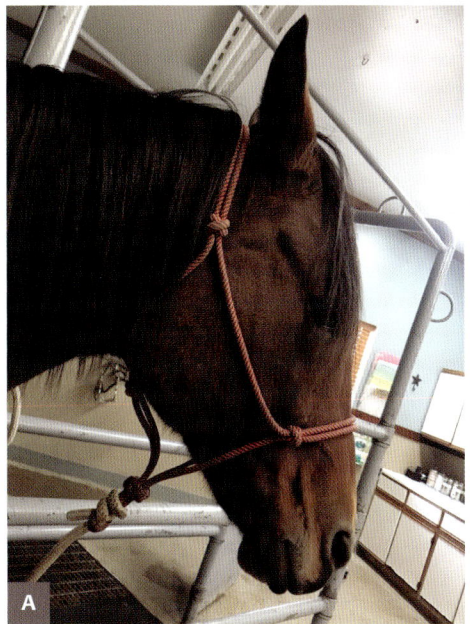 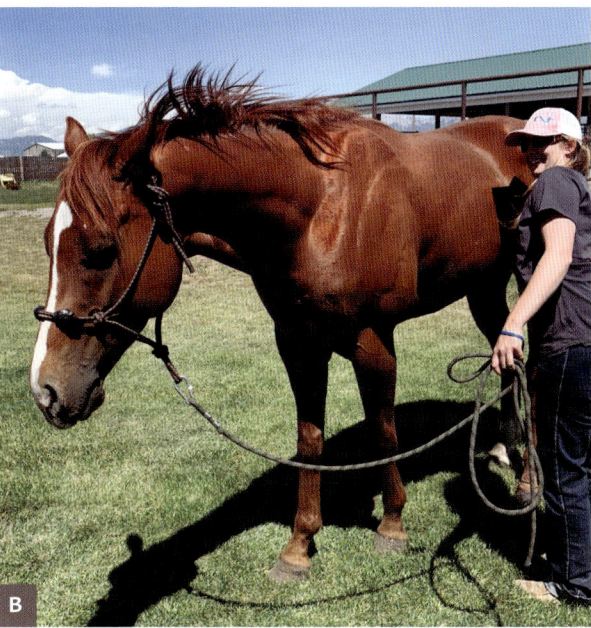

12.4 A & B A tense horse, with wrinkles around his lips, tight eye muscles, and ears held slightly back (A). A relaxed horse, with a drooping lip and relaxed eyes and ears (B). He is enjoying a good belly scratch.

be different. Neglected or abused horses may have been unintentionally taught inappropriate behavior. He may have a deep, ingrained fear or distrust of humans. Because of starvation, he may not have the muscle or brain capacity that he once did.[151] Finally, horses that have never experienced human touch are challenging to work with (figs. 12.4 A & B).

The initial goal of training is to get your horse to accept haltering, leading, physical touch on his body and legs, and hoof care. Without these critical skills, administering medical treatment is impossible. Training is critical for a horse's future. Horses should eventually be trained to accept injections, load into a trailer, enter and stand quietly in stocks, and be willing to go in and out of barns and stalls.

An untrained horse is typically fairly straightforward to teach, as he is a clean slate. A rescue horse who has had a bad experience can be difficult to retrain and have trouble overcoming previous trauma. The memory of the bad experience can stay with him for a lifetime. An untrained horse may need 20 to 30 repetitions to master a task, but a horse who is being *retrained* may require 200 to 300 repetitions to confidently and willingly master the same task. One additional consideration for the amount of repetition necessary: It should be proportional to the severity of the incorrect response as well as the necessity of the knowledge for the horse's well-being.

A horse who only trusts one person is at risk. If an emergency occurs and evacuation or medical care is necessary, it is important that he is adaptable and accepts handling by other humans. It is good to establish trust

Signs of Apprehension or Fear

- Increase in heart and respiratory rate
- Dilated pupils
- Whites of eyes showing
- Head up
- Tense muscles, including those of the head, neck, lips, and eyelids
- Ears erect and tight or pinned flat as a warning
- Snorting
- High-stepping on new footing
- Tail-swishing
- Defecation
- Moving feet

and a relationship with your horse, but it is necessary to establish to the horse that other people can also be trusted and should be respected.

The Fear Response

Wild Mustangs are the most fearful horses. Even non-wild horses that have not been handled will be fearful. An abused horse may have fear to specific stimuli. Fear is not logical. He may be terrified of the bottle of fly spray and at the same time have no problems with getting a bath from a spray nozzle on a hose. Although all horses exhibit fear responses from time to time due to their nature as prey animals, your rescue horse may be more fearful than average. A rescue horse may come with an undesirable learned set of behaviors or an unmoderated and exceptionally strong fear response.

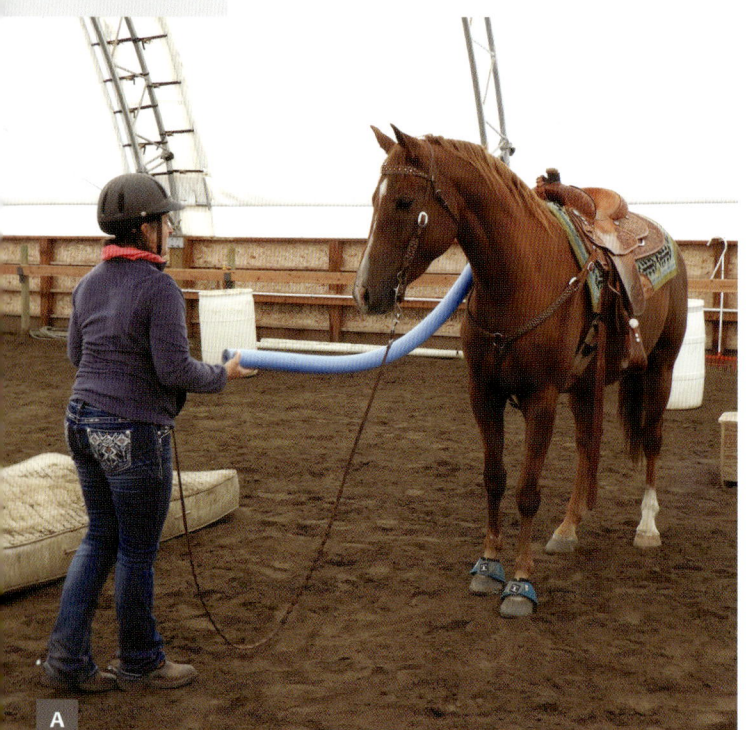
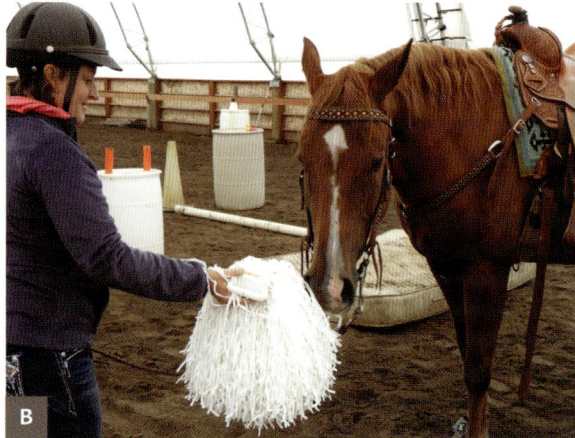

12.5 A & B In photo A, I approach "Spicy" with a novel object. Although he hasn't moved his feet, his head is high, his neck muscles are tense, his ears are erect, and his body is leaning away from the object. In photo B, Spicy is allowed to approach this new object on his own. He is reaching down to initiate contact, and his neck is more relaxed. His ears are held relaxed and to the side. He is sniffing the object as well as using his lips to investigate it.

Recognizing Fear—What Your Horse Is Telling You

If you think of horses as extra large rabbits, it may help you understand the nature of the fears and responses a prey animal has. Rabbits and horses have a lot in common: They eat grass, hay, and carrots, and digest them in a similar way. Both horses and rabbits are always worried that a carnivore is going to eat them. When a horse is fearful, what you are going to generally observe is that he will move his feet, or run away from whatever is scaring him—just as a rabbit naturally runs when afraid (figs. 12.5 A & B).[152]

It is important to be able to tell when your horse is frightened. An agitated and anxious large animal can panic, causing an accident and injury both to himself and his handler. His head will be up, and the muscles of his neck and body will be rigid and taut. If a trusting horse goes forward, but is nervous about an object he is passing by, he may look at it carefully, bend his body away from it, and make a characteristic snort. When he is unsure of footing, he may step uncharacteristically high.

A fearful horse has erect ears, which are pointed to the object or person causing him distress. Beware! Ears pinned flat against his head means that he is giving you a threat that he is ready to defend himself. Tail swishing is also a sign of discomfort or anxiety that is used as a warning signal preceding a kick. His eyelids will be tense and his eyes wide open, with dilated pupils. The whites may show. Observe your horse when he is not fearful, and look at how much white shows. (Appaloosas, for example, have more white visible than other breeds.) Watch for a difference in your horse's eyes when he is afraid (figs. 12.6 A & B).

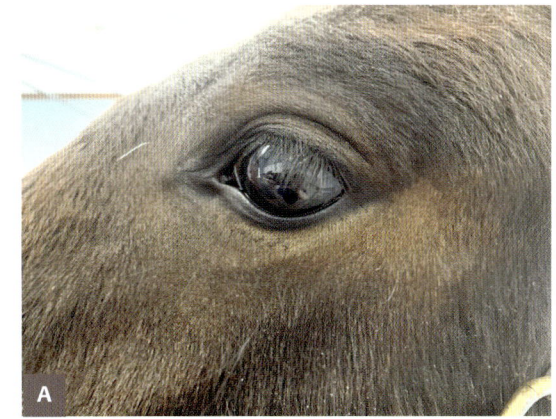

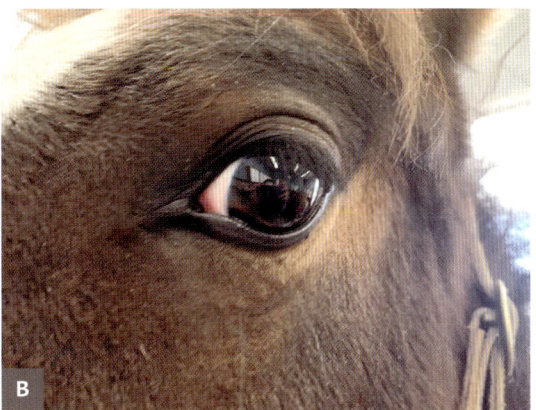

12.6 A & B The horse's eyes will look different when he is calm and comfortable (A) and when he is fearful (B).

The flight response begins in the brain and adrenal glands. The horse's main defense is to run. Before he runs, however, he sometimes lightens his load by defecating. If he does this while thinking about or completing a new task, it is important that you recognize this indication of stress. Then, as the anxiety takes hold, he will move his feet. If tied, he may move from side to side, or he may sit back and fight the pressure from the lead rope and halter. This can result in broken tack or injury. In a small stall or pen, he may face a corner, showing you his defensive, kicking posterior. In a larger paddock, he may walk or even run away.

A single event that scares or hurts a

horse can make a memory response that lasts for his lifetime. For example, a horse who is loaded into the trailer and slips and falls during the process may become fearful of loading. This memory response is especially strong if the incident is the first time he experiences the event. In our example of trailer loading, a horse who has never been loaded before is going to be more fearful and resistant to loading the next time when compared to one that loaded 100 times before slipping and falling.

The spook or startle response is innate in the horse's psyche due to the self-preservation prey response. Predators approach their prey from behind, so your horse is naturally more scared of things that are behind him, intensifying his spook response.

Physiology of Fear

Think about how you feel when you are nervous or afraid: your adrenaline quickens your heart and breathing, you may have tunnel vision, and your mouth may feel dry at the same time you begin to sweat. The properties of adrenaline are the same for all mammals that have been studied. We know horses experience changes in heart and respiratory rates and pupil size.

When a horse becomes fearful, learning is more difficult. Horses are intelligent creatures with an excellent memory. Training takes multiple repetitions for the horse to become fully versed in the pressure → response → release pattern. Pushing your horse outside his comfort zone in a moderated way is critical for learning, but pushing him until he

Long Ears

Fearful donkeys and mules act differently than horses. Donkeys tend to be more solitary in nature. Because of this, donkeys may first hide and assess the situation, and run only when under extreme duress. If they are the only individual in range of a predator, they could reveal their presence by running, whereas a horse only has to outrun the other members of a herd.

The behavior of the mule is between that of the horse and the donkey. "Standing and waiting" before running is one reason why people absolutely love their mules—the mule is less likely to spook on a trail ride and run away with his rider than a horse. This does not mean a mule or donkey never spooks. When he does, his fear reaction is less obvious to you because his feet aren't moving. He may flinch in place or stop and take in his surroundings before going forward any more.

The "standing and waiting" behavior is also why mules and donkeys have a reputation of stubbornness. When they become fearful during training or when asked to complete a task, they may not move at all as they decide about a potential threat or stressor. This behavior is misunderstood as being stubborn.

When stressed, if the donkey or mule is further pushed, he will eventually respond and defend himself, sometimes violently. Lack of recognition of his standing behavior as a fear response is one reason why donkeys and mules have a reputation for being explosive.

explodes with a fear response is likely to result in the horse only learning to be afraid.

Ramping up the fear response in a horse is pretty easy to do, and if you teach your horse to stress out in novel situations, you are doing your horse a disservice and creating a danger for yourself. Think about ways to prevent fear from ramping up. The more consistent and fair you are, the easier it will be for your horse to believe you when you say, "Hey, trailers are no biggie; you can do this!"

Recognizing Relaxation— What Your Horse Is Telling You

Look at your horse often and ask yourself how he might be feeling. Observe his head: A relaxed horse's head is down and he may be exploring his environment. As he relaxes, he may lick his lips or make chewing motions.[153] This is a characteristic behavior that results from a change in central nervous system input. Many trainers look for this behavior because it indirectly indicates learning.

When a horse is thinking about going forward, he may sniff the footing or floor, paw at the ground, lick, mouth, or bump his nose on the enclosure, or otherwise explore the area or footing. People often misconstrue these signs as hesitation and reluctance. If he is engaging in these behaviors, your horse is unsure or mildly anxious, but he is trying. At this point, waiting is the most effective tool you have. When the horse is not allowed to process and think about his options, and we instead make a premature and strong demand that he get going, the defensive and fearful part of his brain can be switched on. Instead of taking five minutes for him to think about his options and go where we want, it can take an hour to get him pushed where we want.

A Violation of Trust

This is the story of a yearling filly with a unique problem who was hauled over 500 miles to see one of the specialty surgeons at the hospital where I worked. She was a trooper through her arrival at the new location with all of its loud noises and busy areas. Her behavior for treatments, general anesthesia for surgery, recovery, medications, and being in a new stall with other horses coming and going at all hours was stellar.

When she was being discharged from the hospital, her owners asked for sedation to load her into the trailer. I asked them if they had had trouble loading her at home to bring her to the hospital. These people were respected and successful trainers. They told me that "…she loaded real easy at home, stepped right in, but, well, you know, Doc, it is always more difficult the second time."

I was baffled by their lack of insight and inconsideration of the filly's perspective. They took a young horse who had never been off the farm or away from her herd, and asked her to get in a scary, dark, lonely box. When she did, they shut the door, started rolling, and rattled down the road for 12 hours. When she arrived at a new place, she did not have any of her known herd-mates, and then underwent general anesthesia and intense medical care with new handlers. The entire experience must have been terrifying. No wonder "the second time is difficult." These trainers completely violated her trust the first time they loaded her in the trailer. And, even though they are professionals who work with horses every day, they had not figured out a better way to help their horses learn to travel with less stress.

> **Signs of Relaxation and Comfort**
>
> - Steady, slow breathing
> - Head down
> - Relaxed muscles, including those of the head, neck, lips, ears, and eyelids
> - Sighing
> - Licking lips or making chewing motions
> - Eating
> - Willingness to approach people or objects

Changing Fear

Overcoming fear is not an overnight event, and some horses require way more breathing room than others. Be fair, be consistent, be predictable, and pay attention to what your horse is telling you. Great horse people can get horses to do amazing things using a variety of techniques, but mostly they are great at reading their horses.

A lot of the work around training horses is to wait for them to make up their mind to decide to do what you are asking of them. These are willing creatures. In my work, I see horse people of all skill levels, and I frequently observe people mistime, misunderstand, and miscue their charges. This is just while asking relatively simple tasks such as leading the horse from the parking lot into the veterinary hospital or barn, and walking into the stocks. I am frequently surprised that the discombobulated ask actually results in getting the horse to go where the person wants him to go.

HELPING OTHERS IMPROVE THEIR TRAINING SKILLS

Experience helps avoid errors, but gaining experience involves the accumulation of errors. Every horse person in existence has made a mistake with a horse. If a training technique is not working, be open to trying something else or trying a different way.

Rescue group volunteers and other horse people should be patient with each other. We are all there to help the horse, even beginners. Most people want to learn more about training and handling. Just like with horses, kindness will go a lot further in teaching the lesson than harsh criticism. Volunteers are valuable! They keep the rescue effort going, and we don't want to lose them due to interpersonal communication mishaps regarding training techniques, theories, and errors. There is room for everybody to learn, and the more people learn, the better off all our horses will be. Using kindness toward other horse people also leads to gentle handling and training techniques that are respectful of our horses.

MUTUAL UNDERSTANDING

Horses are prey animals. This affects how they absorb and respond to sensory information (sight, hearing, and smell). Training a horse takes patience and effort. Understanding what your horse is telling you is central to progressing in your training skills. Getting the horse to understand you through the use of basic training concepts such as positive reinforcement takes many repetitions. Kindly helping other people learn horsemanship skills helps ensure more horses learn through gentle techniques.

CHAPTER 13

Restoring Trust:
Developing a Relationship

READINESS REVIEW

Before beginning the tasks in this chapter, make sure you have completed tasks from previous chapters:

- Established ownership.
- Established quarantine.
- Had a veterinary examination and any ailments are improving or resolved.
- Understand basic equine physiology and behavior as applied to training.

SOCIAL INTEGRATION

It is normal for horses to have a period of social adjustment any time a new herd member arrives or leaves. The social order, sometimes called the *pecking order*, is not always top-down dominance, and may have nothing to do with size. For example, when my lead Quarter Horse mare passed away, I thought I would watch two older mares spar for the top rung. Curiously, one of them stepped back and allowed her low-ranking daughter to step up and run the show. I was surprised to watch my smallest mare boss the larger horses around. This is a perfect example that size is not always directly related to herd dominance, and that herd rank is not linear.

Generally, mares will be at the top of the herd rank. Older horses are also more likely to have a higher social standing, especially if they are long-established herd members. Young horses and passive geldings will have low social status. New members have the lowest status and are initially driven away with pinned ears, bites, and kicks.

For a new member, herd integration takes six to eight weeks. It is important to have a realistic expectation of time frame, because sometimes owners perceive that a horse hasn't settled in and begin seeking a new home for him. The least dominant horse of your current herd is the one most likely to chastise your new one the most severely and for the longest period. The new herd member may not end up on the bottom, but he has to earn his place over time. This is the natural course of horse socialization in a domestic environment, and the social dance can continue for a couple of months.

Allowing horses to meet vocally and visually before physical contact occurs can sometimes alleviate or reduce injuries. While your new rescue horse is in quarantine, it is possible for him to be within sight and vocal distance of the remainder of your horses. Once the quarantine period is over, allowing horses to meet with a fence between them limits physical contact, but doesn't always ensure that there are no injuries. Once they are calm together at the fence line, they can then be put in the same pasture or paddock. Another way to reduce herd introduction strife is to put your new horse with only one other herd member at a time until he has met each individual. This prevents groups of other horses from "ganging up" on the new one. How you approach the introduction depends on your new horse, your current horses, and the arrangement of your pastures and fencing. If your horse is at a boarding stable, you may have very little control over the introduction. Even though introducing a new horse can be scary, the majority of the time they remain unscathed.

DEVELOP A FOUNDATION OF TRUST

Your horse's relationship with humans begins the very first day you interact with him. Time you devote to brushing him, petting him, and getting to know each other is important. Your horse is depending on you for food and water, and compared to his former situation of neglect, the fact that you show up with regular rations goes a long way to establish trust. The horse you acquire may have never had a good relationship with a human, so you may have to invest more time and energy than you expect to break down his barriers. Early training as he recovers is the foundation for any future training or riding (fig. 13.1).

Routine and Respect

Your routine should be kept as consistent as possible from day to day. The time period early after acquisition is critical for kind and dependable care and handling—give the horse the opportunity to develop trust and respect for his caretakers. Think of respect from the horse in this way: He is depending on you for his needs. You consistently provide for those needs. In exchange, the horse obeys your requests. He should not be pushy or mean; he should be cognizant of your presence and space. He should also learn not to fear you.

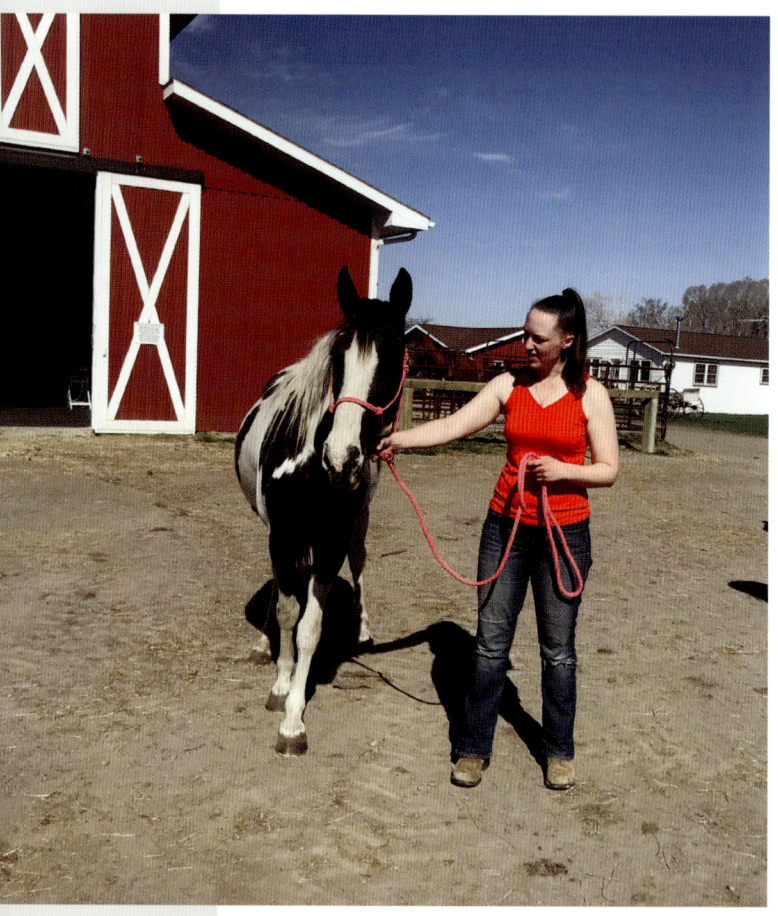

13.1 Crystal with her newly adopted rescue mare. They have known each other for less than an hour, and both are probably wondering how this relationship will go.

A shy or timid horse will need socialization and reassurance, while a bold or pushy horse can hurt somebody. If you punish a curious horse, he will become fearful. If you reassure a pushy or bold horse, he can become dangerous by invading your space. Seek to understand the individual you are working with in order to achieve a relationship with respect. Each horse—even each situation—requires different inputs from you as a handler and trainer (fig. 13.2).

Behavior and Weakness

If you acquired a thin, weak horse, understand that his behavioral reactions may be blunted. As his BCS increases, his brio can increase, changing him to a vigorous, active, reactive, fearful, or aggressive horse. This is why it is so important to gain his trust early and establish ground rules and handling skills.

There is no reason to stress a weakened horse excessively, but it is a good strategy to use this "calmer" time period to reduce the horse's fear and establish boundaries. Your goal is to have a horse who accepts the halter and being led, fits into your daily routine, and enjoys grooming.

Rebuild Muscle

As a horse is gaining weight, turning him out in a larger enclosure for some self-walking and moderate amounts of walking him in-hand are appropriate for helping him rebuild muscle. Think of this as physical therapy. His body has self-digested his fat stores as well as his muscle. You must work to build the muscle back up, without burning off the excess calories that he needs to gain weight.

Horses who are thin and weak should not be asked to do any lateral movements or exercises that require coordination and

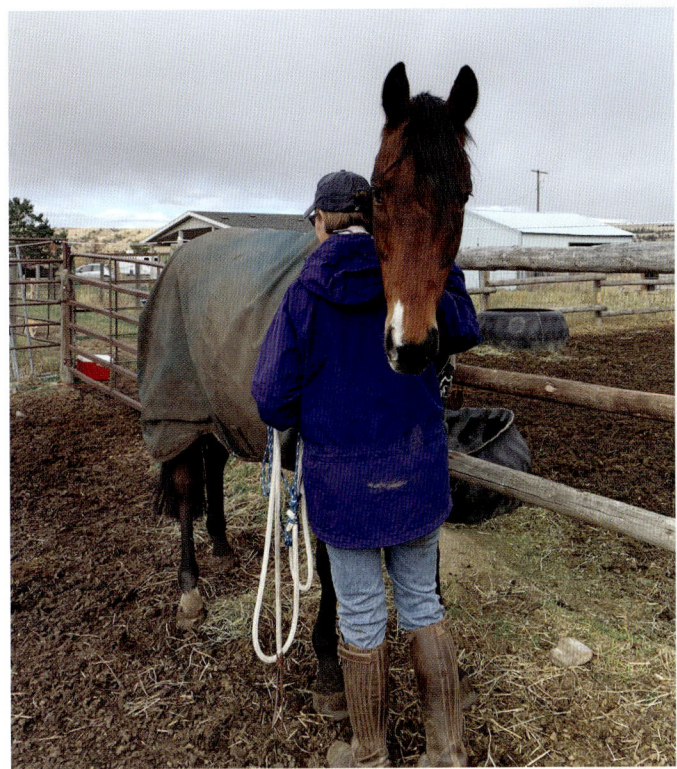

13.2 Meggan and her horse have a special bond.

musculature. For a horse with a BCS of 1 or 2, there should be no arena obstacles or ground poles, no circling exercises, and no trotting. Once the horse has gained weight and has a BCS of 3, trotting and obstacles can be slowly introduced. Wait to introduce cantering until the horse has a BCS of 4 or more (see chapter 11, p. 152).

You can work on refining your horse's halter training and confidence when he has a BCS of 2 or more. Walk him as many different places as you can. As he gains condition (BCS of 3 or more), hand-walking can begin to include working on a hill or over ground poles or *cavalletti* (poles to step over, sometimes raised 4 to 6 inches off the ground) to build muscle mass and coordination. Limb elevation required by such exercise develops his core muscles to maintain postural balance as he places his feet. Walking him on trails and taking him places outside of his normal daily routine helps you understand how he is going to react in new situations before you ever consider riding him.

Consistency and Fairness

Rescue horses value the ability to predict how you will act. The more consistently and fairly you behave, the more comfortable your horse will become. There are many aspects to being consistent and fair with your horse.

Consistency does not mean that you always walk very slowly, never wave your arms around while you talk, and never raise your voice above a whisper. Consistency means that you establish expectations and that the set of expectations is the same each time you interact. For example, if you expect your horse to not step on your feet, and he does, your response should be the same each time: Push him away. If he steps on your feet and one time you hop around in agony, and the next time you push him away, and another time you laugh it off in front of your friends, then you haven't been consistent. Your horse will not be able to meet your expectations because what you expect is a moving target.

Fairness does not mean that you never reprimand bad behavior. Fairness means that when you ask a horse to do something, you have considered all the options and made every effort to set him up for success. You ask him to train incrementally, and you reward him when he does well. For example, the first time you ride your new horse, you would not take him out on a 25-mile trail ride on steep mountain hills all alone. Instead, you would fairly ride him in the arena until you and he understand each other enough that you both feel safe. Then, you could go on a brief 1- to 2-mile ride with a confident friendly horse as a companion. Next, you may be able to go out alone, and work your way up gradually to tackling longer distances.

To be consistent and fair, you work to maintain an even keel, matter-of-fact approach. You are confident your horse can do what you ask, and he will develop confidence in himself as he progressively succeeds in the tasks set before him. You don't exaggerate your excitement, nor act angry in your corrections to him. You are steady, with your emotions under control and balanced. It takes practice to achieve and maintain this balanced emotional state.

TRAINING STRESS

Work to expose your horse to as many new objects and sights and sounds as possible, keeping in mind that you may be working in quarantine. Brush him and show him crinkly bags and horse toys. Look around and be creative with the tools and the environment you have. Understand that his response to an object at home may change when you are away from home: The weather, the time of day, and the other horses around him are different. Experience is cumulative, so the more consistent your requests are under a variety of circumstances, the better he will be over the months and years ahead.

Training a rescue horse will be stressful at times. Learning involves struggle, but it is worth it! An unruffled approach can allow you to manage the stress in both you and your horse as you add tasks to his repertoire. Your horse is going to learn that you aren't going to be flying off the handle at him, so he doesn't need to feel fearful or defensive.

Stress is needed for learning, but your understanding of when to moderate and stop the stress is critical for safety. When stress intensifies and the horse's natural flight instinct is switched on, injuries or accidents are more likely to happen. Each horse has a different threshold of stress that leads to fear, so understanding your horse as an individual is important.

Novelty and Anxiety

When you don't know a horse, his history, or anything else about him, begin as you would with a foal. Assume everything he sees is novel. Approach slowly. Watch his eyes, ears, and movements. He won't speak with his voice, but rather with his body. Work hard to listen to him. Prepare yourself that this horse probably won't react as a foal or young horse would. A foal approaches the world with curiosity. A mishandled and under-confident horse will exhibit fear.[154]

An example of a high-anxiety-producing object is a whip. The whip, flag, or "carrot-stick" should function as an extension of the horse person's arm. The carrot-stick has a heavy lash that is much more difficult to "pop" or sting a horse with, and a flag can be used to wave at a horse without ever touching him. (fig. 13.3). These items are used to move the horse in ways that develop your relationship as a leader and to clarify your cues. Horses that have experienced improper use from a person whipping them excessively or without a reason that the horse can understand will see the whip and engage in avoidance behavior. The minute you move a whip, some horses

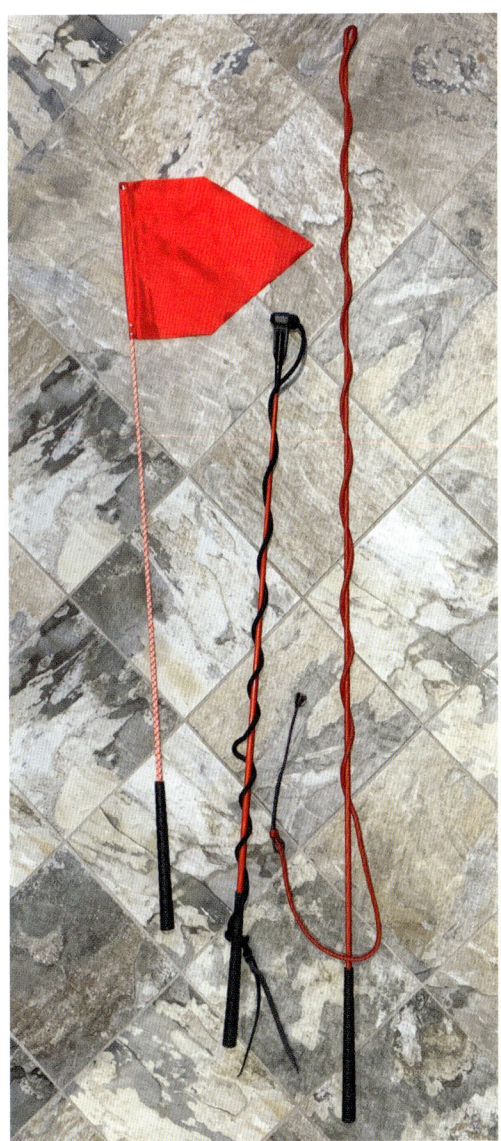

13.3 Three "arm extensions": On the left, a flag, in the center, a carrot stick with a heavy lash that is difficult to "pop" a horse with, and on the right, a traditional longe whip.

will almost instantaneously snort, widen and show the whites of their eyes, and try to get away. The horse's reaction can be sudden and very strong, even to the point of pulling back and breaking the halter and lead rope when tied. A few horses learn to defend themselves and become dangerously aggressive toward the whip and handler.

Using approach-and-retreat and positive reinforcement can allay the horse's fears so that common tools can be useful for you as a trainer.

Fear of Whips: If your horse shows intense fear of the whip, immediately put the whip down. Then, set yourself up to work to restore his trust in you, and demonstrate that the whip is not harmful in and of itself. He should accept that the whip or stick is allowed to gently touch him on his withers, back, and neck. Wind the string or lash around the base and secure it with a knot, then rub him with the stick portion only. Positively reinforce his acceptance with treats, petting, and praise. He should accept it touching all four legs on both the inside and the outside.

When working with a flag or a whip with a string or lash, finally, unfurl the end and gently wave it around while standing near him. Use a movement that is to the side and not aggressive to him. Stand at the level of his shoulder a few feet away from him and face parallel to his body. Don't face as if you are approaching him with it. Again, positively reinforce his acceptance. Finally, he should accept the lash touching him and swinging across his back and around and under his belly.

Depending on what the horse's past

Some Stuff Your Steed May Be Afraid Of

- Baby strollers
- Barking or running dogs
- Other riders falling off their horses
- Weed whackers
- Lawnmowers
- Garden hoses
- Tractors, golf carts, or other vehicles
- Flapping caution tape
- Deer or wildlife—especially when they are running or appear suddenly
- Donkeys, mules, Miniature Horses, llamas, pigs, cows, sheep, geese, chickens or any other unfamiliar farm animal
- Port-a-potties
- Swinging doors
- Horses or humans suddenly entering arena doors
- Sudden noises such as humans "passing gas," sirens, or ripping sound of Velcro
- Birds or large butterflies appearing suddenly in his field of vision
- Logs or ground poles
- Large rocks or boulders, especially when in shadow
- Wind-blown leaves, weeds, small candy wrappers, or other litter
- Canoes, balloons, umbrellas, or other new objects
- Cats (they still move like predators)
- Children or babies
- Flags
- Garbage cans
- Mud puddles
- Noisy raincoats
- Shadows
- Saddles, blankets, and other tack

experience is it can take one session or one hundred sessions for him to have calm acceptance.

Scary Objects: In addition to being afraid of a whip, horses that have been mistreated may also be afraid of the farrier, of trailer loading, or of going into buildings. Anything that is in a strange location, breaking up the scenery, or has new noises or erratic movements can be terror-inducing. Odors, such as smoke, can also incite fear. As a prey animal, a horse is naturally afraid of any object that he doesn't know about. It can be difficult to sort out if he is afraid of the new object, or when he is afraid because he has been abused with the object. Generally, the more novelty a horse is exposed to in a kind approach-and-retreat manner interspersed with positive reinforcement, the less fear reaction he will exhibit with more and more new objects. Horses that are fearful due to abuse have an excessively strong fear reaction. A high-intensity fear-driven horse is dangerous because he is predisposed to either defend himself or to hurt himself or his handler while trying to escape.

OVERCOMING FEAR

When fearful, your horse will be tense, his eyes will be wide, his ears will be focused, and he will move his feet. If he moves himself even 1 or 2 inches away from the object that is scaring him, his prey-animal brain automatically clicks, "Aha, I succeeded! I got away!" Try to withdraw the object before he moves. If he does move, withdraw the object as soon as his feet hesitate or stop. Timing is critical, so work hard to make your timing as accurate and responsive as possible.

Sometimes rescue horses will overreact. And sometimes, no matter how well you have planned, things will go wrong. Do a little extra planning with a fearful horse. If things fall apart, take a deep breath to calm yourself, think about another way of asking the horse, and try again. Even if he shows unreasonable fear in the beginning, when he realizes that you are consistent and fair, his fear will slowly melt away.

If you cannot think of a different way to proceed with the task at hand, choose a different task that the horse knows well, and go to it. This will allow him to succeed, and you can conclude your interaction or training session on a positive note. Later, consult others and seek new ideas for approaching the difficult or fear-inciting task.

Medically Addressing Fear

It's critical that you work to train your horse for compliance for medical procedures and hoof care. However, the need for an immediate medical procedure or farrier visit may arise. Medical necessity may not follow your training schedule, so your horse may not yet be prepared. You may need to employ tools or drugs to help facilitate critical or emergency procedures.

Twitch: This tool is applied to the horse's nose and used to distract and calm the horse (fig. 13.4 and see sidebar). Twitches exist in a variety of configurations. As with acupuncture, the horse will relax due to the release of his own chemical signals.

Other types of twitching can be used in a pinch. Some people use an *ear twitch*, where the ear is held tightly and rolled. I don't recommend this as it can cause a horse to be ear-shy or fearful of humans

The Twitch

Think back before modern sedation drugs were available and when horses were necessary for work and transportation. Veterinarians and horse people were obliged to work on horses with very few tools. The twitch was widely used throughout the 1800s and perhaps earlier.

The twitch comes in a variety of configurations, from a basic V-shaped humane twitch, to a one-man twitch with a ratchet handle, to a handle made of wood or plastic with a loop of rope or chain at the end. A twitch is applied to the end of the horse's nose, where it is squeezed or rolled.

Whatever the case, the twitch serves as a distraction for minor procedures. Although some people view twitches as barbaric, they keep handlers safe. Most horses respond positively to the twitch because it stimulates the release of natural endorphins. Studies have shown that a twitch works much like acupuncture and the release of endorphins is real and significant. *Endorphins* are signaling chemicals used by the brain to relieve pain and enhance happiness. These endorphins help the horse stand still so that veterinarians can safely do their job.[155, 156]

One study evaluated teaching horses to accept clipping the hair on their ears with or without a twitch.[157] When a twitch was used, horses underwent the procedure more calmly. After the first time, the group that had been twitched was still more calm when the procedure was performed a second time *without* a twitch.

After the procedure is complete, it is important to remove the twitch immediately, and praise the horse.

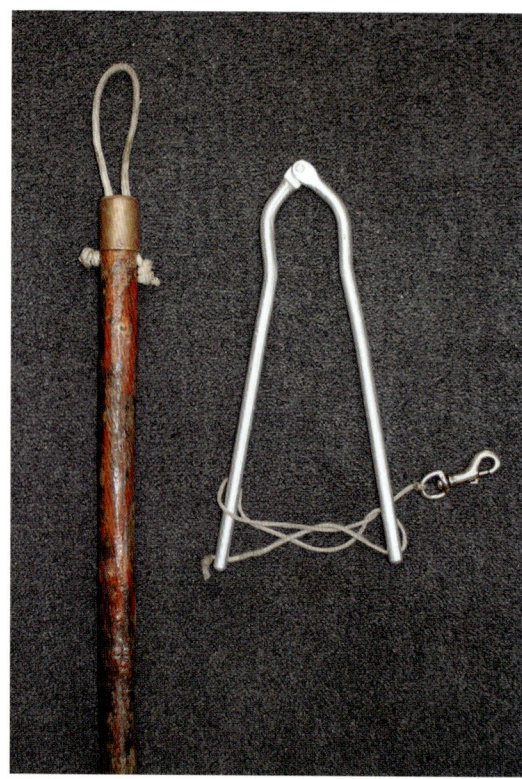

13.4 Two different twitches.

touching his ears. However, a *neck twitch* is an acceptable alternative. For a neck twitch, a handler grasps the skin of the neck and rolls it tightly. This is enough of a distraction for many horses to stand and accept injections or other mildly noxious procedures.

EAP: The equine appeasing pheromone (EAP) is available commercially as Confidence EQ®. Pheromones are airborne, invisible, odorless substances that are absorbed in a special part of the nose and cause a response from the animal. EAP is secreted by a mare as her foal suckles, and signals to the horse that everything is safe and comfortable.[158] It comes as a small packet of gel that is rubbed near the opening of your horse's nostrils. In my experience, it may not work on every horse, but on many horses the response is notable and results in a calmer patient.

Drugs: Drugs should only be used under the guidance of a veterinarian. Dormosedan Gel® is a sedative medication that is given by mouth and absorbed through the gums and lips. Unfortunately, it does not work very well when it is fed to the horse with grain because it gets swallowed that way, instead of absorbed. At the recommended dosing it has a calming effect, but the horse remains steady on his feet.

Other drugs can be employed, so consult with your veterinarian if you think an injection of sedatives is needed for your horse.

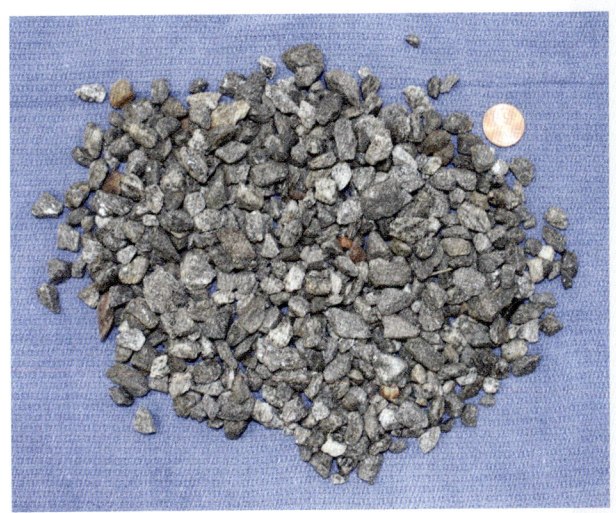

13.5 A draft horse ate about 30 gallons of this gravel, which had to be removed surgically.

MEALTIME ANXIETY

A rescue horse may be worried about his next meal, and he may kick his stall, paw, or pin his ears. An anxious horse may do best in a quiet place, where he can see and hear other horses, but feels safe in his own space and does not need to defend his food.

There are many strategies to minimizing equine mealtime anxiety, and each horse is different. What works for you, your horse, your stable setup, and your feeding routine may not be what works for others. Because every horse and situation is unique, you may need to use trial-and-error to tweak the process. Over time, your horse should feel more comfortable and secure. Pay attention to his body language and listen to what he tells you he needs.

It may be safer to place food in the stall and then bring the horse to it, but you must have his absolute trust and respect. This eliminates pawing, aggression, stall kicking, and other unwanted behaviors while the horse is waiting for his meal to be served. You can lead him into the stall, or open a gate and allow him to enter the area with the food.

Your rescue horse will need at least four to six hours of protected time per day alone with his meals. This may be divided into two sessions of two to three hours each. Group feeding is not a good option for a horse who is slow to eat because of dental problems, a horse with mealtime anxiety or aggression, or one who is being fed more food than other horses in your herd. As a newcomer to the herd, a recently rescued horse is unlikely to be high enough in the social hierarchy to be allowed to eat his extra ration.

Once a horse has experienced starvation, he can be mentally changed forever. Extreme mealtime anxiety can be reduced, but for some it is never eliminated. This type of horse is likely to eat indiscriminately, ingest foreign material, and will be prone to obesity due to overeating (fig. 13.5). Science on horses' psychology is elusive, but a

The Portly Paso

Talking about weight can be a tricky issue. In this instance, I was asked to evaluate a Peruvian Paso mare, Peanut. She was 12 years old—in the prime of her life—and wasn't able to keep up on the trail.

"Sometimes," her owner Martha told me, "Peanut seems slow. Other times she limps on a front leg. It's not always the same one. Once in a while, I think she is limping on a back leg. I'm not really sure what the problem is."

Peanut was obese—she was a petite 14.2 hands with refined bone structure. But she weighed in at almost 1,050 pounds when she should have been around 850. She had fat deposits making her neck "cresty," fat rolls behind her shoulders, a deep crease down her back, and large fatty lumps on either side of her tail head. Peanut had a BCS of 9; additionally, Martha was herself obese. When evaluating her gait, Peanut was lame in three of her legs.

Martha needed a larger horse, and the horse needed to be fit, not fat. I finally mustered the courage to suggest that petite Peanut retire, and a more stout horse be purchased. We also talked about fitness and body condition scoring. Matching horse and rider size is an important part of maintaining your horse's long-term health and well-being.

57-year followup on the human starvation experiment reported that patients had abnormal eating habits and carried extra weight for months to years after the conclusion of the experiment.[159]

Speedy eating can stem from a period of starvation, so some horses *bolt* their food. A medical consequence is that inadequately chewed pelleted feeds can lead to choke.

Strategies to prevent bolting include adding grain or pellets on top of the hay so

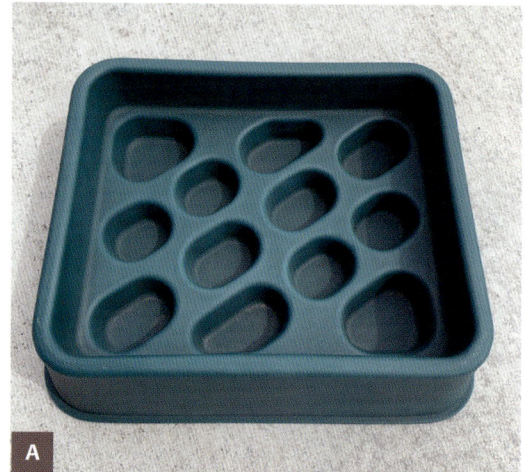

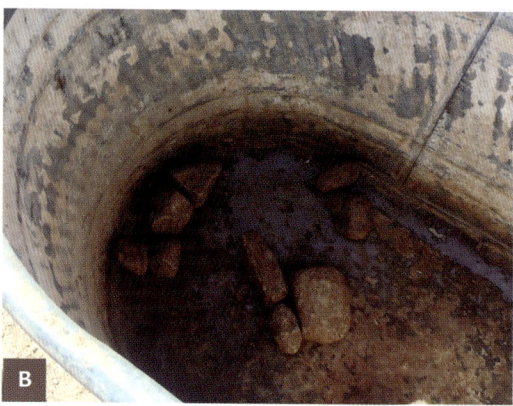

13.6 A & B Feeder strategies to slow down a horse that "bolts" his grain include this sturdy plastic contour feeder (A). A water trough can also be used as a feeder with large rocks in it to slow a horse down when he is eating grain (B). He must eat around the rocks.

that the horse must pick through the hay to slowly eat them. Grain or pellets can be fed out of a feeder with contours, and bricks or large rocks added to a conventional feeder will slow the horse down as he eats around the obstacles (figs. 13.6 A & B).

When your horse doesn't spend enough time chewing his food, the roughage will be swallowed as a larger particle size. As the larger pieces travel through the digestive tract, there can be repercussions. First, absorption is less efficient from large particles. Therefore, badly-needed nutrients may pass through unused. Second, the roughage is more likely to build up at certain locations in the digestive tract. The consequent impaction is a subcategory of colic and can require intensive medical treatment to resolve.

Slow-feeders for hay can moderate the speed of the horse's eating process and so help prevent obesity and encourage chewing (figs. 13.7 A–C). But sometimes they can cause injury, and no design is perfect. Some are more durable than others, so choose a high-quality one with a smooth design. Thinner plastic feeders tend to become worn

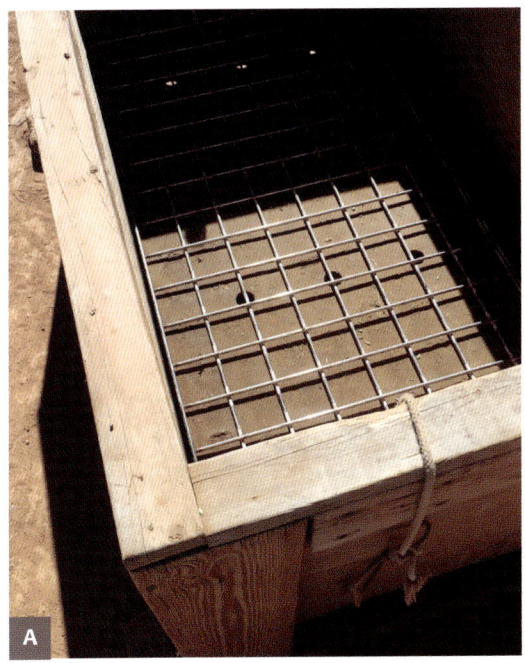
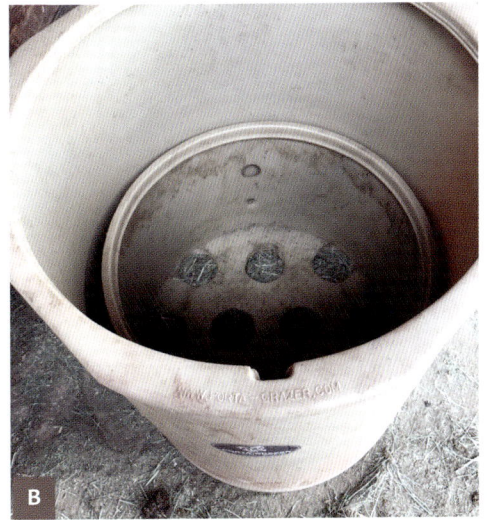
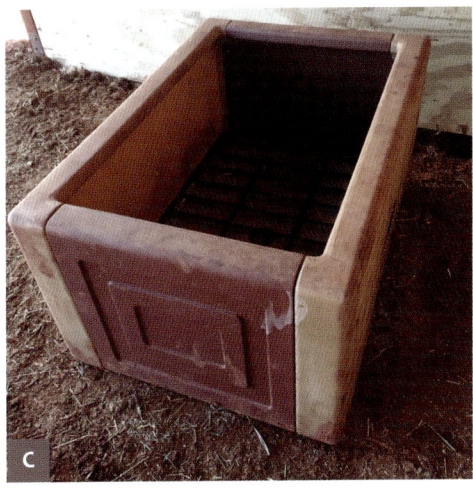

13.7 A–C Slow-feeders of varying types for use with hay include the homemade wood feeder with a metal grate shown here (A). The grate can be removed from the top and hay put underneath it. The grate prevents horses from eating large mouthfuls, slowing them down. Some other options include a commercial feeder of durable plastic with round holes (B) and another with a metal grate (C). The grate slides out through a slot in the top, hay can be added, and the grate replaced.

out or break, slow-feed nets or bags can be dangerous if they are shredded or ingested, and metal grates can damage teeth. Sharp edges are a hazard to gums, lips, eyes, and other soft tissues of the face.

HANDLING FEET AND LEGS WITH TRUST

You want your rescue horse to be sound and comfortable, therefore, it is critical that he allow you to handle his feet and legs. Many horses that come from a background of neglect have not had proper foot care. This can be due to financial constraints, lack of training, bad behavior due to pain, or a combination of all of these factors. A thin, weak horse may not be able to balance and support himself when picking up a foot.

Picking up the Feet of a Trained Adult

First, it is important to practice how to safely cue a trained horse to pick up his feet. By learning this method, you have an understanding of the goal you are trying to reach. Make sure you are comfortable with all of these steps on a trained horse before you try to teach your rescue horse.

Normal Nerves: Horses have a reflexive startle response, and when a horse is surprised with touch on his lower leg, he can kick you. The reaction is hard-wired into the horse. To avoid this, we touch the horse's barrel or withers and maintain contact while moving to touch his legs. During the training process, the touch may be an extension of your arm, such as a carrot stick (see p. 173).

Proper Pick-Up: In a well-trained adult horse, it is best to pick up his front feet by first greeting the horse and then touching or petting him on his withers. To pick up the left front foot, face his hind end. Start at the withers and maintain contact as you run your hand down the back of his left leg and bend over. When your hand is below the horse's knee, grip the tendons gently. A trained horse will pick up his foot for you.

To pick up the left hind foot, again face the horse and touch his withers. Staying in a safe position is critical. Maintain contact and run your hand to his left hip. Put both hands on his left hip. Your left hand will remain on his hip while your right hand maintains firm, yet gentle contact and moves down

---

Shivers

A condition known as *shivers* occurs in horses. Draft breeds or draft crosses are most commonly affected. When a horse with shivers picks up his leg for a human, he will raise it reflexively high, and may shake, shiver, or tremble for a few moments before he can relax. These horses cannot control the body's response, much like how your leg will kick when the tendon below your kneecap is struck.

If these horses are reprimanded or punished, they become anxious. The more anxious the horse becomes, the worse the nervous problem becomes. It is critical to recognize when your horse has this problem, because understanding the seemingly exaggerated response will help you be patient and kind. The manifestation of shivers is minimized when human and horse remain relaxed.

the back of his leg. When your right hand is below his hocks, grip the tendons on the back of his leg and perhaps give a pull of his leg forward at the fetlock if he needs more encouragement. A trained horse will willingly and non-threateningly pick up his hind leg for you. Once you have the leg and foot off the ground, your left hand can then be used to help hold his foot while you pick the debris out of it.

There are two main reasons for keeping contact with the left hip while you are picking up the limb: you can push the hip and shift his weight over, and you can feel tension in the horse's body. If he suddenly moves, your contact with him will cause your body to move away and keep you safe.

Training for Hoof Care

Picking up your horse's feet is a test of trust because his main defense is to run away from predators. By allowing you to hold his leg, he becomes defenseless and unable to run. He must trust that you are not going to harm his life-saving leg.

An untrained adult horse who does not understand how to pick up his feet takes patience and deliberation to train. Don't try to pick up any leg until he trusts you enough that you can walk out to his pen, put the halter on him, and lead him. At each training session, try to introduce only one new movement or concept to the horse. Break the process down into the simplest baby steps possible.

Get Assistance: It is best to find a capable and confident assistant to help you by holding the lead rope and halter to restrict the horse's movement. While he is being trained, it is not yet safe to tie your horse to a fixed object, as he may panic and hurt himself or you.

Have the person helping you stand on the same side that you are working on. From that position the helper can directly observe you and your horse, and have a better chance of moving the horse's hind end away from you. If the horse tries to kick, your assistant should pull the halter toward herself, which will cause the horse to swing his hip safely away.

Finally, it is not worth getting hurt over. If you feel you and your horse will not be able to work through this segment of training or if you notice that your horse's behavior is worsening rather than improving, get professional assistance. Don't give up, though, and leave your horse untrained.

Touch First: Begin by touching your horse with a carrot stick or other extension of your arm (see p. 173). This keeps you at a safe distance as he learns about being touched. Gradually work with your horse so that he accepts you brushing his legs. Use a soft or medium brush. A brush that is too stiff could incite his kicking reflex if he is poked by the bristles.

Shift Weight: When the horse accepts touch, ask him to shift his weight away from the foot you are touching. You can lean into your horse's shoulder to shift his weight to the other front foot. His foot is not moving when he shifts his weight; he is simply leaning away from you. Make sure you recognize and reward him when he leans to the other leg.

Lift a Front Foot: When the weight shift has been consistently occurring, you are then going to ask your horse to lift his foot off the ground on cue. Use all the signals that you would use for a trained horse. Then help your horse pick up the foot. There are a variety of reinforcing techniques that can be used to increase your ask. You may tap the back of his heel bulbs with a hoof pick until he is annoyed enough to pick up his leg. If you gently pinch his chestnut it will cause him to pick up his leg. You can also pull his fetlock up and backward until you have lifted his foot. Whatever the case, you only need him to release his foot for a split second. Put it back down almost instantly, and give him immediate positive reinforcement. The first time he picks up his foot, don't try to hold it up, or keep it up, or take it away from him. If he has never held his foot up for a person before, trying to hang on to it for too long will scare him. When he is consistent and understands the cue on the front legs, then work on the hind legs.

Training for Hind Legs: Once the horse has some understanding of the game of picking up his feet and trusts that no harm will come to him, you can turn your attention to working with the hind legs. You are one step ahead of where you were when you started working on the front legs. To reinforce or increase your cue, use one hand on his hip to shift his weight off the hind leg. Then, pull the fetlock up and forward until the leg is ever so slightly off the ground. Use lots of positive reinforcement.

Repeat the exercise of picking up one leg two or three times, then work on the other leg. That is plenty for one day. The next training session, go through the same moves, and pick up each foot two or three times.

Keep It Up: Once your horse consistently picks up his leg, you can begin to keep the leg for a bit longer. Increasing the time the foot is held is a gradual process. Remember, this training is for a lifetime. It is more important to achieve consistency than to achieve a lot in one training session.

As you are lengthening the time you hold his leg up, consider your whole horse. If he has arthritis, it may be painful for him to flex his joints for longer and longer periods and to hold all his weight on the other leg. If he was malnourished, he may be too weak to balance on only three legs.

Keep it for one second, then for two seconds, then for three seconds. When you can keep the leg up for 10 seconds, start picking out his feet. First, use your hand to get him used to touching all parts of his foot. Then, pick with your hoof pick and brush.

Preparing for the Farrier: It is ideal for you to mimic the way a farrier will hold his leg. Practice holding a trained horse's front leg between your knees, and resting a back leg over your thigh. When you are comfortable, start showing your horse how to be comfortable in this position. Being in that position for a second or two is a good starting point.

To break things down even more for an especially nervous horse, it isn't necessary for the farrier to achieve a full trim. If he or she only uses the rasp on the first visit, but ends on a positive note, that is a win for you and your horse. If the farrier is only able to trim the front feet, that's fine. Choose a patient and kind farrier who understands positive reinforcement. Pay him or her generously for the time it takes to drive to you for half a trim. Take care of your farrier so you can have the best care for your horse.

Setting His Foot Down: As your horse becomes comfortable with having his feet handled, start working toward how you put them back down. Search for the moment when he is relaxed to release a leg. Always set the foot back down gently. Don't drop it suddenly.

Go Slowly to Obtain Consistent Results: Gradual and incremental training steps seem slow, but actually progress faster than if you try to make great big leaps and bounds. A quiet and calm progression produces a solid and reliable behavior response from the horse. It takes time and patience.

Using a Rope: While working with your untrained horse, you may find information about how to use a rope to pick up his feet. These techniques can and do work for experienced trainers. However, it's more complicated, so mistakes are likely. The plus is that using a rope can keep you out of harm's way should your horse decide to kick. Only use rope techniques if you are comfortable with the description and have help. Practice your rope-handling skills on a calm, willing, and trained horse before deciding to use them on your untrained horse.

A BASIC FOUNDATION

In the earliest stage of training, you may only be working to consistently halter, lead, and groom your horse without frightening him. Learn to recognize when he is fearful. Be as even-tempered as possible. Work gradually so that he will accept touch on all areas of his body and pick up his feet for you.

CHAPTER 14

Fearless:
Halter Training Adult Horses

READINESS REVIEW

Many horses that have suffered from abuse or neglect are already halter trained. When that is not the case, make sure you have done the following before beginning the tasks set forth in this chapter:

- Understand equine physiology as it applies to training.

- Established a daily routine of food and water as a foundation for trust.

- Have a sturdy, safe enclosure.

- Make sure your horse feels comfortable in his living situation.

Horses that cannot be touched are the most challenging to train. These include wild Mustangs and neglected, untrained domestic horses. You may not have any idea how old an adult equine is—after all, you cannot touch him to examine his teeth. Each horse presents unique challenges. First, I'll discuss what behavior you might expect from a mature horse, and the critical step of initially approaching your horse.

Halter selection and fit is important. When you are able to put a halter on your horse, you can get him moving with pressure-and-release training techniques. Once he accepts direction, teach your horse to stand tied. Tools and techniques in this chapter may take minutes for one horse, and months for another. Each learns at his own pace; keep working with yours until he is confident being handled by humans.

If you feel you aren't making progress or your horse is not responding to your concerted efforts, seek assistance. No horse is at higher risk for suffering or resale than an adult horse that is not halter trained.

HORSE PERSONALITY

As an adult, your horse's personality is already defined. A rescuer should "carefully evaluate the personality of an older horse before committing to him, because he's not likely to change."[160] That is, trained or untrained, some horses are naturally more flighty and fearful compared to other more stoic and thoughtful individuals. Observe an unhandled horse carefully before you bring him home.

Pay attention to his body language. What does he do when you enter his enclosure? A horse who runs to the corner and pins back his ears defensively will be more difficult to train than one who looks at you

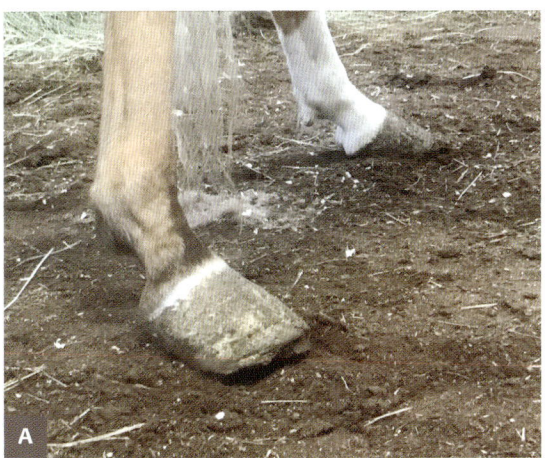
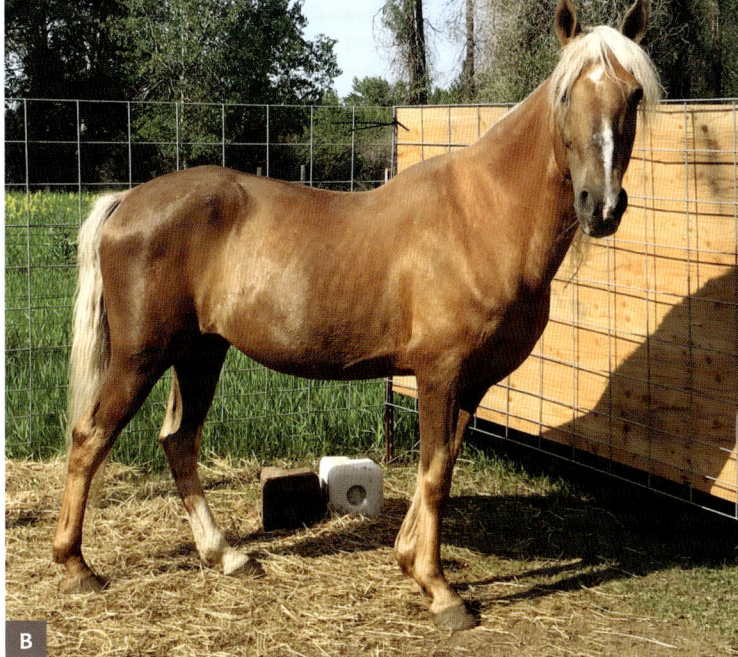

14.1 A & B The severely neglected hind feet of a thin stallion who was confiscated for neglect (A), and the same horse, several months after castration, with improved condition (B). An adult horse that looks at a person with curiosity like this is more likely to enjoy interacting with humans once he is halter-trained.

with curiosity. Many older horses have a calm, patient attitude that results in thinking through problems, and adults usually have a longer attention span than youngsters (figs. 14.1 A & B).

Illness and starvation can make a horse seem quiet and kind, but this can change as his health improves. Approaches to horses outlined in this chapter can be used for debilitated horses. When your horse has a BCS of 1, 2, or 3, the techniques here for befriending your horse are appropriate. Use the situation to your advantage and teach him to accept the halter right away.

THE FLIGHT ZONE

The *flight zone* is a lot like a personal space "bubble." Its size varies with each individual: A wild Mustang may run when a human is 50 yards away, and a domestic horse may be willing to let a human be within inches. Whatever the distance the animal's comfort level is, when a human or predator enters his flight zone, he will flee. His movement will be influenced both by fear and by body language.

Using the flight zone, you can move your horse, even though he is not halter trained. There are three basic movements:

1. When you move toward the horse's hip, he will move forward (fig. 14.2 A).

2. Movement toward the front of the horse (in front of the shoulders) causes him to either back up or turn away from you (fig. 14.2 B).

3. The *balance point* is near the horse's shoulder or withers. Stepping toward the balance point is your best chance for touching your horse.

Part II: Training Horses in Need—185

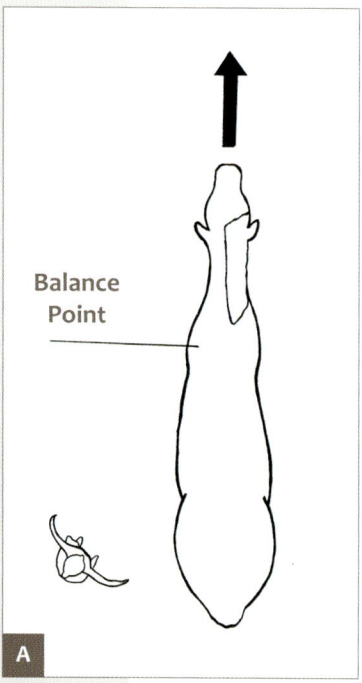
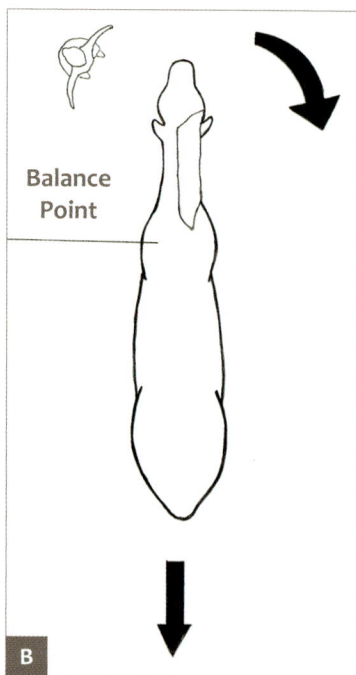

14.2 A & B Two diagrams showing the movement of a horse using his flight zone and body language. The balance point is the line of the shoulder or withers. Your movement toward the horse's hip will drive him forward (A). Your movement toward him, but in front of his shoulder will cause him to either back or turn away (B).

When you acquire an untouched horse, the flight zone will be used to quietly herd or move a horse across his pen and into a trailer for shipping. The goal is to not chase or excite him, but rather to allow him to investigate and enter the new enclosure or trailer as willingly as possible. Remember, when his fear response is turned on, it will be much harder to disassociate fear from the task of trailer loading later. Plan ahead so you have plenty of time because getting a previously untouched horse into a trailer may take hours.[161]

Enclosure Guidelines

Halter training will coincide with quarantine, so your horse's pen should be relatively small and made of sturdy material.

For Mustangs, Bureau of Land Management (BLM) requirements are that fencing for horses 18 months and older is between 20 by 20 feet and 50 by 50 feet in size. The horse needs enough room to move around, but too large an enclosure will make the gentling process more difficult. Fences and gates must be at least 6 feet high, but 5 feet is acceptable if horses are already gentled, younger than 18 months, or if you are working with a burro. Finally, the material the fence is made of cannot be strands of wire: Two-by-six boards, pipes, or heavy-gauge woven mesh is acceptable. Barbed wire, electric wires, and high-tensile wire are not acceptable.[162]

These are good guidelines for any untouched horse. If your horse is debilitated or sick, he is unlikely to challenge a fence, but if he is healthy and vigorous, he might.

REDUCE FLIGHT ZONE

Before you are ready to touch your horse, he must accept your presence. Neglected domestic horses are generally more used to the idea of a human being nearby. However, Mustangs may remain extremely fearful for long periods. Matter-of-factly going into your horse's pen or stall with feed and water can allow your new horse to get used to your presence and movements.

Enter your horse's pen, and get as close as possible to his flight zone, but retreat before he moves his feet. Figure out how close you can get before your horse moves, and work to reduce his flight-zone distance. Move deliberately and pay attention. His body will tell you when you have reached the point at which he is no longer comfortable with your presence. Some trainers say that the horse will fidget. Watch for him to move or swish his tail. Look for his weight to shift from one leg to another or for him to lean away from you. As you watch your horse, watch his eyes. If they are wide or he is trembling, he is fearful. A fearful horse will run away from you. When you corner a fearful horse, he is likely to defend himself and injure you. The first order of business is to convince your horse that you are a friend and that he has no reason to be afraid of you. Simply feeding the horse in his pen may be the beginning of the process, but you must work hard to get beyond that step.

Don't hide or sneak up on the horse; move in full view with purpose. If he moves away, don't chase him, but instead wait until he settles (stops moving) and try again. Get as close as you can, and stop your approach before he moves his feet. If you can get within arm's reach, you are in really good shape. If you cannot, keep working to get closer every day. It may take weeks to get within arms' reach, but it is feasible with patience and attention to the horse's body language. Work to get close while he is eating. He has positive reinforcement, and he has a reason to stand and allow you to approach.

Round Pen

An alternative approach to the befriending technique just described is to work with the horse in a round pen until you have communicated to him that you want him near you. There are dozens of trainers who have extensive presentations on round-penning techniques, so I will not cover this topic further.

If your horse has any medical problems, round-penning is not appropriate. Because round-penning a horse requires him to be able to trot or canter for extended periods of time, many rescue horses are not fit or healthy enough for these techniques. Medical problems that preclude round-pen use include lameness, respiratory or breathing problems, generalized weakness or lack of muscle, or any other problem that would prevent athletic activity. A horse should have a BCS of 4 or more before he is worked in a round pen.

INITIATE TOUCH

The best place to start touching a horse is on his withers. It is a neutral body location, and a point at which horses mutually groom each other (fig. 14.3). Rubbing or scratching that area is pleasant for the horse, and he should be taught that your touch is pleasant. Rubbing or scratching your horse's withers and neck is primary positive reinforcement.

From the withers, maintain touch along his neck, shoulder, and eventually to his cheek and head. Try to touch him under the chin and over all the areas on his head where the halter will touch.

Some horses will show interest in you as you feed them. You may be able to bribe your horse to take grain out of a bucket you are holding and initiate touch while he is eating. You may be able to coax him to take food out of your hand. Any contact is progress. However, you will have to push his boundaries to make it past this step. Keep

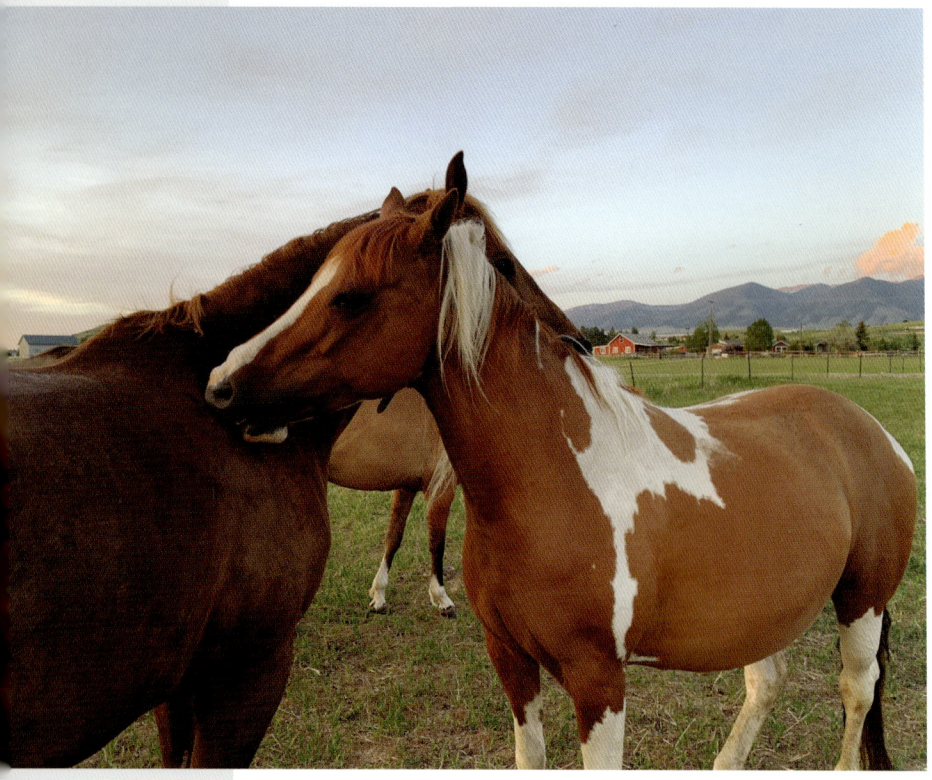

14.3 Horses like to groom each other on their withers and neck. This is the area where they enjoy being petted or scratched, and it lines up with the "balance point" of their flight zone, so it is usually the best place to begin touching a horse.

working until you can easily walk up and touch him.

A few horses will panic when they are touched. Some trainers use an extension of their arm to help horses learn that human touch "does not equal death." The extension may be a pole made of lightweight, flexible material, such as bamboo or PVC. For a difficult horse, you will need to work within a confined safe area (for example, a solid-sided pen) to reach out and touch his withers with your extension.

Working to teach your horse to accept touch involves time, energy, patience, and effort from you as the trainer. Offer treats, petting, and verbal praise often. Do your best to keep your even-keel approach and don't lose your temper in frustration. If you become angry and incite a panic response from the horse, getting him halter trained will be that much tougher. Quick movements will scare him, so stay calm and deliberate.

HALTERING AND HALTER TYPES

There are several types of halters including flat leather, flat nylon, rope halters, and combinations thereof. Each has a purpose.

Flat Halters

Flat halters are constructed of either nylon or leather. One that breaks in an emergency is the safest choice. Breakaway halters are nylon halters designed with a thin leather piece that breaks when strained, keeping the horse safe should an accident occur. He will be released instead of remaining tied or hanging by his neck. Most all-leather halters will also break, whereas flat nylon and rope halters are less likely to break.

Flat halters are comfortable for the horse. One of the reasons they are comfortable is because the point of pressure is spread over the width of the halter. To understand this concept, think about pushing a point of a pencil into your hand compared to the feel of the flat eraser. The flat halter has a more blunted feeling, much like the eraser end.

Rope Halters

The rope halter is more like the point of a pencil. It is thinner and transmits pressure to only a small area, so rope halters are more effective at relaying subtle cues than flat halters are. Many horses are more respectful of their handlers when a rope halter is used. Rope halters are handy in certain situations because they *don't* break under pressure. For example, when you are tying your horse to a highline in the backcountry, you might want to ensure that he doesn't get loose.

A rope halter has a crown piece that goes over the horse's poll from right to left and then ties to a loop on the right cheek piece. When putting a halter on the horse, tie the knot of a rope halter properly (figs. 14.4 A–D). The knot should be tied over the loop on the cheek piece (fig. 14.5). When tied incorrectly, the result is an unstable knot that can loosen, allowing the halter to slip to an incorrect fit (fig. 14.6). It can also tighten if the horse pulls hard, rendering it impossible to untie. When tied correctly, the pull is transmitted from the cheek piece loop to the crown piece of the rope

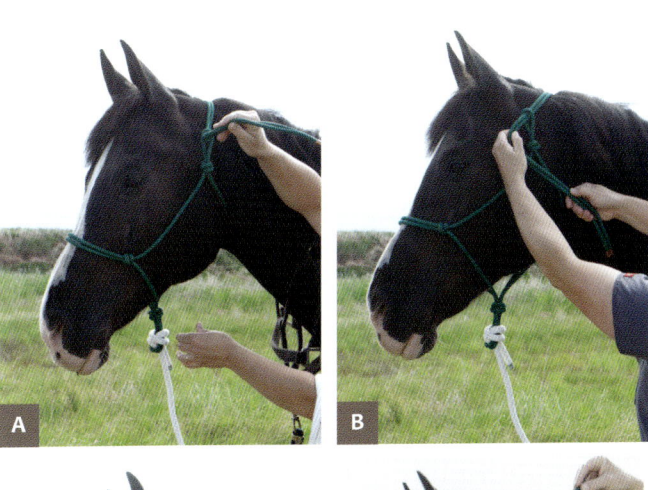

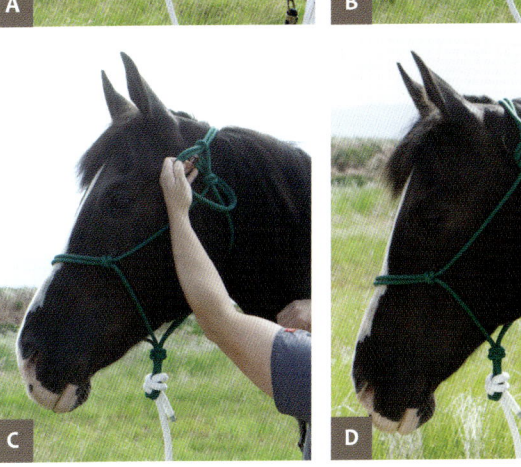

14.4 A–D Tying a rope halter properly: First the poll piece goes though the loop (A). Then a "reverse D" shape is made (B). The poll piece goes around the back of the cheek piece loop (C) and through the "D" shape (D). The knot is made from the poll piece, but is tied over the loop of the cheek piece, not back on itself. A good way to remember this sequence (courtesy of Janice Cartwright at Montana Horse Sense) is the crown piece should go "through to you, toward the eye, then around and through to the sky."

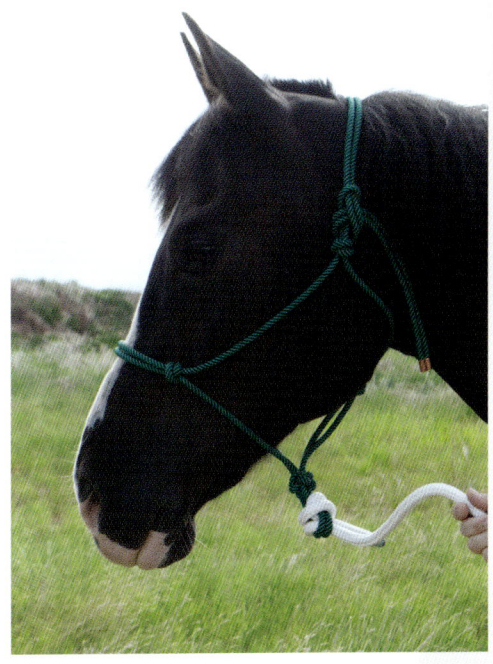

14.5 Here you can see a correctly tied knot on a rope halter.

Part II: Training Horses in Need—189

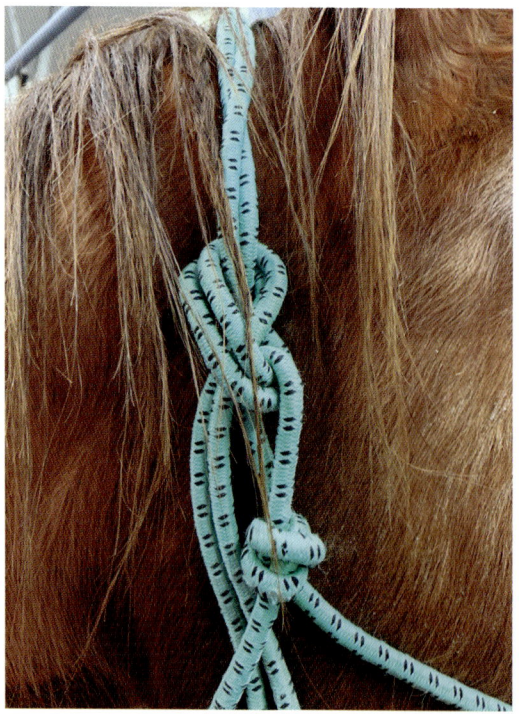

14.6 A rope halter tied incorrectly.

halter. Therefore, it is always possible to undo a correctly tied knot, even if the horse has pulled on the halter very hard.[163]

It is supremely unsafe for a horse to wear a rope halter while he is loose in his paddock or pasture. The rope halter is more likely to catch on things because it has a loop under the chin where the lead rope attaches. Many rope halters have the lead rope incorporated in a permanent manner, so obviously it is not a good idea for the horse to be dragging a long rope around. A long rope is more likely to catch in a fence or entangle the horse's legs.

Halter Fit

Whichever halter you choose, select one that fits well. Halter fit guidelines apply to all types of halters. A loose halter (a gap your fist would easily fit in) is dangerous. A tight halter (you cannot get two fingers between your horse and his halter) is uncomfortable, and a tight halter never allows a release of pressure, so cues you are trying to transmit to the horse are lost.

The halter should lie halfway between the eye and the nostril. Other landmarks to pay attention to are the nasoincisive notch and the facial crest. The nasoincisive notch is the indentation above a horse's nostrils where the soft tissue of the face meets the thin bones of the nose (figs. 14.7 A & B). Pressure on a halter below the nasoincisive notch can result in fractures to the fine nasal bones.

The facial crest is the bony prominence on either side of the horse's face or cheeks. It is parallel to the front of a horse's face. If the halter rides up above the facial crest, it is too high on your horse's head. At this position, you lose your leverage and your cues lose effectiveness.

APPLYING THE HALTER

Once your horse's fear is decreased and he will accept touch, allow him to see the halter. He should get used to how it looks in your hands. Allow him to sniff and investigate the halter at his own pace by leaving it in his pen. Looking at the halter without a human present will help convince him that the halter is not a threat.

When he is comfortable with you touching his withers, his face, his chin, and his neck, and he is used to seeing the halter, start using the halter to pet him. You may be able to place it on his back and slowly move it forward, eventually working to his neck and his poll.

Sometimes people place the halter over

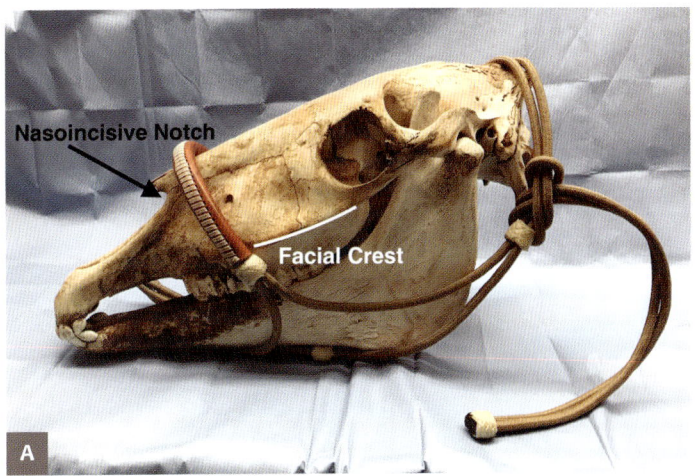
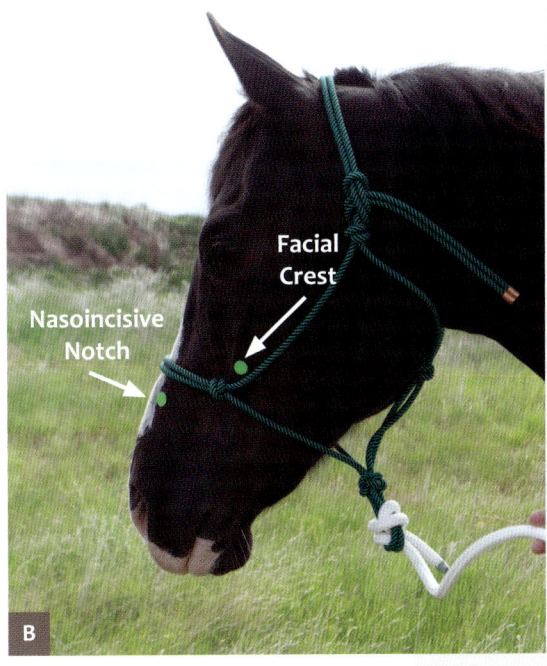

14.7 A & B Here you can see correct fit of a halter on the horse's skull. The halter should not rest over the facial crest nor below the nasoincisive notch (A). The halter rests halfway between the eye and the nostril. Green dots are placed on the end of the facial crest and over the nasoincisive notch (B).

the bucket of feed, and when he eats will use the halter to move his head and eventually work to fasten the halter on him. Even if the halter isn't attached, it can be used to move the head out of the bucket, introducing him to the concept of giving to the pressure of the halter. If you are adopting a Mustang, BLM will apply a halter if you provide one.

Once the halter is on, many people leave it on the horse for days to weeks. If you choose to do this, it is best to have a flat halter with a breakaway function. This allows him to get used to the feel of it on his face and touching him. It also allows you to continue to work until your horse is comfortable with being caught and haltered. You may also leave a short "catch rope" on the halter. Leaving halters on calm, trained adult horses is not ideal. In this instance, we are bending the rules to get this horse some help, and to make sure we can continue to work with him in his small, safe, obstacle-free pen.

While the horse is already wearing a halter and you have some measure of control, work to approach him and put another halter and lead rope on. The second one can be put right over the top of the first. This allows you to practice the process of catching and haltering him, while maintaining control. In this way, you avoid inadvertently having him learn to get away or having to go back and start the halter process all over. Reward the horse with petting or a treat each time you put a halter on.

Try to end each session with some success. This doesn't mean that you are going to march out to the pen and spend all day until your horse is halter trained that evening. It just doesn't work that way. It does mean that if you don't get the halter on today, you are closer than you were yesterday. Maybe today you could touch him with

> ## Lost
>
> It's really impossible to predict the future. The cute and kind sorrel overo horse, Gaucho, had been owned by the family for their son since Gaucho was three years old. The family hunted, camped, and packed in the remote backcountry of the Rocky Mountains. It's common to hobble pack horses out overnight to allow them to graze the good mountain grass. One night, a wild animal came through camp, and Gaucho and the rest of his herd scattered. Although the other horses and mules were caught, Gaucho was terrified and unreachable. Eventually, the family's time away was up, and the weather was bad. The family was very sad to leave him behind.
>
> Gaucho ended up being alone in the wilderness for over two years. His hobbles had come off, and he was living on his own. There was plenty of grass and water, but no horse companionship. He was rarely seen, and each time a person tried to catch or capture him, he proved uncatchable.
>
> Eventually, though, he was haltered and rescued from the wilderness. Now, he is a senior horse, and has a kind home where he teaches riding lessons (fig. 14.8). He is still a little tricky to halter in his paddock, but treats and kindness have improved his catchability over the years.
>
>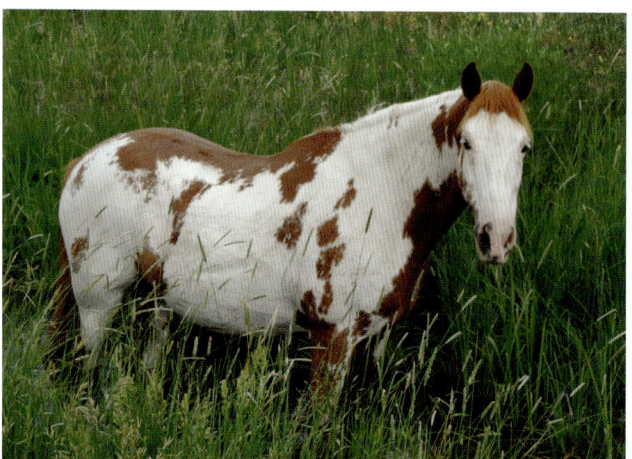
>
> *14.8 Gaucho was lost in the wild for two years before finding his way to a caring new home.*

it while yesterday you could not. Maybe tomorrow you will get it over his nose. Ten or fifteen minutes each day is enough time to achieve success, as long as you make progress.

Halter Training

At all costs, you want to avoid a fight with this horse. He is bigger, stronger, and more agile than a person. Use leverage and patience. Applying pressure to the lead rope sideways is less likely to cause the horse to fight back and panic as he would if straightforward pressure is applied to his poll. Avoid resistance because it can lead to injury to horse and human.

Using a longer (20-foot) lead rope gives you more flexibility to hold the horse's head and at the same time drive his hip forward using his flight drive. Safety first: Keep the lead rope folded, never wrapped or looped around your hand or wrist.

Before the step, take the stand. If you apply a small amount of pressure and your horse travels backward, stay with him, and as soon as he stops running, release the pressure. If he will stand, then work to get him to turn his head toward you. Soon, you will work up to moving his feet.

Apply pressure to the lead rope, wait for him to move a foot, and then release the pressure. Applying pressure sideways and getting him to move sideways is usually much more successful than applying pressure forward. A horse's natural urge to lean back into pressure is strong.

Once you can ask for one foot to consistently move, ask for two. Soon, he will understand. Lead him across the pen for his dinner. Lead him to your treat bucket and reward him. It is harder for him to lead away from the herd or barn, so sweeten the deal with a food reward at the end.

A competent assistant can be helpful in teaching a horse to lead. You may hold the halter and lead rope, while the second person walks behind and encourages forward movement. You can also have a partner lead another herd-mate in front of your horse, and have him follow, building confidence.

Work in a small pen first then as your horse becomes less fearful and more apt to give to pressure, work in a larger enclosed pen. I advise staying in an enclosed area until you are sure that he is unafraid of humans and understands halter cues.

TYING

Some already halter-trained horses may not accept being tied. Even very good horses can have quirks and "not tying" is one of them. They can pull back aggressively, breaking the lead, ties, posts, or halter. You want to make sure you discover this foible in a place where the horse cannot injure himself or any people.

In order for a horse to learn to stand tied, he must first understand the concept of pressure-and-release from a halter. If this seems to be the case for your horse, first test him somewhere safe (i.e. not the cement or asphalt barn aisle). Take him to a stout post in an enclosed area with soft, sandy footing. Mentally prepare him for being tied: A tired horse is ready to stand still and rest, while a fresh horse will want to move. Consider using the Blocker Tie Ring™, which allows the lead rope to slip through and prevents the horse from panicking (fig. 14.9).

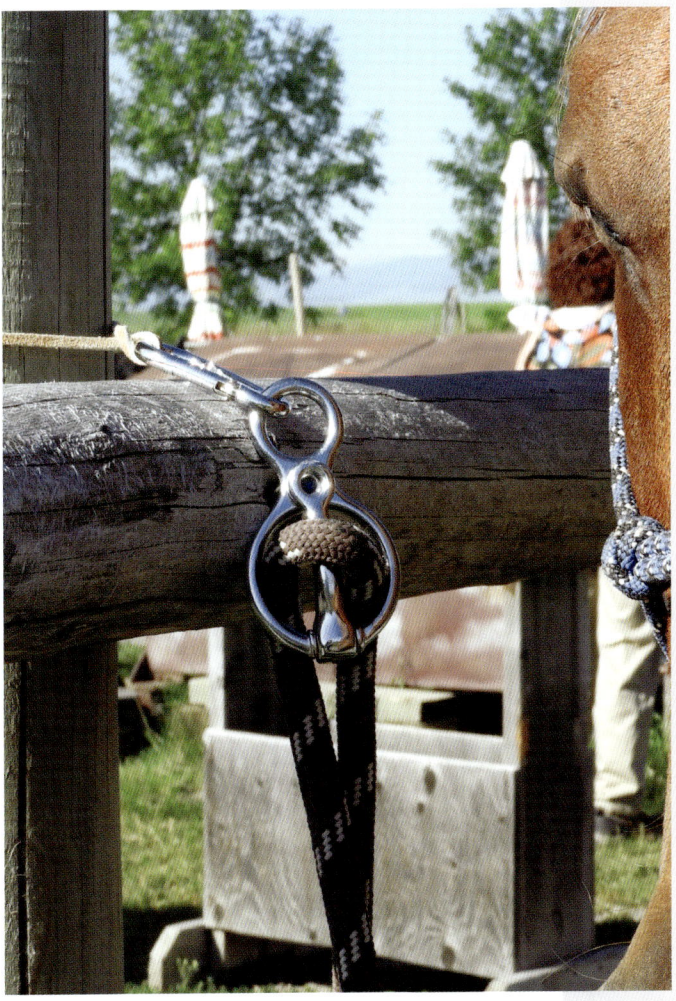

14.9 *A Blocker Tie Ring™. The metal piece in the middle is held by a magnet, and friction pressure holds the horse's lead in place. With no knot tying, the horse is less likely to panic or sustain an injury due to a fast-tied halter knot.*

A horse who doesn't tie is inconvenient, troublesome, embarrassing, and downright dangerous. Remember, your horse must have absolute trust and confidence in you if he is to stand there. By tying him, his natural defense to run is eliminated.

Evaluate the safety of where you tie your horse and what you tie him with. Look for nearby objects that could startle him. Watch for ropes and tack that he could get tangled in. If the object moves, (for example, a jump standard or a wobbly fence) you should not tie a horse to it. If he pulls away and breaks or moves the object, it will "chase" him as he runs, inciting a fear response, and endangering himself and bystanders as he runs around dragging the object. Don't tie your horse with a training halter that has a cable, chain, or additional metal rivets built in to it, as they can cause serious injury.

When beginning, tie him for only a short period of time, and stay with him using positive reinforcement. As he remains comfortable, step away for just a few seconds. Then step back to him, give more positive reinforcement, and untie him. Incrementally increase the amount of time he is expected to stand tied.

THE SICK HORSE

Imagine treating a leg wound on a horse who is starved, not halter trained, and terrified. Health care should be a serious motivator for you to get this horse halter trained as soon as possible.

When a horse is debilitated—for example, a thin horse who also has a severe pneumonia—he will actually be much easier to handle. Sadly, he may not have enough energy to fight. But as I've mentioned before, when his health improves, his attitude may change and he may become more difficult to handle.

When a fearful, active horse requires medical care, options are limited. It is much like wildlife medical care: It is a question of stressing the animal to get near enough to administer medications weighed against the risk of not administering medications. One last-resort option is using a "dart gun" to administer sedation from a distance. Another option for the horse is confining him to a small area and roping him. Roping doesn't leave a pleasant memory for the horse; rather, it is an action that will turn on his fear response and make him less likely to trust humans.

Both the dart gun sedation and the roping require specialized technical skills. Additionally, these options are risky for handlers, and we don't want any humans to get hurt. Remember, this is not a healthy animal. This situation is a choice between stressing the animal and possibly causing more injury or harm, versus the odds that the horse will recover with his own immune system and medications in feed. The horse may continue to be unmanageable, leaving humans to watch helplessly as his health declines.

A CRUCIAL STEP

It is of grave importance that horses be halter trained as soon as possible. While it may be frustrating, time-consuming, and tricky, it is a crucial step toward bonding with your horse and moving forward with health care, training, and a relationship. A horse who is not halter trained is at risk for unnecessary suffering. Halter training an unthrifty adult horse requires a different approach than halter training a healthy, fearful adult horse. Make sure your enclosure and halter are safe and functional. Hiring a trainer to help you may be the best option for your horse in the long run.

CHAPTER 15

Patient Training:
Ground Skills for Medical Care

READINESS REVIEW

Before beginning the tasks in this chapter, make sure you have these baselines:

- Your horse is halter trained and understands pressure-and-release when asked to move forward.
- The halter you have selected fits correctly.
- Your horse allows you to groom him.
- You are able to pick up your horse's feet.

Neglected horses can have a whole host of ailments. Even if your horse seems healthy when you get him, this is no guarantee of future wellness. As we've already discussed, an annual physical examination and vaccines are necessary to maintain health. This chapter focuses on groundwork and handling that is of critical importance to medical care. When you pre-train your horse before veterinary visits, it helps him remain relaxed. This decreases the stress level you both will experience if he gets sick, and will make routine veterinary visits more pleasant for everybody.

If you know your horse is *needle-shy* (fearful of injections), doesn't accept touch in some areas, or has any quirks regarding treatment and handling, tell your veterinarian at the beginning of your appointment.

REVIEWING APPROACH-AND-RETREAT

The *approach-and-retreat* training technique is key for introducing anything new to a horse. You want to approximate the end goal with successive steps closer to it. The first step may not look anything like the final goal, after all it's only the beginning. For example, if you want a horse to walk over a tarp, you could follow this sequence:

1. Leave a folded tarp in his pen or paddock for him to inspect.

2. Move the tarp to your round pen, but not do anything more than move the horse around the perimeter of the pen with the tarp nearby.

3. Start allowing the horse to rest near the tarp when working with him in the round pen.

4. Feed the horse grain or treats in several different areas near and on top of the unfolded tarp.

5. Feed the horse grain or treats while moving and flapping the tarp so he gets used to the sound it makes.
6. Hand-walk the horse in circles around the unfolded tarp, both to the right and to the left.
7. On some of the circles, walk across the corner of the tarp with the horse.
8. Walk the horse all the way across the narrow span of the tarp (some horses will initially jump over it).
9. Walk the horse all the way across the widest length of the tarp.

As your horse develops confidence with each step, you progress to the next. When he balks or shies, go back to the previous step (for example, if he is unnerved walking across the corner of the tarp, make more circles, then walk across a corner again until he improves). The whole process could take minutes or months, depending on the horse.

The key to approach-and-retreat is to watch the horse's expression, how he moves, and where his focus is. All horses will experience new places and be asked to complete new tasks. Working up to each task gradually and positively, results in better long-term compliance and horse happiness.

ADVANCED LEADING SKILLS—TIGHT SPACES AND NEW SITUATIONS

Leading in new situations can be stressful for both the horse and the handler. In rescue, factors such as a short relationship between you and your horse, and illness add to the stress. Some horses have never entered any man-made structures. When they are asked to go into a barn or stall, load in a trailer, go to a hospital, or stand quietly in stocks this may be their first experience with each one of these things (fig. 15.1). It is important to give your horse reassurance and positive reinforcement whenever possible through these tasks. Not only do you want to take care of him today, but you want to set the stage for making future care possible.

As soon as medically possible, your horse should be taught more advanced leading skills. Your rescue horse should not only follow his handler when unafraid, but should also be trained to go forward willingly even in new and scary situations. Horses should be taught a cue to go forward, and have a

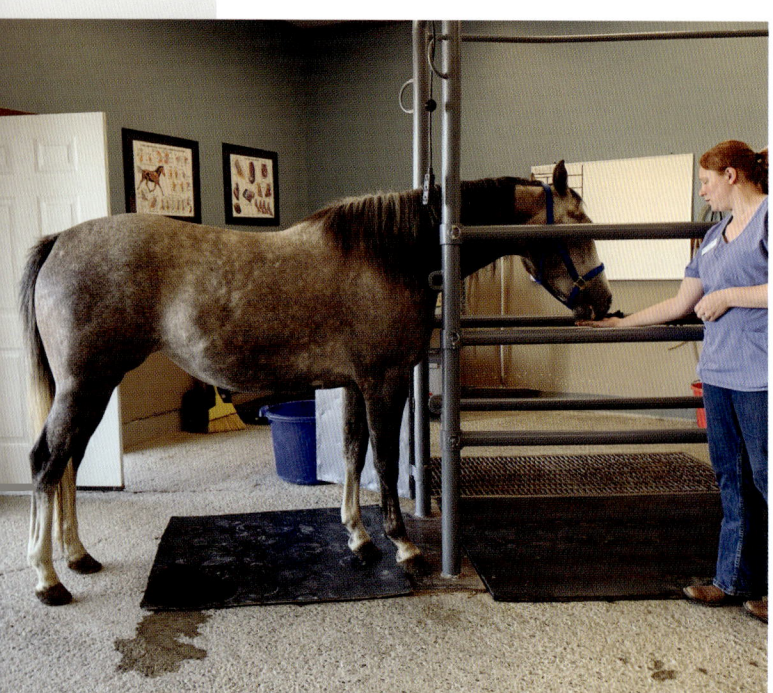

15.1 Angie gives a patient positive reinforcement while this horse is led into the stocks.

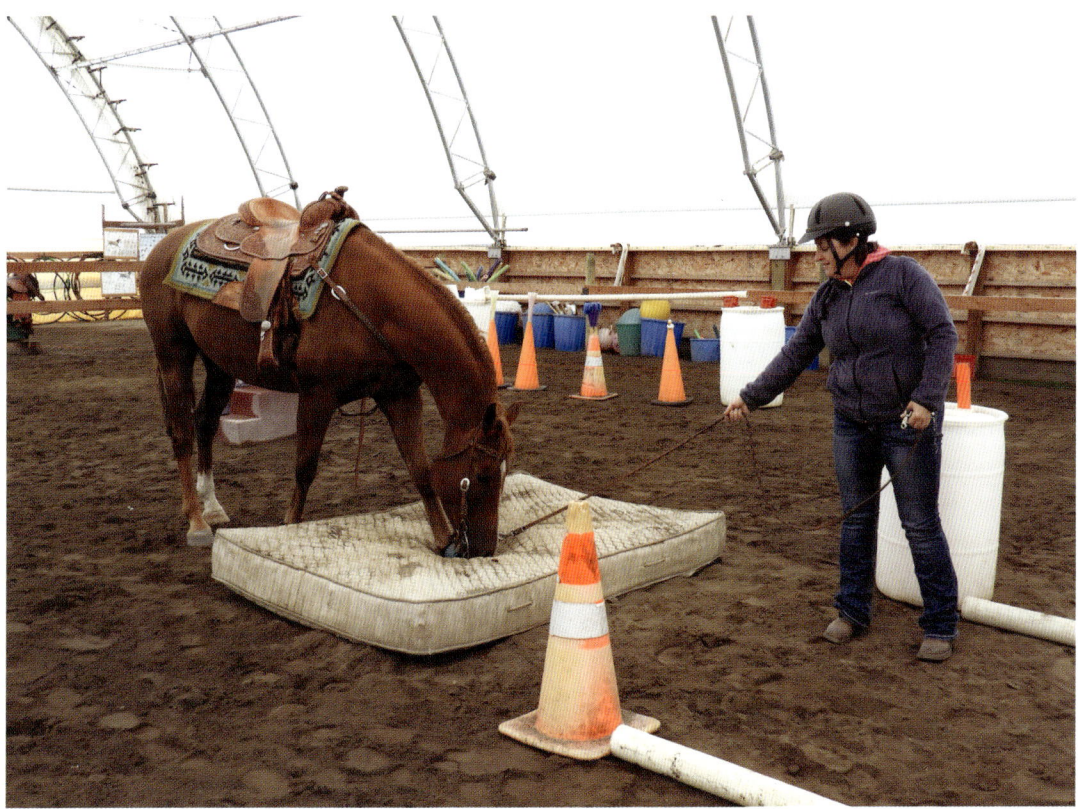

15.2 *Spicy evaluates new footing by pawing and sniffing it.*

consistent and trusting response to it. The cue should include a sound (cluck) and a physical cue (pressure on the halter).

Thinking About His Options

It is difficult for horses to enter buildings or transition to new surroundings because their eyes do not perceive their surroundings the way our eyes do (see p. 155). Confined spaces limit the horse's running defense. He is putting his life in your hands—a responsibility that you should not take lightly.

You should have an excellent understanding of when a horse is considering his options and is thinking about doing what you ask. If a horse is licking, sniffing, inspecting the ground or trailer floor, or pawing the difference in footing, he is showing you he is thinking about his options and checking them out for safety (fig. 15.2). This is the time to be patient and reward your rescue horse for his effort. Remember, you don't know his whole story or what previous bad experiences he has had. Be patient, and the trust you have developed with him will help him be brave and go forward.

If, during the thinking process of going forward, the horse's brain is disrupted by pushing him too hard or too fast, this is the moment when he will balk. When he balks, he may stand still, raise his head, evade the entrance by going sideways, or back up. If he is struck, his worry may intensify to fear.

Rushed—A Leading Story

Starlight was a yearling and Jeannette had raised her from a foal. Starlight had never left the farm, but now she was sick, and had to visit the veterinary hospital.

The hospital was being remodeled and was under construction. Starlight was unloaded from the trailer, and Jeannette walked her right up to the big, metal garage door, which then suddenly began to move and make noise as the door opened. The filly flinched, but then went forward over a drain grate, raising her feet high as she tentatively stepped onto the new footing inside.

Within 20 yards of entering the strange new place, a door to a mechanical closet swung open, missing her by only a few inches. She flinched again, but continued to go forward as asked.

As Starlight moved apace her fast-walking handler, another door opened and a human with a flapping white coat came bursting out of it in front of her, bustling off to some critical task. Starlight jumped in earnest and hesitated momentarily.

Jeannette gave the halter a tug, and led Starlight around the corner to the scales to weigh her. Jeannette began to pull hard on the lead rope as Starlight made a U-turn in the hallway to approach the new footing over the scale. The scales had a slight movement underneath the filly's feet and a large bar bordering the edge that prevented escape. Veterinary students and staff were surrounding her. Starlight stepped obediently forward onto the scales, and stood while her weight was recorded, although she was trembling. Starlight was then whisked forward and around the corner where she high-stepped across another drain into a room that had stocks. She had not been reassured or allowed to think at any single moment or obstacle along the way.

I thought this young horse had handled herself exceptionally well. She had respected the space of all of the humans around her and had continued to go forward. Jeanette had begun to tug on Starlight as the filly finally started to decide that going forward wasn't resulting in fewer scary experiences. Starlight balked at the stocks and planted her feet.

I was able to slow the scene down a little bit by asking Jeannette to fill out some paperwork while I held the filly. Meanwhile, I allowed Starlight to sniff the stocks and inspect the floor. She cautiously stepped forward a little bit at a time, and was finally in. After a few minutes of petting, Starlight was calmer, and the doors of the stocks were closed in front of and behind her.

We don't want to unintentionally reward a fear response in a horse. In this instance, Starlight needed a bit of reassurance that the hospital house of horrors was going to be okay. She needed time to slow down and think for herself. The first experience a horse has cements in his memories for an incredibly long time, and you don't want that experience to be frightening.

You are less likely to get him into the trailer or stocks today. If you do succeed but the experience is unpleasant, you will be less likely to get him to enter that area again on another day. Being patient may seem difficult and time-consuming, but in the long run it will result in a more compliant horse, saving you time and hassle later.

Reward the tiniest effort—the look, the sniff, the one-inch foot movement forward. When a horse is presented with a new obstacle, he instinctively wants to please. Give him the chance to do so by allowing him to explore his environment and think about his decisions.

Advanced Leading Skills

When you walk with your horse, you don't want him too far in front or too far behind you. You want to be right at the throatlatch area, where his head and neck intersect.

Because of tradition, horses are most comfortable being led from the left. Get your horse comfortable with being handled from his right as well. Work on the following exercises:

- Lead in a tight figure-eight pattern.
- Lead him at the trot as well as the walk.
- Turn and face him, asking him to back up.
- Lead him away from the herd or barn, both with a companion horse and alone.
- Take him over new obstacles, such as ground poles, logs, or tarps.
- Lead him up and down hills.
- Work over new footing: in gravel, in grass, over bare dirt or sand, and over asphalt.

Spend five minutes each day leading him in new places and new ways. Testing and expanding your handling skills will also carry over to leadership when riding. He should trust you, so that even if he looks or snorts at the new sights, he is willing to go forward.

Small Spaces

Trailers: Consider that your horse may have a strong fear memory associated with the trailer. If he was gathered as a Mustang, then run through a chute system away from his herd and family and into a trailer, his first trailering experience was probably terrifying, so it will be challenging to work around that memory. Another scenario to consider is the weak horse who had to be transported while down or fell while traveling. He may now be physically stronger, but he will remember how afraid he was, lying helpless in a noisy, moving trailer.

There are scores of articles, numerous books, and countless trainers who work to address the "trailer-loading" problem. Having watched many people with horses getting in and out of trailers coming and going from the veterinary hospital, I have observed some common themes. The following three rules will help horses be compliant while trailering:

First, allow the horse to inspect the floor and give him a moment for his eyes to adjust to the change in light when loading him in the trailer.

Second, always reward the horse when he gets in.

Third, allow him to ride comfortably, keeping in mind that each horse is an individual. If a horse is unable to relax in the trailer, he may be reluctant to enter it.

These rules may not solve 100 percent of trailering problems, but they go a long way to helping equine obedience when trailering.

Training Horses That Don't Know How to Load: You will need to guide your horse into the trailer, which you will not be able to effectively do unless he is halter trained. He will need to lead forward willingly and back up. The approach outlined below for trailer training is incremental. Prepare yourself to take time to do this. While some horses are naturally compliant and learn quickly, fearful horses could take months to learn properly.

Don't travel with your horse until he has a BCS of 4 or more. If he has a BCS of 3, he will build muscle as he learns to step in and out of the trailer. He will need that muscle and higher BCS of 4 to balance comfortably when the trailer moves. Stressful loading and a long ride could completely exhaust a thin, weakened horse.

Eliminate the Fear Factor: Your first step is to make sure your horse feels comfortable in the trailer. Positive reinforcement is critical for this. Think again about Pavlov's experiment where dogs were taught that ringing a bell meant that food would appear (p. 160). The dogs salivated as soon as the bell rang, whether or not they could see the food. This is a response that became innate, or hard-wired in the dogs' brains. This is the response you want to create for your horse in the trailer.

Begin by parking the trailer where the horse can access its entry point. Do the best you can to keep it safe. You also want to be able to access him. If you park your trailer in the field with your horse, he may be fine or he may eat your trailer lights and wires and lacerate his leg on the coupler in the front. It often works best to back the trailer to the gate, and then safely latch the gate to the trailer, so he only has access to the trailer entry. Your horse needs to be able to inspect the footing or enter the trailer, but not necessarily access any other part of it. Each trailer and pen or paddock will have a different setup, but your goal is always to make it as safe as possible.

Feed your horse near the trailer for a few days to a week. Then, begin putting his ration just inside the trailer on the floor. He will need to eat while standing outside, just putting his mouth and head inside to eat. When his head is in the trailer, his view of the outside world around him is limited.

Next, as he remains comfortable, put the food nearer and nearer the front of the trailer. At first, he may extend his head and neck to grab each bite. Then, he will be eating with one foot in, then two, and eventually all four legs and his entire body.

Teach Him Unloading First: Once he begins stepping in the trailer, you should start feeding him in it with his halter on. This is because at some point, most horses need help to back out of the trailer, especially one that is designed where they cannot turn around (such as a two-horse straight-load). Trailer unloading can be a source of stress for a horse. Because of the trailer design, he may not be able to observe his new surroundings as he backs out of it, and the footing feels new and unexpected.

Horses carry more weight on their front legs, so backing a horse out of the trailer is usually safer and more stable than unloading forward. When a horse unloads front-end first, he is more likely to slip on his hind end as he exits the trailer. However, if he has an injury or there is a problem, you want your horse to be willing and able to exit the trailer in whatever way he is asked. A few horses learn to fly dangerously backward out of the trailer and do better with the front end unloading first.

The first time your horse unloads forward he may leap out of the trailer. Make sure the footing is good, stay out of his way, and allow him to use his head for balance and choose where he puts his feet. Reward him when he achieves success.

Previous experience of half-loading and half-unloading himself, as he had to do when he was fed in the trailer, smooths the backward-unloading experience. He has had the time to think about how to get himself in and out of the trailer without a person getting in the way.

Nonetheless, the first few times he is asked to back out, he may get "stuck" at the back of the trailer with one leg going out, swiping at the ground, and then getting right back in. If you can park your trailer in such a way that it is more level with the ground (such as backing up to a hill), this will help alleviate the problem. If the ground is slick, his leg could slip underneath, so make sure the footing is good, especially in the beginning of training. Again, after you get him unloaded, give him lots of rewards. As he develops confidence and coordination, he will be able to unload in less-perfect circumstances without trouble.

Ninety percent of the trailer loading work is complete—your horse is now unafraid and knows how to unload. Continue feeding him in the trailer, but ask him to get in. Depending on your setup and comfort level, you may hand-walk or cue him to send him in to his eating (and traveling) place. All you are doing is adding a cue to the action he is already anticipating. Another step is to start closing him in with the divider or trailer door during his meal. Don't leave him in too long—you don't want him to become anxious.

Drive On: Once you have a horse who loads, he needs to learn to travel. It is helpful to have a well-seasoned buddy horse travel with him. Load the buddy first then load your horse into his spot. Give him a positive reward. Start the truck. Give him another positive reward. Ever so gently, roll the trailer forward a few feet and stop. Most horses will startle or stumble. Repeat this step several times, until he is more stable and not fearful. Reward him, allow him to stand and eat in the stable, non-moving trailer for a few minutes, and then unload both horses and leave the lesson.

If this goes well, transition to driving 5 or 10 slow and cautious miles and returning home. Short trips prepare him to balance himself when the vehicle starts forward, turns, or brakes. Each horse is different, so you will need to gauge his comfort level by observing how he acts. If all is well, he is ready for longer trips. Shorter trips also prepare a horse's muscles, so he will have better fitness for longer rides.

Finally, make your horse's trailer-loading and traveling skills solid by practicing in a variety of trailer types and in all conditions. He should load when it is dark, raining, snowing, and when the wind is blowing. If a natural disaster or emergency occurs, your horse is ready to be rescued once again. It's easier to load a horse if he enters the trailer while it is oriented toward the barn or herd, but make sure that he can load when it is faced away from his home as well.

Some horses continue to have anxiety about the trailer despite practice and training. Two common causes for this are: first, the way they are facing, and second, their feelings in an enclosed area. Some individual horses simply don't like to ride facing forward and will kick the trailer while in it, stomp around, or be hesitant about loading. The reason they don't like to face forward is unclear. They may not feel stable or balanced, or perhaps it is because they cannot see out. The feeding process can reduce the anxiety of this type of horse to some extent, but allowing him to choose his position in the trailer or to ride backward can help. Whatever the reason, I've known several clients that have a horse that stopped kicking the trailer wall and started loading much more willingly when they were shipped facing backward. A few horses seem to be claustrophobic, and you may need to haul this type of horse in a trailer with more room or an open configuration to help him feel comfortable.

Entering the Hospital Environment: Compared to trailering, entering the hospital environment is simple, but still worth thinking about. Prepare your horse by making sure he trusts you, and lead him over new footing and in many environments. Know that the hospital has many sights, sounds, and odors he will take in. You may not be aware of some of the things he can hear and smell. If he is a horse who has been in an open field or range and has not entered buildings, you need to work to get him accustomed to entering a barn and stall.

Entering and Being Restrained in Stocks: Stocks are made for keeping humans safe while performing mildly to moderately uncomfortable or noxious procedures on horses. For example, a horse who moves his feet to escape having blood drawn may stand perfectly contentedly in the stocks. If, however, a horse tries to exit the stocks by jumping over them, kicking, lying down or falling over, he can sustain serious, life-threatening injuries. Make sure your horse is trained to enter and exit confidently and quietly.

Stocks sometimes have a change in footing underneath them, such as rubber mats. Stocks also are confining. Most horses will hesitate and need to inspect the stocks before going forward into them.

The key is to convince a horse that stocks are safe. He must be allowed to sniff the sides and floor, to explore what is there, and to paw or step cautiously on to the new footing. Once he goes in, give him positive reinforcement. You may also allow him to walk forward and out. Show him that this is no big deal.

When he is reasonably confident walking through the stocks, have him pause and stand in the stocks without shutting the doors. Feed him some alfalfa cubes or treats for a few seconds after he stands there. Ask him to walk out. Then walk him back in, and shut the doors. The doors may be out of his visual range, so he will not know or understand that they are shut until he bumps them with his chest and rump. You want him to be calm so he doesn't panic when this happens.

If a horse has a nervous nature or is prone to panic, your veterinarian may sedate him *before* asking him to enter the stocks. Once he is in with the gates shut, feed him carrots, cookies, or grain to help establish a hard-wired response: stocks equal yummy food. If you hard-wire a different response (stocks equal painful procedure), you will have a tough time getting him to go in.

PHYSICAL EXAMINATION

Once you have your horse in the veterinary clinic, here is what you can expect for a basic physical examination:[164]

- An overall appraisal (evaluation of body condition, conformation, asymmetry, and distribution of fat or muscle)
- Taking a rectal temperature
- Using a stethoscope to listen to his heart, lungs, and gut sounds
- Evaluation of gums and teeth
- Evaluation of eyes and ears
- Touching the horse's skin and body, including under the belly
- Assessing limbs and digital pulses, including picking up his feet and palpating the tendons, ligaments, and joints of his legs.

Your horse will need to tolerate a complete stranger looking over his whole body while he stands still for about five minutes. When he will let you practice an examination, see if he will let a confident, kind friend do one as well. It's also good to know your horse's vitals when he is healthy. It's good horsemanship to work on all of this at home in advance.

As you work on specific tasks, you may find difficulties. Communicate this to your veterinarian. For example, "Hey, doc, I've been working with him trusting me around his tail, so be careful when you take his temperature." If you have never taken your horse's temperature, and he decides to kick, both your horse and your veterinarian are going to wind up feeling a little resentful. He won't like a complete stranger "violating" him, and veterinarians definitely don't like being kicked.

Physical Touch

When you mime a physical examination with your horse, you want to approximate each training goal. Test your horse: Does he stand still? Will he let you touch his whole body, including his flanks, his belly, and lifting or handling his tail? He should stand still a second longer, and let you touch more of his body. Work gradually, kindly, slowly, and make it a positive experience. Pet or rub him gently in an area he enjoys, working gradually to more sensitive areas. Rub his head and face all over. Touch his ears. Give him an occasional treat for positive reinforcement to let him know he is doing well.

Evaluating Gums

Here are some steps to examine your horse's gums: Hold the lead rope in your left hand. Slowly and gently, put your right hand on the bridge of your horse's nose. Then move your thumb to the corner of his mouth. If he accepts this, use your thumb to gently lift his upper lip and touch his gums. If you can only touch the bridge of his nose and lip, but not lift it, calmly reassure him and work on the task every day. As he allows more touch, praise him often.

Rectal Temperature

If you need to work on desensitizing your

horse to taking a rectal temperature, have an assistant hold your horse for you. For safety, both of you should be on the same side of the horse. Start by touching your horse's shoulder or withers with your left hand, while you hold your thermometer with your right. Maintain firm, but gentle contact with him as you move toward his rump. Gently touch his tail with your left hand, and slowly lift it. Stay to the side of your horse, in as safe a spot as possible.

If your horse's tail is tight and tense, then stop and work only to this step for several days or weeks until your horse is more relaxed and comfortable. Don't suddenly grab his tail or surprise him with your touch.

The next step is the tricky part: inserting the thermometer. What I have found works quite well is to touch the horse with the thermometer on the muscles of the rump, and then maintain contact as you slide it over to his anus.

With any portion of your physical examination practice, as soon as your horse tells you that he is uncomfortable or nervous, back up to the previous step, reassure and reward him, and try again. Continue to apply approach-and-retreat techniques paired with positive reinforcement, and work your way closer to the final step.

Nervous Nellies

If your horse is nervous or energetic, don't pick a fight. Instead, do a moving workout with him first. Your horse will find it much easier to stand still for examination if he is a bit tired. Give your horse the opportunity to do the right thing, and begin with post-workout grooming. If he is still not interested in standing, do some more groundwork, working more excessive energy out.

Companionship for Reassurance

Another factor to help your horse stay calm during veterinary visits is to have a buddy for reassurance. If your horse is anxious away from the herd or from his best horsey friend, then work on training for examination with the friend present. Although you also want to teach him that there is no need for anxiety when away from his herd, you can only train one thing at a time. Train the buddy-sour problem differently, and apart from training for physical examination. In fact, social isolation trumps pain, and a horse is more likely to show a response to isolation than to pain when both occur at the same time.[165]

This all boils down to your horse trusting you. Your horse could be traumatized if he is scared, in a new environment and not feeling well, but you can improve his experience with your veterinarian if you practice acceptance of touch and physical examinations at home.

ORAL MEDICATIONS

You may need to administer medications to your sick horse. Most courses of treatment are once or twice daily, and may be from five days to the lifetime of the horse. At the very minimum, your horse will need periodic deworming throughout his life.

Medications are available in a variety of forms. Some drugs are made into small tablets or flavored powder that can be fed to the horse as a top-dressing on his grain ration. Others are formulated as a paste, or come as tablets that can be soaked in water to make a paste. If you have to soak these medications yourself, adding a bit of corn syrup (for example, Karo) can help sweeten the mixture. Don't use molasses because it can absorb or inactivate some drugs.

To administer paste to your horse, you've already built the foundation: he accepts your hand on the bridge of his nose and lifting his lip with your thumb. The transition to administration of oral medication or deworming paste is a step or two from there.

Start by standing beside your horse. Although horses are more comfortable with us on their left side, a horse who has had a bad experience or learned to avoid medications coming from the left might have better behavior if you start on his right. If your horse resists or you don't feel comfortable, test both sides and start with the side that seems less challenging.

Positive reinforcement enhances compliance, "A spoonful of sugar makes the medicine go down." One way to achieve this is to practice with a delicious treat, like applesauce. You can rinse and refill oral dosing syringes or dewormer tubes with applesauce. Use these yummy treats in combination with approach-and-retreat to perfect your skills and your horse's compliance.

You may use one hand to either hold your horse's halter or you may cradle his head keeping a hand over the bridge of his nose. Use your other hand to touch the side of your horse's face with the tube of medication, rather than your thumb. Move the tube to the horse's lips, and then gently use it to part his lips, and put the tube in the gap between his teeth—over the bars (fig. 15.3). Push the plunger and give the medication. You may need to hold your horse's nose up to ensure that he swallows rather than spits the medication out. Last, but not least, reward the horse with lots of "good boys" and petting.

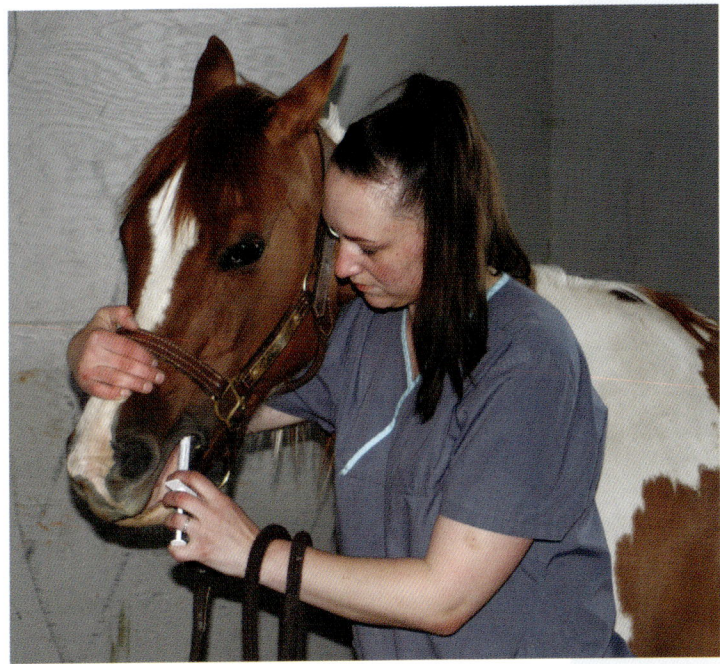

15.3 *Crystal, a veterinary technician, administers oral medication to a pony.*

INJECTION TRAINING

Routine healthcare for horses includes vaccines, which are usually injected into the muscle (intramuscular, or IM). Some vaccines for respiratory diseases such as influenza or strangles are administered into a nostril (intranasal, IN). Finally, your horse may receive sedation or medication in the vein (intravenous, IV) or have blood drawn for diagnostic testing. Every horse should, and will, receive injections in his life.

Most of the time, injections are routine and should result in no harm to the horse. Some horses experience mild muscle pain or swelling for a day or two after they have received an IM injection.

The most commonly used and accessible vessel for IV drug administration is the jugular vein in the horse's neck. The carotid

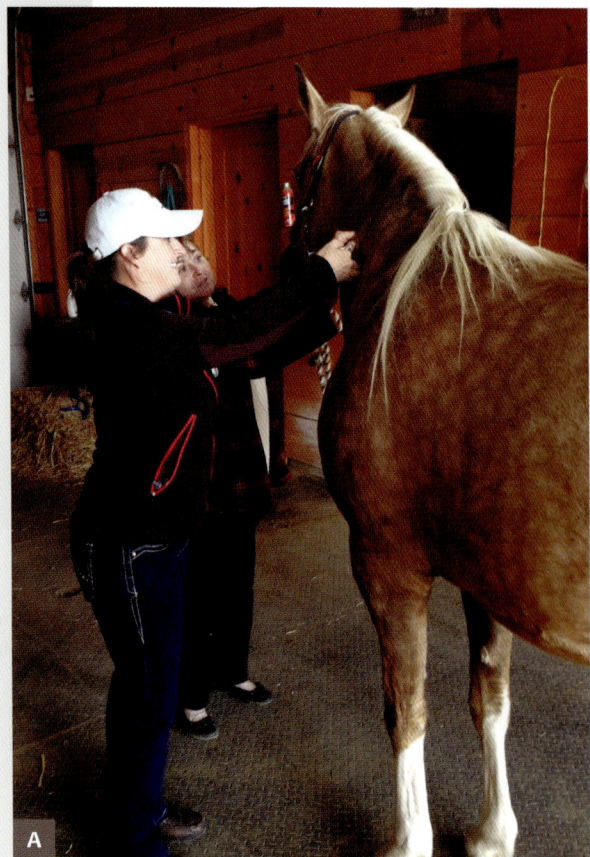 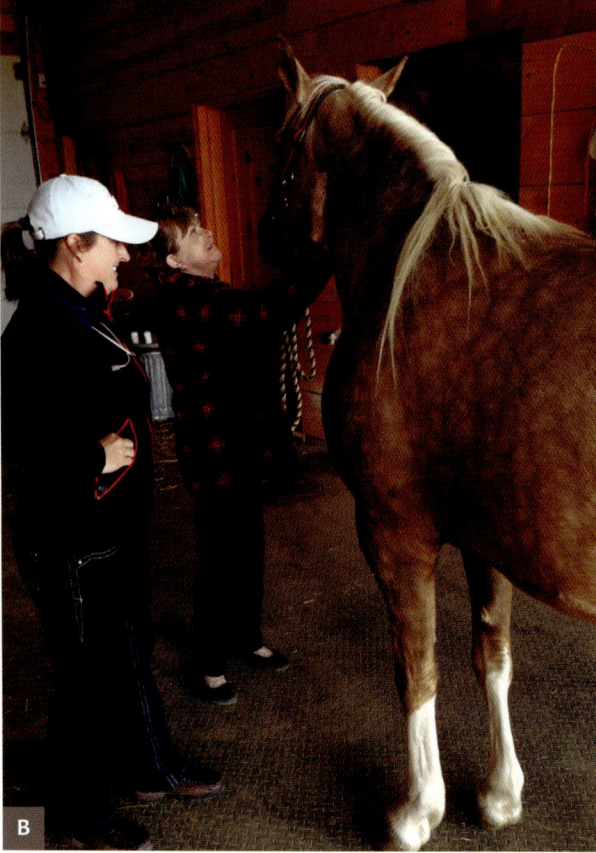

15.4 A & B *I administer a vaccine in a horse's neck muscle (A) and the owner automatically gives her horse positive reinforcement with petting and kind words (B). This keeps the experience as pleasant as possible for her horse, so that we will be able to easily administer vaccines again next year.*

artery is underneath (deep to) the jugular vein, and this anatomy can result in the rare adverse event of injecting medication into the artery instead of the vein. Generally, the horse will survive, although he will fall over, paddling in seizure-like activity. When it subsides, the horse may lie anesthetized for about half an hour. When a horse misbehaves to avoid an injection—he may shake his head, tighten his neck muscles, and dance around trying to avoid the needle—it is more likely that your veterinarian will need to try that injection more than once and more likely that an adverse event will occur.

This is why training the horse and familiarizing him in these areas of treatment is crucial.

As the forgiving and people-pleasing creatures that they are, many horses allow us to treat them as unfeeling pincushions. But they are exquisitely intelligent and know exactly what is coming. Have you ever seen them twitch a fly off? If they can feel that fly, they can definitely feel that needle.

If a horse has never been injected, using grain as a distraction can be helpful. After the injection has been given, reward the horse and rub, scratch, or pet the area that received the needle stick. Even if a horse accepts injections with no objection, I strongly advocate that he should receive petting and scratching along with a treat after every injection (figs. 15.4 A & B).

Retraining Needle-Shy Horses

Needle-shy horses have a strong fear and avoidance response to needles and injections. When they weigh 1,200 pounds and they don't want to accept something, it is about impossible to coerce them into it. They are dangerous to their handlers, and may also injure themselves.

Some horses become nervous as soon as they see the syringe. People use all kinds of tactics for these horses, including hiding the syringe and covering the horse's eye so he won't see the person with a needle and syringe. The horse may interpret this as a cue—his eye is only ever covered when an injection is about to occur.[166]

There are many strategies that can work to inject a needle-shy horse. Success may be achieved by approaching the horse without the needle and syringe and petting him and reassuring him first. Then, for some horses, the twitch can be applied. Horses that flinch and balk when injected with the smallest of needles don't seem to feel it when they have circulating endorphins from the twitch.

For horses that are moving their feet or running away as an escape mechanism, putting them into the stocks for the injection may be all that is necessary for them to quietly accept the needle stick.

As I said earlier, even if his behavior wasn't perfect, the horse should be overloaded with reward after the injection. It's not just about rewarding behavior, it's also about making the overall experience more positive for your horse.

Desensitize Your Horse to Injections—Long-Term Training

Long-term desensitization training is needed for your horse if he is fearful of being injected. You want to apply enough stress so you can get close each time, but less stress than it would take for the horse to move his feet. Retrain or desensitize him on both the left and right sides of his neck.

Hold a syringe and needle and positively reinforce standing still—that is, as long as his feet aren't moving, give him food or pet him. This step alone may take several weeks to accomplish. Next, ensure that he accepts being touched on the muscular region of the neck where injections are administered. It is even better if he will accept mildly noxious stimuli, like a poke with your finger or a pinch. It works like this: rub, rub, pet, pet, poke, treat, rub, rub, pet, pet, pinch, treat.

Progress through all the steps of an injection using approach-and-retreat tactics, and stop and reward the horse often. Hold the needle and syringe in your hand, and perform the rubbing, petting, poking, and pinching routine from above.

Once a real injection is administered, it is critical to reward the horse with positive reinforcement afterward and to continue with the rubbing, petting, and poking or pinching as above. Don't end the handling or training session right after sticking him, because the last thing that occurred will be the thing that he remembers the most. It's hard to re-train these horses. One horse I worked with took five years to have a different (and safer) response, although she improved incrementally throughout that period.

When working on a needle-shy horse, the first injection can be sedation drugs in the muscle. These drugs also blunt the pain response. Then, I can administer the necessary vaccines or draw blood for testing. It is not ideal to use this for the lifetime of a horse, but I also want to make the experience as positive as possible. He will need veterinary care with routine injections for the rest of his life. We are setting your horse up for 20 more years of either success or stress and fear.

Your job as a horse owner is to prepare your horse for injections in advance, and when your veterinarian is there, reassure your horse. Make sure you administer positive reinforcement, and your horse's forgiveness and patience doesn't go unrewarded.

Preparation for Intranasal Treatments

There is one last piece of training that will help your horse accept intranasal vaccines as well as when a tube needs to be passed through his nose and into his stomach (commonly used to treat colic). To prepare him, make sure you can touch his nose and just inside his sensitive nostrils.

You already have the foundation for this: Start with a hand on the bridge of his nose, with your thumb near his nostril. If you can do this, work up to him allowing you to touch the inside of his nostril. It's not necessary to poke your finger too far up his nose, you just want him to accept being touched in this sensitive area. It is impossible to make up for the fact that the nose cannula with the vaccine or the stomach tube is uncomfortable. But, we can make the horse think that usually we are going to touch his nostril, and then he will get a cookie.

BUILDING TOWARD HEALTH WITH A RESPECTFUL HORSE

As a veterinarian, I prefer to be presented with a well-mannered patient. As a horse person, I have found that the busy hospital environment is scary for my patients and their people. A caring approach, positive reinforcement, and a respectful horse make any procedure less stressful.

It is important for your horse to lead confidently into new places, including the tight quarters of the stocks or a trailer. He should accept all aspects of the physical examination, including taking his temperature rectally, and he should accept injections. A needle-shy horse can be a serious danger to people. While an exhaustive training methodology is outside the scope of this book, you should know what to expect from a veterinary visit. More importantly, preparatory training at home will allow us to work as a team to maximize our capacity to heal your equine companion in an efficient and successful way.

CHAPTER 16

Getting Going:
Groundwork

READINESS REVIEW

Before beginning the tasks in this chapter, make sure these baseline skills are solid:

- Halter training is refined, and the horse leads readily in a variety of places and conditions.
- Allows you to groom him and pick up all four feet.
- Is desensitized to a variety of objects.
- Is comfortable socially.
- Has a BCS of 4 or more, and otherwise has a clean bill of health.

The strict definition of groundwork is handling a horse while he is not being ridden. Whatever period of time you have had your rescue horse, you have already been doing groundwork. The more you both work together, the more understanding you'll develop. In this chapter, I will address groundwork as it is used in preparation for riding. Your goals are to strengthen your relationship, establish your leadership (and, therefore, his trust), and build your horse's muscle and fitness in preparation for riding. You will also introduce him to tack. Before you reach this stage, you may have owned this horse for two weeks, two months, or two years.

SAFETY FIRST

Safety in horse work and training is critical. As you start this more intensive training period, if you must be alone when working with your horse, set up safety checks. For example, phone a trusted friend when you start, and set a time to call her back. Set a timer for yourself and stick with it. If your friend doesn't hear from you, she knows to search for you. Let your friend know where you are, especially when leaving home.

Even if you don't have access to a small area, it may be feasible to start working your horse using a longe line (pronounced *lunge*). A longe line is longer than a regular lead rope (20 to 30 feet in length). Fold the excess line; don't loop it. Soft, round material is safest. I know somebody who lost a finger when her horse zipped away and rapidly pulled a flat nylon line through her hand!

A capable assistant at a few critical steps is helpful. Continue to read your horse and pay attention to what he is telling you as communication between the two of you is the primary factor in staying safe.

If you don't feel confident about your skills, work with a trainer or professional who has experience starting rescue horses. A well-trained horse is more likely to retain a permanent home, so work to get your horse trained, even if it means seeking outside assistance (fig. 16.1).

HEALTH STATUS OF THE HORSE

A horse is not healthy enough for groundwork until he has a BCS of at least 4, as prior to that time, he is too weak and lacks muscle necessary for athleticism. A starved horse's body metabolized his fat stores for energy, and used up muscle in the process known as *muscle wasting*.

There are instances where athletic horses have a BCS of 4 and are under saddle and ridden. I don't recommend this for rescue horses. There is a significant difference between an extreme athlete that can hardly eat enough (think endurance horses, racehorses, upper-level eventers, and Michael Phelps) and a malnourished individual that is finally on his way out of a metabolic vortex (think neglected horses and refugees). A horse with a BCS of 4 that is gaining weight is healthy enough to be trained how to carry a saddle, but not a rider quite yet.

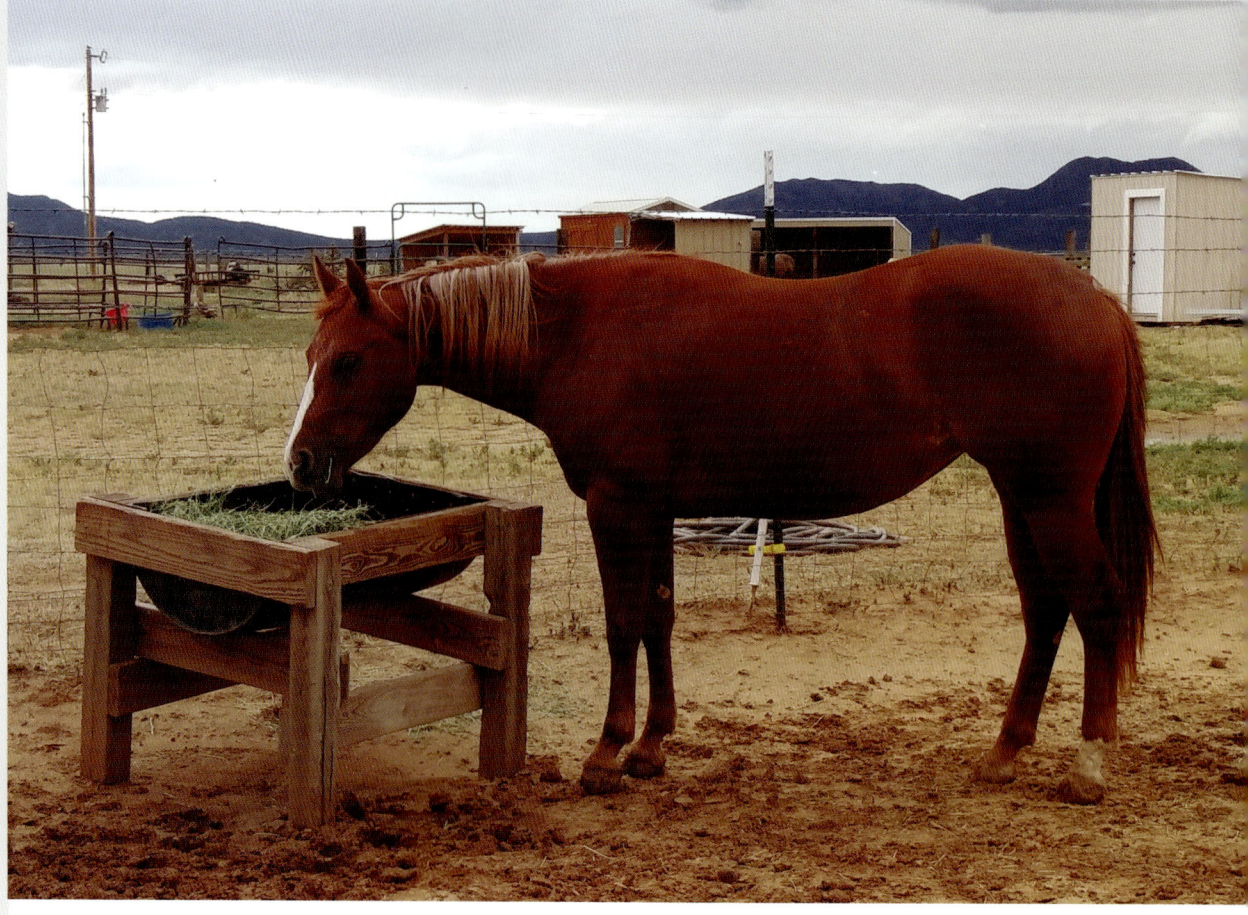

16.1 Here is the orphaned foal you saw in fig. 7.17 as a two-year-old (see p. 114). In this photo she is healthy and ready to start work.

If your rescue horse had foot problems, make sure they are completely resolved. You wouldn't go on a 10-mile hike in high heels; he should not be expected to do proper work or learn if his foot conformation is unbalanced or painful.

Asking your horse to progress through groundwork is critical for his mental training as well as his physical fitness and muscle building (figs. 16.2 A & B). When you prepare him for riding, you are either checking his previous level of training or training him from the beginning. In either case, going through each step is important. If he had previous training, groundwork will increase his fitness, polish your communication with each other, and expose any gaps in his knowledge.

Progressing through groundwork prepares his muscles, tendons, and ligaments for more exercise and riding. Through gradual strengthening, these tissues are protected from injury. This time period also serves as a soundness trial. If he is unable to remain sound during this phase, he will not hold up to riding. If you observe lameness, call your veterinarian.

Considerations of the Mental Status of the Horse

Before starting his training, your horse should be comfortable socially. Each rescue horse's exercise and groundwork program should be individually tailored, focusing on the areas where he needs the most help. For the most part, working with this horse as if he were an untrained two-year-old is a good idea. His response will set the pace of your training.

An abused horse needs patience during his training time to recuperate and come

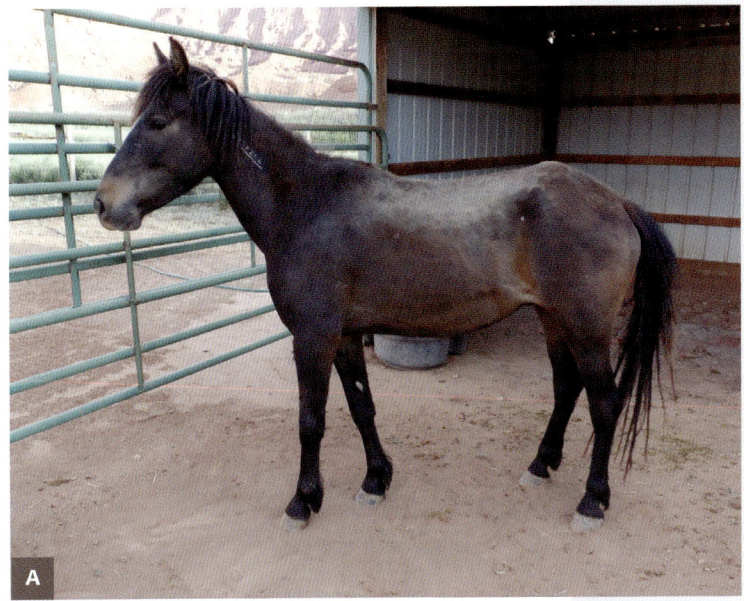

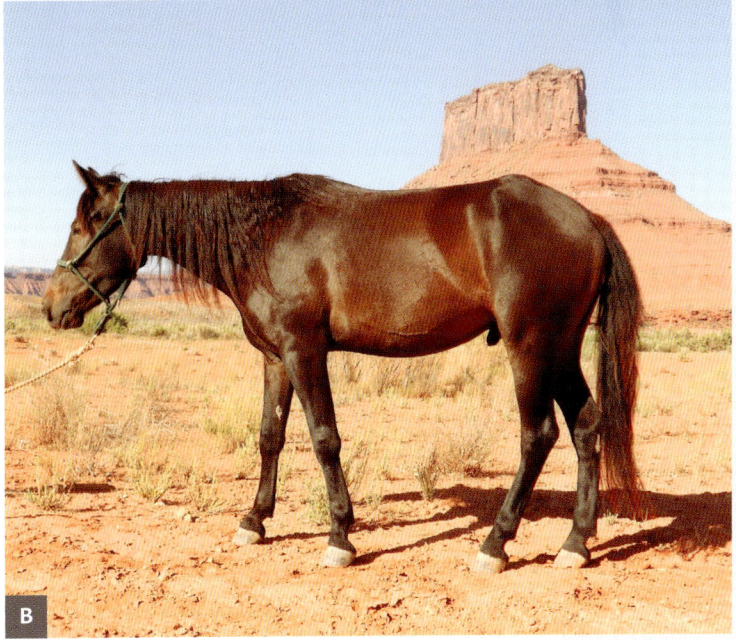

16.2 A & B This thin Mustang soon after acquisition is not ready for intense training (A). The same horse with 90 days of weight gain. It is reasonable to start groundwork with this horse, but he is not yet ready to ride.

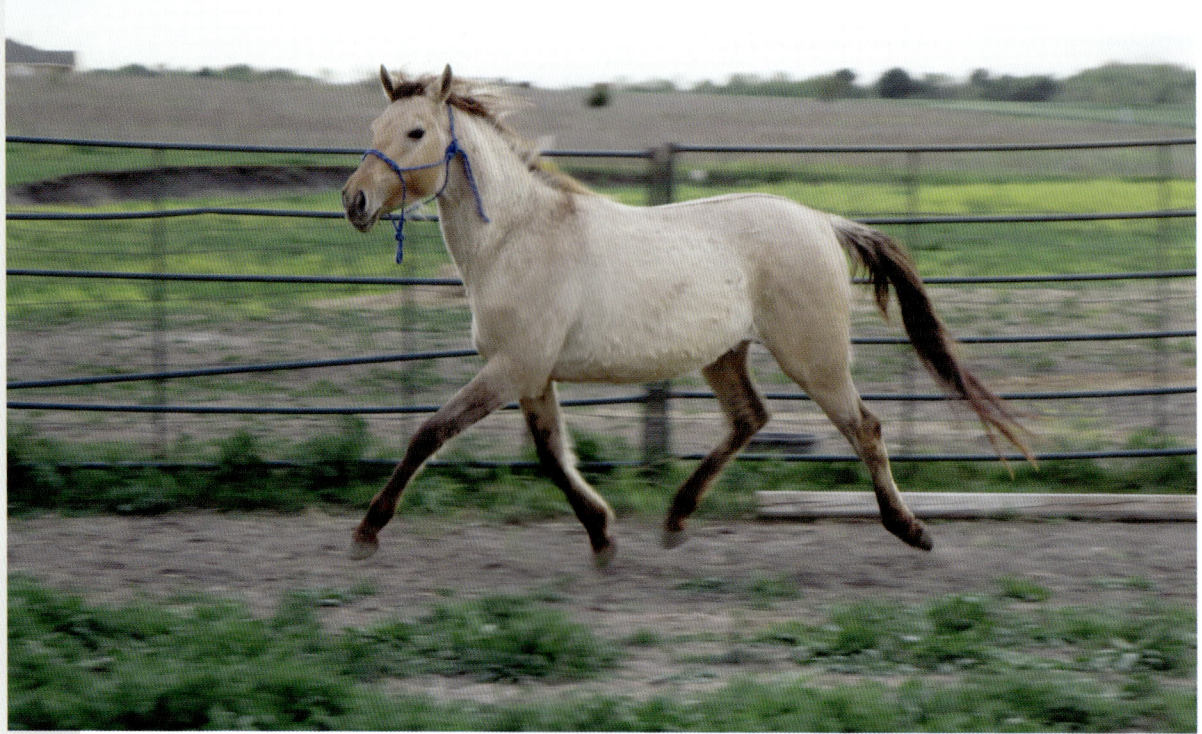

16.3 *This rehabilitated horse, "Justin Time," is ready for groundwork. A volunteer and rescue group leader went to pick up three horses, a gelding and two fillies, from a neglect case. They took a three-horse trailer, but when they arrived, they also found an emaciated young stallion. Stallions can be harder to place in foster homes—not everyone can care for them or handle them—but the rescuers took one look at this horse and could not imagine leaving him behind. The rescue group leader agreed to foster him until he was adopted. He was named "Justin Time" because they rescued him just in time. He gained weight and was gelded. Just a few months later, he was in good enough shape to be adopted, and very quickly he found the perfect home. His adopter adores him—they ride over obstacles together and she is training him to drive!*

out of his shell. You won't know if or where his fear response will show up, so test him with many situations. Try to work with him at home and away from home, with and without other horses, while wearing different types of hats (for example your helmet, ball caps, and cowboy hats), and in both indoor and outdoor arenas. Ask him to go over obstacles such as bridges, ground poles, tarps, and different footing. When you practice with kindness and patience, he will learn to trust you. You'll also identify specific triggers that can make him wary or nervous. If any are identified, pair approach-and-retreat with positive reinforcement to habituate him to objects or triggers.

LONGEING

Extensive horse training is outside the scope of this book, so I will not address either specific methodologies or trainers in-depth.

What I will do is talk about building muscle, coordination, strength, and partnership in concert with basic training techniques that can be applied to any discipline.

As your horse gains weight and becomes more responsive to halter training, it is fair to begin trotting exercise. Many horsemen employ modern natural horsemanship techniques, although longeing is a training technique that has been around for hundreds of years.

Longeing Movements

To begin longeing with an untrained, unknown, or unfit horse, begin in a small area or round pen. If there isn't one available to you, using a corner of your horse's enclosure can be helpful to maintain your horse's position (fig. 16.3).[169]

The basic premise of longeing is that the horse moves in a larger circle around the perimeter while the handler moves constantly toward the horse's hip in a smaller circle, thus driving him forward (fig. 16.4). You are using your body language and position to encroach on his flight zone, naturally asking him to move forward. You limit his forward movement and maintain the circle using a physical barrier (either the fence or the longe line).

Watch your horse's ears and eyes. His mental focus is where his ears are pointed. If he keeps the inside ear toward you, he is focused on you. Work until you have his focus.

Generally, horses are better at longeing to the left than to the right, because most traditional horse-handling occurs on the left. Horses are more practiced at responding

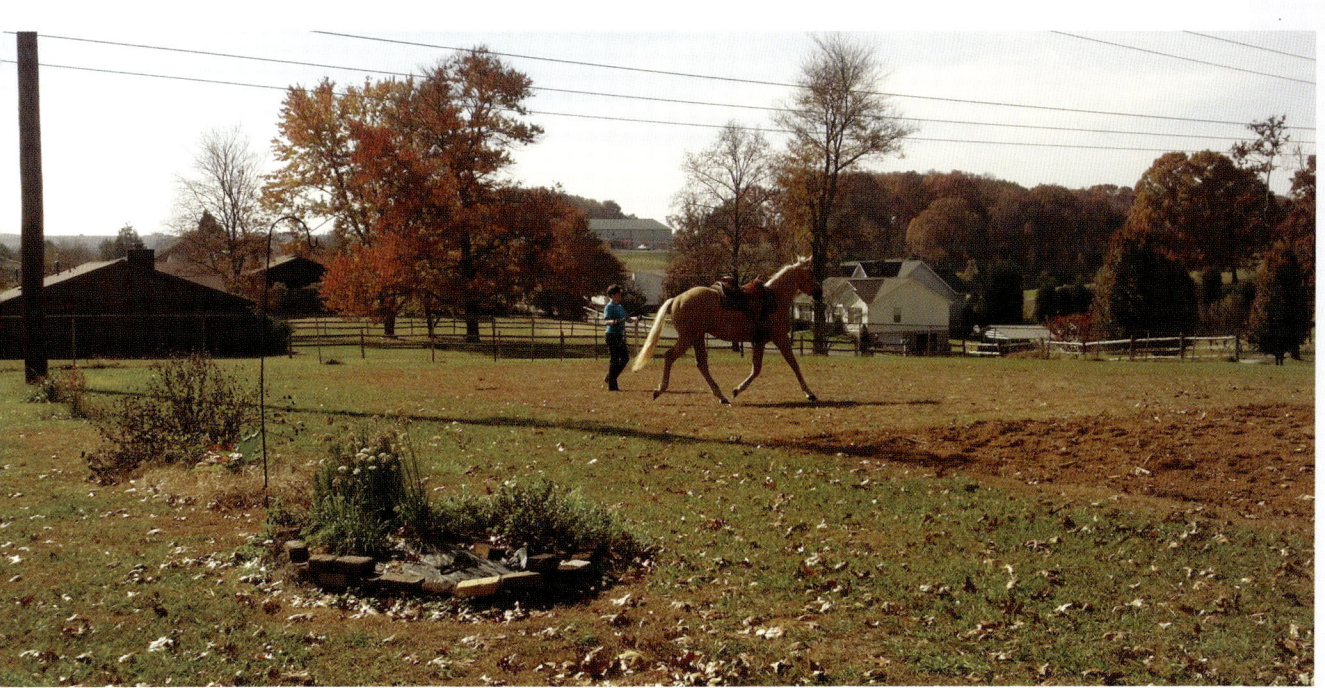

16.4 This adopted gelding was started under saddle without the benefit of a round pen. Here, he is longeing nicely.

to cues from the left. In a left circle, the left side of the horse's body is on the inside of the circle, and is the side you are facing. The right side of the horse's body is on the outside of the circle. Your ultimate goal is to have your horse work equally on both left and right circles.

Begin with a small circle at a walk using a 14- to 20-foot lead rope or longe line. Ask your horse to move forward while you step toward his hip. You may need to twirl the end of your longe line, or use a carrot stick, flag, or whip as an arm extension to communicate clearly (see p. 173). Keep stepping to his hip as he walks around you. This is not a leisurely, grazing walk, but a working, active walk. Both you and he are moving forward. Having a line on your horse in the initial period, even if you are working in a round pen, will give you more control of his head. If he tries to kick at you or run away from you, pulling his head toward you and toward the center will move his hip to the perimeter of the circle and away from you. Don't ask him to trot until your horse clearly understands what is expected of him at the walk (see Increasing Speed, p. 215).

Halting When Longeing

Perfect your selected maneuver at the walk before adding speed. To stop your horse, square your shoulders and face toward your horse. You want to step in front of the line of his shoulder and give a verbal cue ("Whoa"). Make your body's communication with him as clear as you can. Use your body rather than the longe line as much as possible.

There are at least three methods to stop a horse on a longe line. First, the horse is asked to stop square, and some trainers even have him back a step or two while staying on the outside of the circle on the line. While he is attached to the longe line, he will not be able to physically stop and reverse direction by turning to the outside of the circle. However, he can turn to the inside at the end of the longe line to change direction (second method). The third method is to have the horse come into the center and then go back out. No single method is the only correct way. Many successful trainers use one or more of these different techniques. In the beginning, choose one way and teach your horse to consistently understand it. Choose the way you are most likely to use in the future. If you aren't sure, then choose the way that works best for you.

My preference is that after the horse stops, he is allowed to rest for a moment. He should have his attention focused on the handler. Then, when the handler asks, he should be able to either begin in the same direction, or turn and reverse toward the inside while staying on the perimeter of the circle. To get him to turn, reorient your shoulders toward his hip, and back up a few steps, moving your body in the direction he was going. This is his invitation to come to you—you are "pulling" him to you with your body language. He will turn to you. He should not go past you, so if it seems like he is going to move beyond you or invade your space, reposition yourself and again ask him to stop.

In the beginning, you'll need to use the halter and longe line to direct him and clarify what you are asking. If you want your horse to be versatile, train him for all three maneuvers (stopping square, turning in while staying on the perimeter of the circle, or coming in to you before being sent back out on a circle in the other direction). To achieve this, communication with your horse must be precise.

After he is turned, switch everything your hands are doing (your ambidexterity as your horse's trainer will improve—don't worry). Now, the right side of his body is on the inside of the circle, and you are walking in a small circle to the right as he goes forward. The longe line is in your right hand and the whip or carrot stick will be in your left.

Increasing Speed

Increasing speed means an increase in circle size as well as the level of difficulty. As your horse becomes confident at the walk, begin asking him to trot. A 14- to 20-foot line is fine for trotting, but when you progress to canter/lope, you will want a 25- to 30-foot line. Hold the slack, excess line in the same hand you are holding your longe whip or carrot stick.

To increase your horse's speed, use a common verbal cue such as kissing or clucking. Reinforce this cue by becoming more active with your body. Make your steps quicker, and "chase" him a little bit with your arm, whip, or end of the longe line. Because he is unfit, he may only be able to go a few strides before he tires. Save energy for doing this both directions. You want to push him to do more than he wants to do on his own, but you don't want to completely exhaust him.

Canter: Your horse will need to be fit enough to longe on the correct lead in a circle: He should be able to willingly trot at least three circles in each direction before you start asking for a canter. Make sure the area you are working in is large enough to accommodate your horse's size.

When a horse canters, his footfall pattern is either "left-leaded" or "right-leaded." To see the left lead, watch his left front foot. It is the last foot in the canter stride to hit the ground. When it lands, it is in front of where the right foot landed. The left hind foot should also land well in front of the right foot. In basic training, the horse should be on the lead in the direction he is going. When he is circling left, he should be on the left lead.

Not Trotting

Gaited horse breeds include Tennessee Walking Horses, Paso Finos, or Peruvian Pasos, and others. Some of these have distinct physical features, but some (like the Missouri Fox Trotter) look a lot like a Quarter Horse or stock horse breed. You may acquire a gaited horse on purpose or accidentally. None of these horses trot. Instead, they have a gait specific to their breed.

A trot is a bilaterally symmetrical gait, with opposite diagonal pairs of limbs moving in synchrony (for example, left fore and the right hind). When watching a gaited horse, you will notice that his gait does not pair up on opposite diagonals. Instead, the footfall pattern is the same as the walk. He is very smooth, in part because at least one foot is always on the ground (unlike the rough trot, where the horse and rider bounce up and down—a rhythm that can be difficult for riders to learn to "sit"). If you have one of these gaited horses, you can use the word "gait" in place of "trot" for most training instruction.

Rowdy Ranger: A Need for Training

Ranger was a gorgeous, young, palomino grandson of a famous stallion. Two brothers owned Ranger as an investment. They intended him to be their prized stud horse. He had been managed by living alone—as many stallions are—and was not properly socialized with other horses. As a cute, young horse, the brothers had not disciplined him. When Ranger started going through puberty, he became rebellious and unruly. The two brothers realized that they were in over their heads and now wanted him gelded in hopes that reducing his testosterone would improve his manners. The surgical procedure went fine, and they went home with management instructions and advice to find a trainer to help them.

A few months later, rambunctious Ranger was back to be treated for a severe cut on his hind leg. He was nearly unmanageable and bit one of his caretakers quite badly, leaving a large bruise under her ribs. Ranger's laceration was cleaned, sutured, and bandaged. The brothers were given instructions about recheck appointments and bandage changes.

Sadly, rebellious Ranger returned about two weeks later and the brothers wanted to euthanize him. He was still wearing the original bandage from the day of the injury. The brothers said the horse was kicking them, and they were frustrated and afraid. They believed the horse had no use: he was no longer a stallion prospect, and they felt the nasty scar from the wound made him an unsuitable riding prospect, especially in light of his rude antics. The veterinarians working with Ranger saw a handsome two-year-old with a serious need for some training, and convinced the brothers to simply give him up.

After two months in the hospital, the wound had healed. Ranger's team of caretakers refused to tolerate him crowding them or showing any signs of aggression. Appropriate handling led to a more respectful Ranger.

Ranger went home with me and was turned out with my herd of three mares. He needed serious socialization. As my mares put him in his place, I started him under saddle. Another veterinarian committed to Ranger. She rides him regularly, and enjoys his playful personality.

Knowing when to get help is an important part of horse ownership, and especially of horse rescue. Kudos to all of the trainers who keep horses' behavior in line—they are an essential part of a rescue team.

On the longe line, he may only be able to maintain the correct lead for a few strides, before he switches his lead in his hind end only. This is called *cross-cantering*. Cross-cantering or falling out of lead is common when working on a longe line, especially with a horse who is weak or unfit. As the horse gets stronger, this fault should resolve on its own. Sometimes horses cannot maintain their lead on the longe line, but can on a free circle or in a larger space.

It's not a good idea to allow a horse to canter on the longe line or in a round pen imbalanced with the incorrect lead in the hind end. As he works, muscle memory is being built. You want to build correct muscle memory, so your horse needs to engage his core and remain on the correct lead. When he falls out of lead, step back, quiet your body language, and (if necessary) reel in your longe line to make the circle smaller until he trots. After a few trotting strides, get active, allow him enough room, and again ask for the canter. Over several weeks, you will find that he will be able to hold the correct lead for more and more strides. If he isn't progressing or seems to be able to only hold the correct lead unilaterally (for example, to the right, but not to the left), it is a sign of lameness.

TACKING UP

Once your horse walks and trots confidently on the longe line, you can start introducing tack. He should accept touch over his entire body from your hand, brush, lead rope, and towel. Some trainers will also introduce noise-producing objects such as a plastic bag or tarp. Introduction of a new object is easier when the horse is a little bit tired from moving his feet, so longe him to the extent of his fitness then add the object. If he is tired, he will have more incentive to stand still. Finally, introduce the saddle pad.

Saddle Pad

If a horse is allowed to investigate and explore objects on his own, he will have more rapid and solid acceptance of them. When introducing any new object, begin by allowing the horse to sniff it then begin touch on his withers or shoulder. Use approach-and-retreat. One of the reasons retreating is so important when training horses is that it helps convince your horse to trust you. You allow him to relax a little and think about or process the fact that the new "scary" object didn't hurt him at all.

Try leaving the saddle pad over the fence of his enclosure or on the ground in his pen (he may play with it, so use a pad you won't mind getting damaged). Allow him ample time to explore it.

Next training session, work him in your longeing routine then as he rests, pick up the pad and allow him to sniff it in your hand. Touch him briefly on the shoulder with it and retreat. Then touch his shoulder and move to his withers, and immediately retreat again. Do this from both the right and the left. When he accepts this easily, you may put the pad quietly over his withers and then remove it (retreat). Put it on his withers then slide it toward his rump. Rub it over his legs and belly.

Start with quiet slow motions, then increase the activity and speed as he remains comfortable. Move or flap the sides of it while it rests on his back. Eventually, you want him to accept you approaching him with the pad and putting it on him like you would do on a well-seasoned riding horse. You must watch your horse. Depending on his personal behavior tendencies and previous experience, he may need 10 or he may need 100 repetitions to be truly comfortable.

Saddle

Although you have allowed him to investigate other objects, you may not want to risk damage to your saddle, but you should allow the horse to investigate it, if possible. For example, you can put it on the ground in the center of your working area. Then lead him to it, allowing him to sniff and look at it, while maintaining control of him with the halter and lead rope. Introduce the saddle after he's accepted everything previously introduced and is a little bit tired from being longed.

The saddle is the most difficult object to introduce because it is heavy and bulky, and it takes effort to get it on and off the horse. It also gets attached to the horse, and the cinch or girth squeezes his barrel—a feeling that takes some getting used to.

Introduction of the saddle is in three stages: first, accepting it on his back; second, applying pressure to the girth or cinch without fastening or buckling it; and third, accepting the cinch or girth being tightened and fastened. Gaining this acceptance from your horse can take 20 minutes, or it can take a week. Take your time, and try to not incite a fear response. You can reduce the amount of scary flapping by removing the *irons* (stirrups) from English tack or shortening the stirrups of a Western saddle.

It is unsafe to tie your horse while introducing the saddle. You can have an assistant holding his halter and lead rope. If you are alone, you may be holding his lead rope as well as juggling the saddle. Don't loop the lead rope around your arm or hand. Remember also that should you accidentally apply pressure to the halter, it could cue him to move. This takes coordination, but it is an achievable task with effort and practice.

Your goal is for your horse to stand still during this process. If he is moving his feet, he is nervous. (Remember: This rule does not apply to donkeys and mules—they will stand still when fearful—see p. 166.) Look at his eyes, ears, and nostrils. His facial expression will give you clues about how he is feeling. Put the saddle on and off until he is relaxed.

Make sure your horse accepts touch and brushing in the area where the cinch or girth will lie. Once you have the saddle comfortably sitting on your horse's back and he is not afraid, place the girth or cinch where it is hanging off the right side of the horse. From the left, reach underneath him and pick it up until it touches him momentarily. Pet and reward him. Repeat this action several times then use one hand to secure the saddle and the other to pull the cinch or girth toward the D-ring or buckle to apply pressure. After you have repeated this several times, and he seems to accept it, you can move on to the next step.

Now, he accepts the saddle sitting on him and you have prepared him as much as possible for the girth tightening. When you are ready to fasten the saddle on for the first time, make sure your horse is a bit tired, as again, this will reduce his reactivity. Put the saddle on, and reassure and positively reinforce his good behavior. Mime cinch tightening again. If he remains comfortable, you can actually tighten and fasten the girth or cinch. Make sure it is tight enough so the saddle does not slip backward or sideways. Should this happen, it will scare your horse and make the next time you saddle him up much more difficult. If you go too fast it will scare him, and if you go too slowly, he can react when it is only half-attached, which will go poorly (it's likely to slip).

If you have prepared your horse, his likelihood of exploding with bucking and kicking is minimized, though not eliminated. Most horses will buck at least a few times, so be prepared. For some horses, being left alone in a stall or a small, safe pen allows them to get used to the idea of moving with the saddle on. Others may stand stock still until encouraged to move. You must use your best judgement with your horse, your available facilities, and your level of comfort or previous experience. You can longe him or hand-walk him first. Whatever you do, get him to move until he accepts the feel of the saddle and is willing to pay attention to you.

From this point on, he should be wearing the saddle daily when longeing until you are confident that he fully accepts it. The first few times, you can still work with the gradual, approach-and-retreat technique of cinch tightening.

Notes About Bucking: Bucking is a dangerous and unacceptable habit in a riding horse. Trainers approach bucking in a variety of ways: Some discourage it altogether from day one. Some allow a horse to buck all he wants, but only for the first few times he is saddled. Some allow a horse to buck and play on a longe line for years, both with and without a saddle. It depends on the horse, the trainer, the discipline, and the living situation. Horses in boarding or intense training facilities may only have the longe line as their "free time" to move and buck. Conversely, horses that are lucky enough to have access to large pastures and social groups have more free time to move as they choose, and are usually expected to have a working mindset when being longed. As usual with horse training, there are many ways to reach the goal of the horse not bucking with the rider.

BEGINNING TO MAKE A DIFFERENCE

Working through this chapter, you have taught or reviewed longeing at the walk, trot, and canter. Your horse also knows how to halt at your request, and turn as you direct him. You have taught him to be completely comfortable wearing the saddle pad and saddle. Your horse's fitness and muscle have increased. Perhaps most importantly, you have honed your communication skills, and reaffirmed trust and leadership. You have done so much to help your horse! In fact, many riders never achieve the type of relationship and confidence you and your horse now have. Look at him and be proud of the positive difference you have made in his life. You are ready to proceed to the final chapter and start riding.

CHAPTER 17

Final Steps:
Riding

READINESS REVIEW

You are ready to progress to your first ride if your horse:

- Has a BCS of 5 or 6.

- Is sound and physically fit.

- Is respectful of, and amenable to, following your leadership in a variety of environments and circumstances.

- Understands how to walk, trot, canter, halt, and turn at your request on the longe line and/or in a small pen; both to the left and to the right.

- Accepts the whip or carrot stick.

- Is comfortable with tack—saddle pad and saddle, including flapping stirrups, saddle strings, and saddle noises (see p. 217).

This chapter explores the final steps in your journey with your horse: preparation for his life as a riding horse. My approach is to go over the basics of getting started, using simple steps and minimal tack, making the process as accessible to as many horse people as possible. If you have gone through all the steps presented in the previous chapters, your horse is mentally and physically prepared for this next phase. Obviously, there are hundreds of books on perfecting riding skills. Horsemanship and training is a lifelong pursuit. Begin riding your horse with the principles and techniques you intend to use throughout his life.

BEFORE RIDING

In the interest of safety, keep your phone with you on your person (not attached to your saddle). It is recommended to wear a helmet and safety vest. Check in with your safety person. It is best to have another person present for at least your first several rides.

Call your veterinarian and ask her to examine your horse for soundness and review other health issues before you ride him. It is possible that subtle neurologic deficits or systemic illness (for example, a heart murmur) are present. Health problems could cause your horse to be unbalanced, weak, or unstable, rendering him unsafe to ride.

Your horse should pass successfully through a fitness program. Being fit will maximize his muscular stability and cardiovascular stamina, allowing him to support the weight of a rider. I recommend a rescue horse have a BCS of 5 or more before riding him. He should have a clean bill of health. He should be able to maintain a walk on the longe line, trot for at least five circles in each direction without breaking gait, and complete at least three circles at the canter in each direction without becoming exhausted.

Many horse rescue groups work with a professional trainer to help their adoption prospects. These horses are restarted in the same way that a young horse is started. Slow, methodical progression is critical for earning a horse's trust, no matter what the age (fig. 17.1). I suggest that you review the previous chapters and, if you have successfully completed the tasks covered there, then you have "started" your horse and are ready to advance to riding him.

For rescue horses, "even after extensive retraining the fear memories can still resurface and cause misbehavior."[35] A person who is motivated to rescue a horse may not be fully capable of handling the emotional baggage that he comes with. There is great pride in training a horse, but it is also appropriate to seek outside assistance. You may progress faster together with professional coaching. It is of great value to the horse for you to recognize when you need help—after all, a well-trained horse is more likely to retain a good home for life (fig. 17.2).

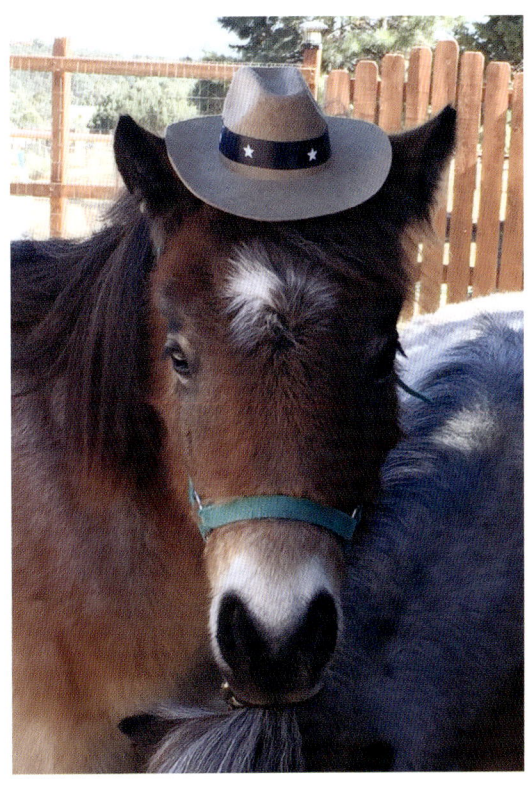

17.1 A miniature horse who is not ridden but is in full work in an equine-assisted psychotherapy program.

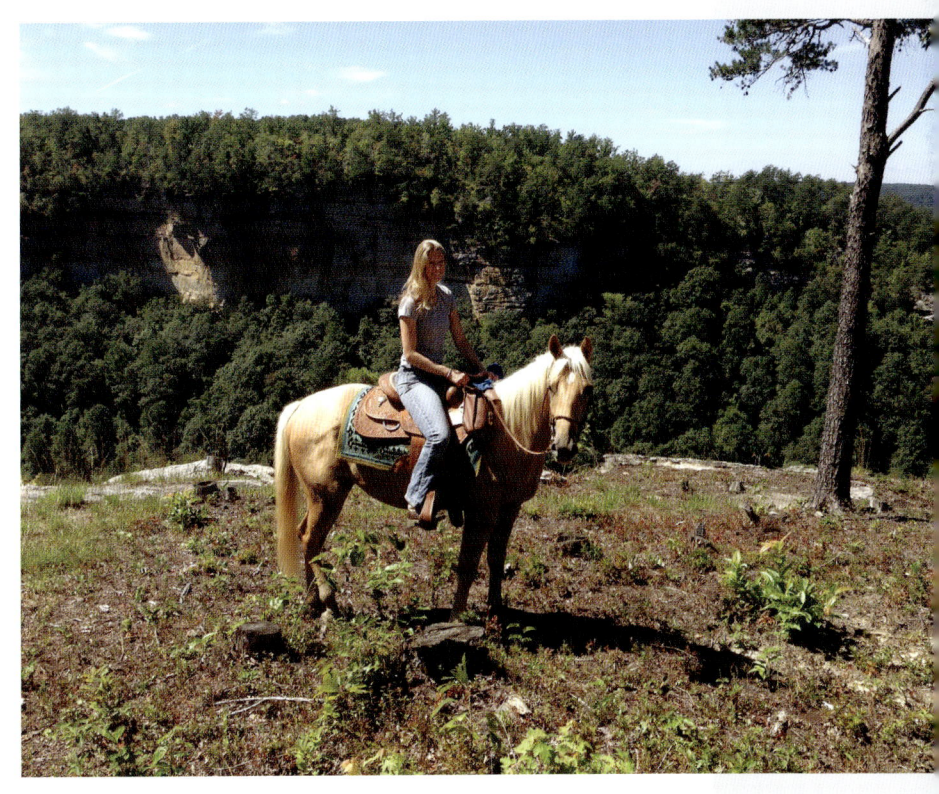

17.2 A horse after he has found a new home and has been started under saddle.

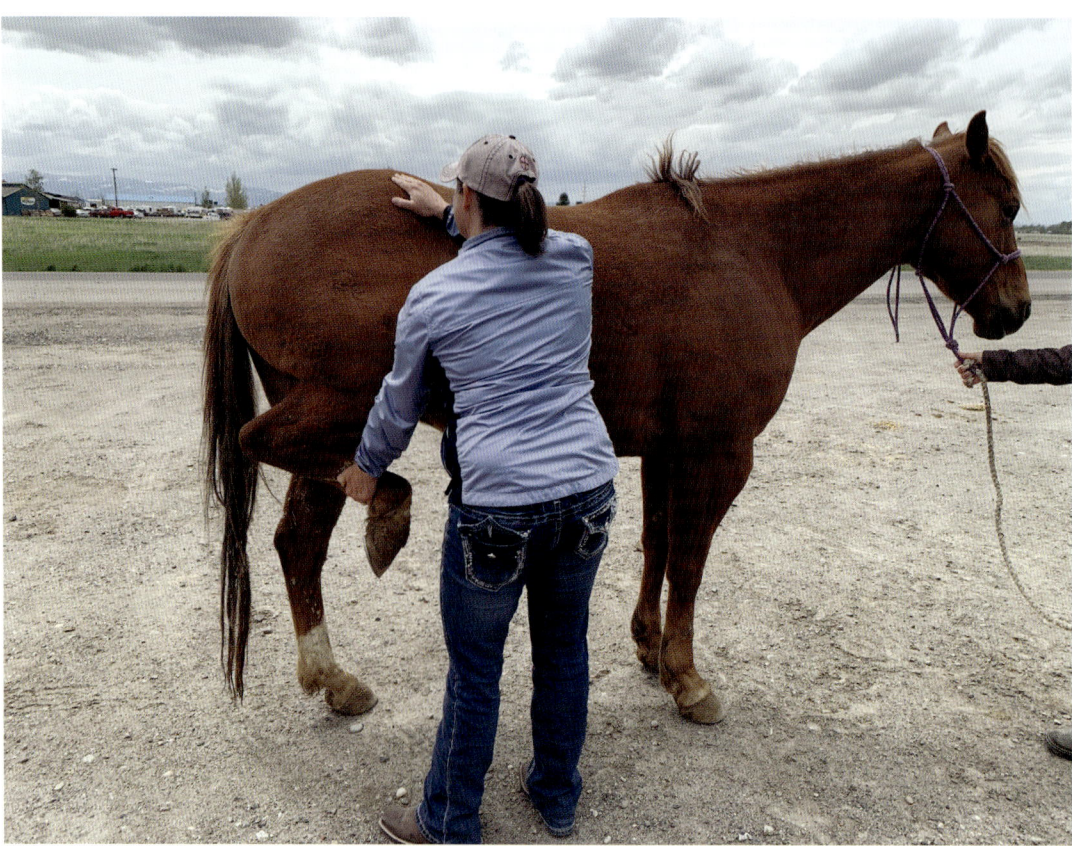

17.3 Flexion tests, like this one, help locate the source of lameness.

Lameness Evaluation

Here is what to expect from a pre-ride lameness evaluation. First of all, your horse will be expected to jog in-hand, and to be able to be longed. Your veterinarian may do flexion tests (fig. 17.3). A flexion test is picking up a limb and putting mild to moderate pressure on specific joints by flexing them for a semi-standardized period of time (for example, 30 to 90 seconds), depending on the joint and the practitioner. Flexion tests help pinpoint the source of lameness.

Your veterinarian will also need to handle your horse's feet and use hoof testers. Hoof testers apply leveraged pressure to specific points of the sole and heels of the hoof. They are useful to pinpoint if and where a horse has pain in his foot.

Because it takes a certain amount of strength, balance, and coordination for a horse to endure jogging, longeing, and standing on three legs during flexion testing and hoof evaluation, it is not possible (or fair to the horse) to perform a thorough lameness examination until he is fit.

TO BRIDLE OR NOT TO BRIDLE

A good horse trainer learns to break training steps into smaller "bites" of learning material. In this instance, separate the introduction of the bridle from the introduction of the rider.

Some horse people put the first few

rides on a horse using the halter and lead rope to steer their horse, thereby minimizing the new things a horse must mentally process. The bridle can also be introduced before and independently of a rider.

Before you start, your horse should be used to having the halter placed on his head and removed with no problem. As an equestrian, you may have already been taught to put a bridle on a horse using either traditional Western or traditional English positioning, which are slightly different. Make sure you are confident with your skill so that you are able to clearly show your horse what is expected of him.

Whichever technique you use, make the experience as pleasant as you can for your horse. Avoid bumping his teeth. As you put the bridle in the mouth of a mare, filly, or young horse, you will not have to contend with canine teeth. For a mature gelding, you may have to beware these large teeth. Bumping them can create a painful, negative experience.

Be gentle with his ears. For mules, you will either partially or fully unbuckle the

Upward Fixation of the Patella

The patella is known more commonly as the kneecap and in horses, is part of the stifle joint. *Upward fixation of the patella* is also known as *delayed patellar release*. The development of this specific lameness is influenced by conformation, but closely associated with weakness.

Horses sleep standing up through a *locking mechanism*. In the hind limb, this involves ligaments and tendons that are structured in a way that ensures a horse's stifle and hock always flex and extend in concert. In the stifle, a ligament hooks the patella over a ridge on the femur. This allows a horse to passively stand, thereby, using very little energy to remain on his feet. This is energy efficient for an animal that needs to be ready to run in an instant, should a predator appear. As long as the ligament is over the ridge, neither the stifle nor the hock will bend. When a horse takes a step, his quadriceps muscles must actively pull the ligament up out of the groove.

A weak horse can have trouble with the active muscle contraction needed to release the ligament, resulting in the patella staying locked.

In the mild form, the horse may appear to "catch" his stifles mid-stride. This will be more apparent, or worse, in small, tight circles. The most severe form involves a horse who has a straight, stiff hind leg and is unable to go forward. If he is backed up several strides, the patella is then able to release, and the horse can bend his leg and move again. Horses who are stalled for extensive periods of time are prone to this problem.

While there is a surgery that modifies the patellar ligaments and reduces the severity of the problem, the first-line therapy is to strengthen the horse. Working up hills, then coming down the hill in a very long, gradual S-shape or working in deep sand strengthens his quadriceps. Work over cavalletti or ground poles is also helpful. And, in the case of the rescue horse, getting the horse to have a BCS of 5 and increasing fitness often solves the problem.

bridle because his ears are larger. Be as kind as possible, but don't allow the horse to evade wearing the bridle.

Hint: In cold weather, warming the metal with a bit warmer or by storing it in a heated tack room goes a long way toward making the overall experience more pleasant for your horse.

Once you have the bit in your horse's mouth, positively reward him with petting and kind words. I will sometimes also feed treats, as do many people. However, some people feel strongly that a horse should never eat with a bit in his mouth.

He only needs to have the bit in his mouth for a few seconds, and then it can be removed. He should learn that it isn't there forever. You may put the bridle on and take it off him several times until he feels secure about the process.

Bridle Fit

The bit sits in a *diastema* (gap between the teeth) called the *bars* of the horse's lower jaw. A properly fitted bit never touches the premolars. The soft tissues of the lips keep it well away from hitting the *cheek teeth* that he uses to grind his food.

Begin with a snaffle bit (those with no shanks, which cause leverage, and usually with a jointed mouthpiece). There should be one wrinkle in the corner of the horse's mouth.

At this point, the horse needs some time to work and play with the very new object in his mouth. A few trainers leave the bridle on the horse for several days. I strongly discourage this tactic because it can rub a sore on the horse. It can also increase the horse's anxiety. He may be confused about how long the object (bit) will be present, especially if it is the first time he is wearing it. Also, if the metal of the bit catches on a feeder, fence, or bucket, it can break the horse's jaw (I have repaired several of these).

The first two or three lessons when the horse is wearing the bridle, you can leave it on him with no reins and longe him as you usually do—preferably free-longeing him in a small pen. If you only have an open space and a longe line, loosen his halter, put it on over the properly fitted bridle, and clip the longe line to the halter. Don't connect the longe line directly to the bit. It doesn't work as well to put the bridle over the halter. The bridle has to be loosened to accommodate the halter, so the bit may not sit in the correct place in his mouth. When the halter is under the bridle, pressure from it can cause the bridle and bit to apply pressure.

After you have worked him several times while he is wearing the bridle, start showing him that you mean to direct his movement with it. Teaching him this before you get on allows the horse to better process the tasks you set forth and learn more clearly. There are many options, so I will present only a few basic maneuvers here.

In-hand bridle work can begin with you standing to the side of your horse and gently pulling the rein, asking him to turn his head and neck. Release when he complies. Do this equally from both sides. Some trainers will also lead a horse in a flexing circle from the ground using the bridle to direct his head.

For further direction, you may also use long, ground-driving reins (fig. 17.4). I really like this method, despite many trainers opting out of this step. I'm a more capable veterinarian than trainer, so I want to do as much training on the ground as I can. That way, when I am finally in the saddle, I have

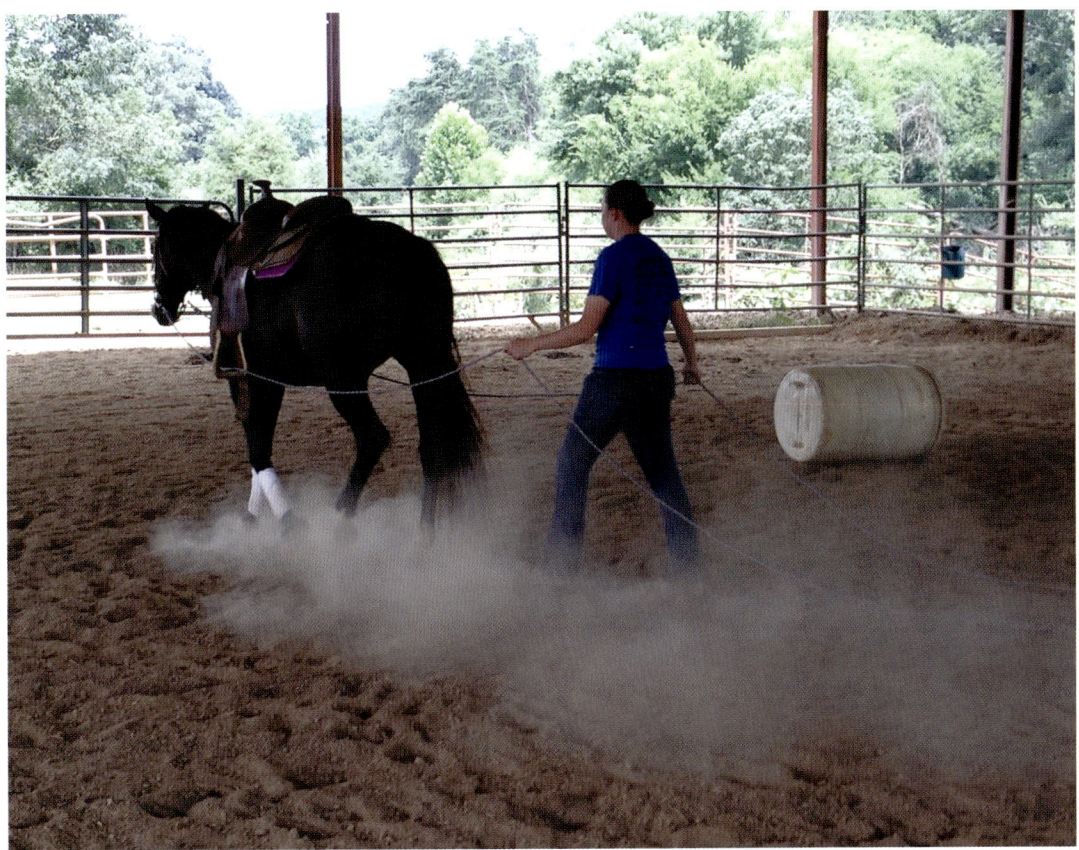

17.4 *This adopted horse, Ella, and her adopter, Storrie, learn to ground-drive in preparation for riding. (You can read more about these two in the sidebar on p. 228.)*

taught my horse as much as possible. This gives him a clearer idea of what is expected, and minimizes what he perceives as new. Also, the enhanced "steering control" ensures that he understands my direction, minimizing the likelihood of him panicking, and me falling off.[170]

First, desensitize your horse to the feel of the long reins around his legs and swinging over his body. When he is unafraid, attach the right rein to the bit and run it through the right stirrup and over the saddle seat. You should work until he will stand quietly for this. Next, move to the left and attach that rein and run it through the left stirrup. You should be standing on the left of the horse, holding one rein in each hand. From the left position, move to the rear of the horse (safely out of kicking distance), and ask him to walk. Cluck or kiss (he already understands your verbal cues from your previous work). If he doesn't move off, work to reinforce voice cues for walking. Usually a gentle waving of the long reins will do, but you can increase your vigor until he moves. A helper at the head of the horse is a wonderful addition to both the ground-driving and the first few rides. Your helper may simply walk beside your horse, not necessarily holding on to him.

> ### We Are the Lucky Ones
>
> Max was a smart, slightly stubborn, gray, three-year-old gelding who had 20 rides on him and a mischievous manner. He had been passed over by multiple adopters and was decidedly not a looker. Narrow chest, unruly mane and tail, odd billowy gaits… but when he made eye contact with you, his gaze was enveloping and warm.
>
> When a potential adopter, Miriam, tacked him up for the first time, the gelding at first insisted that, no the cinch was not a necessary component of this activity, and no he was not interested in standing anywhere close to the mounting block! But when they moved forward into a walk, then a trot, then a canter, Max pricked his ears, floated along, and didn't look back.
>
> With her husband's unwavering encouragement, Miriam decided to adopt him. She was moved by his story, that of a gentle soul, dumped on the side of the road at three months old, rescued and fostered by dedicated volunteers, and now in need of a real home of his own. In the years since, Max has become the steady, predictable horse Miriam wished for. He leads on the trail, stands for the farrier, politely rolls immediately after any beauty treatment, and makes his family chuckle with simultaneous delight and annoyance. He's never in much of a hurry, but on those long uphill sections of the trail, slogging toward the crest, he gives it his all. Max is less interested in the friends he maintains in his herd, and far more dedicated to his human companions.
>
> "They say a rescue animal is acutely aware of his good fortune and tries to please and impress his human," says Miriam. "Although I think Max is mostly oblivious, he never refuses to be caught, never nips or kicks, and never gives us less than 100 percent. We are the lucky ones."

Once he is going forward, you can ask for a turn. It's important for him to be moving forward before turning because it's much easier for him to continue motion and change the direction of it (one thing at a time), than it is for him to turn and begin moving forward at the same time. If he is not moving forward when he is asked to turn—especially in this early period of training, he is more likely to struggle against your cues rather than giving to your requests.

You can work on walking and steering lots and lots of circles and serpentines. Change direction repeatedly and deliberately until your horse is comfortable with the concept of being steered directly from the bit. Next, you can work on stopping, and teach him how to back up.

By teaching him the basics of going forward, left, right, and backward, and giving to the bit from the ground independent of a rider, you decrease the chances of encountering dangerous resistance while in the saddle.

MOUNTING

As with other training steps, there are many methods you can use. The first time you mount your horse, the most important thing is to avoid scaring him and imprinting a negative experience. You are going to break this process up into tiny baby steps, as you have done with all other training steps.

Remember that predators approach the horse from above and behind him, so you will be positioning yourself like a predator. Although traditional horsemanship dictates that you will be mounting from the left, work on everything from both the right and the left. If your horse had a bad experience or developed a bad habit with mounting from the left (for instance, he runs away or bucks with a rider), sometimes you can overcome this by using his right side for mounting.

Use these steps of desensitization for mounting:

1. Accustom the horse to the person visible above him.

2. Let him experience movement at his sides or flanks (in preparation for leg movement there).

3. Put weight in the stirrups.

4. Mount and get off without moving.

5. Mount and ask the horse to move.

Some techniques to get the horse used to the idea of you being on him include: sitting on the fence nearby or above him, standing next to him on the top step of a mounting block, or sitting on another horse and ponying him. The horse in training will get used to the idea of where the rider will be—it will get his eye used to seeing you above him.

Desensitize him to movement and flapping by jumping up and down at each side of him, and flapping the stirrups or saddle fenders. Then, press your weight using your hand into the stirrup. Grab the saddle horn or pommel and move the saddle side to side. You may have done a lot of this desensitization when he was learning to wear the saddle, but reviewing it is a good idea before your first ride. If it seems that he already had some training, I recommend going through these steps anyway, because you want to expose any "holes" in his training, quirks, or bad habits.

Make sure he is fine with being touched on his rump while he is wearing the saddle.

Desensitize him by brushing and petting this area. You want to ensure that if your foot touches his rump while you are getting on and off you don't incite a startle response.

When he seems quiet and ready, put a foot in the stirrup. You've done so much desensitizing that this should be one more baby step in the order of things you've asked your horse to tolerate. If you can enlist an assistant to help hold his head and control his movement, that's great. Otherwise, keep your left hand on the left rein. You want to be able to apply pressure to stop movement if needed, but don't apply pressure prematurely, which could *create* movement. Using a mounting block is a good idea because it minimizes the distance your body has to move to get on your horse, and is easier on his back.

Put your left foot in the left stirrup and stand, leaning over your horse. Don't yet swing a leg all the way over. Instead, use your voice to reassure him, and pet or touch him on both sides of his body. If he moves away, you can step down and off him. Repeat this five or six times on both the left and the right. (Obviously, on the right, you are going to hold the right rein, have your assistant stand on the right side of the horse with you, and use your right foot in the right stirrup.) For some horses, they accept this very quickly and easily. Others may need this exercise repeated daily for three or four days.

Once he is confident that you are going to be getting on and off him on both sides, and he is not afraid, you are ready to swing a leg over. Get him used to the idea that you are up there, and that you will be moving around a bit on him, and that you are going to "retreat" or get off him. Once he feels totally secure, add movement. You have

The Final Phase

I am reminded of an adopted horse who had been donated to a university teaching program as "rideable." Ella was a pretty, black, 16-year-old mare with a little star, and a quiet, kind disposition. She had been used for the last several years teaching veterinary students how to do intravenous injections, bandage legs, and ultrasound the reproductive system.

When a young woman named Storrie adopted Ella, she wanted to use her for light trail riding. Storrie had little horse experience but had been learning through the university's Animal Science program and felt she was ready for her own horse. She purposely adopted an animal that was kind and quiet, and that also had a record that said she had been broke to ride at the time she was donated to the university. Storrie and Ella already had a relationship since Storrie was employed as a weekend caretaker for the university's herd. But, she was having problems riding her mare.

Storrie asked for help, "I'm having trouble with Ella. She doesn't want to turn right."

Ella was clearly comfortable with being haltered, led, standing in cross-ties, and even being saddled up. However, when the bridle and bit were placed on the mare's head and in her mouth, she became anxious. She chomped and chewed and turned her head this way and that. Ella was trying to figure out what this strange object was that Storrie had placed in her mouth. Being a beginning rider, Storrie didn't recognized Ella's discomfort with the bridle as a signal that the mare was not broke—and had been riding her anyway.

Storrie came into the arena and mounted Ella. The sweet-natured mare reverted to a fear response. She was reactive to legs touching her sides and, therefore, Storrie was riding with her legs sticking out and forward to avoid touching her. Ella was communicating that she was most definitely not broke to ride, but she had a good relationship with Storrie and tolerated her presence on her back. Storrie was told to dismount at once.

Since Ella was comfortable with tack, Storrie was taught basic groundwork techniques and worked on them for several weeks. This deepened the duo's relationship and helped Storrie learn to read Ella's body language. Then, the two progressed to ground-driving with long-lines. Finally, time was spent on the ground desensitizing Ella to the saddle fenders and stirrups and moving her hip and shoulder away from pressure from the ground.

After the groundwork, Storrie was able to successfully ride the sweet-natured mare at the walk, trot, and canter around the arena. Ella remained relaxed, and ultimately helped Storrie with her goal of trail riding with her friends.

broken this process into so many small steps, this is just one more.

When you and your horse are comfortable with you being mounted and walking in the same circles and serpentines that you were previously doing from the ground, you can progress by adding in a few trotting steps here and there. Use the same voice signal you use from the ground. Apply pressure with your legs until he trots, then release the pressure.

As with everything you have done, you are going to use gradual approximations to reach your goals. Once your horse is comfortable trotting, you can work up to cantering. When you feel you have control at the walk, trot, and canter in a smaller pen, you can move outside to a larger area. You probably have goals, and will refine your riding skills with a trainer, lessons, and continued work. As you have already employed the approach-and-retreat technique for your horse's training foundation, you will continue to use the same technique approximating each task

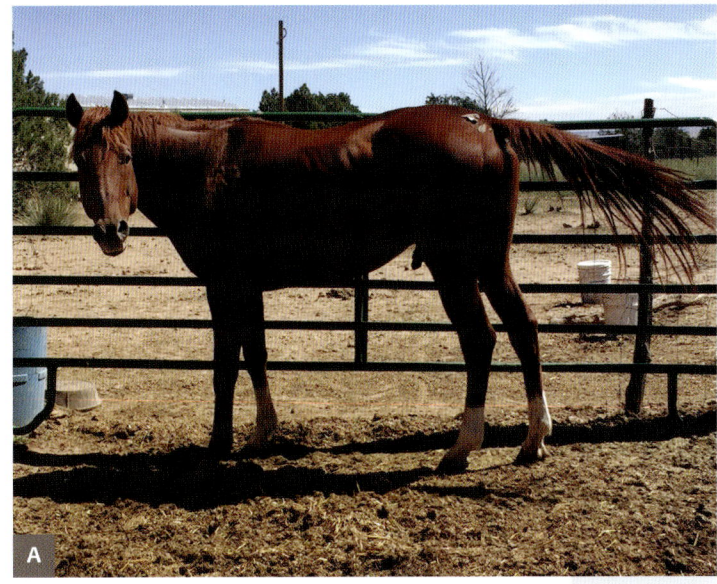

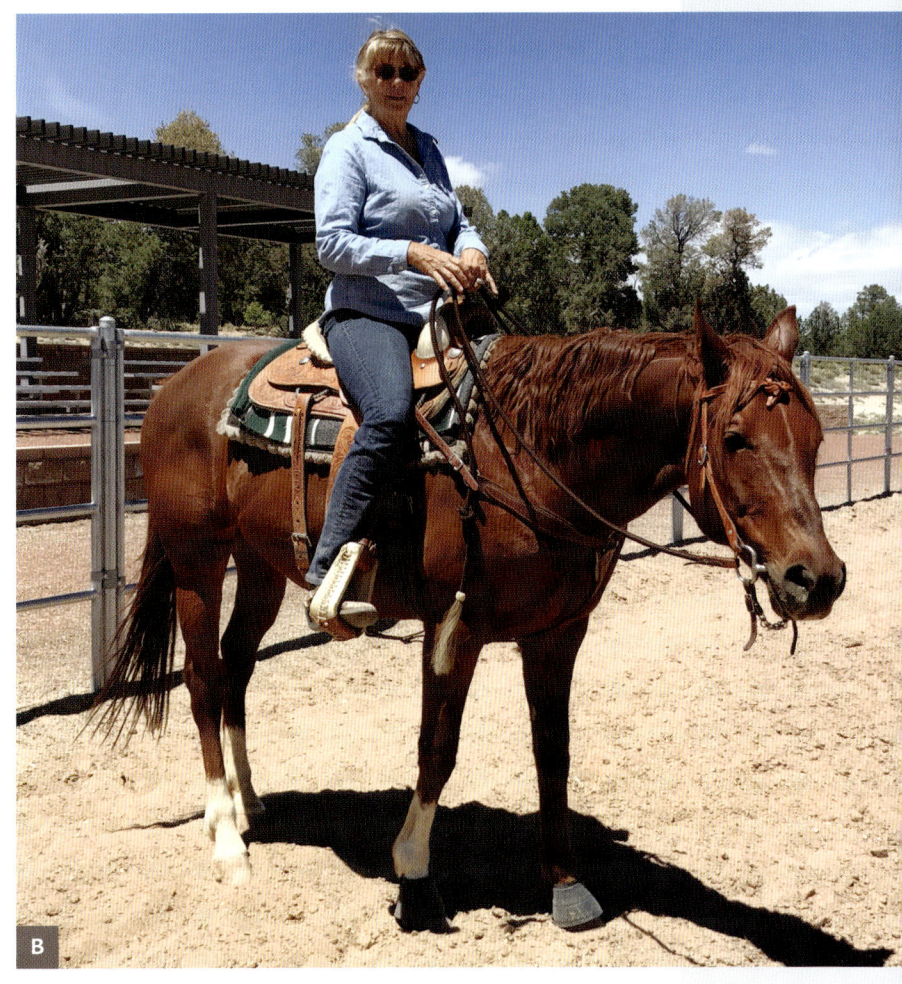

17.5 A & B This cryptorchid stallion, "Nevada," has improved but is still thin (A). The glue from the hip tag at the sale is still visible. His health and strength have improved so that prolonged general anesthesia needed for castration are possible. The Equine Protection Fund of New Mexico covered the cost of the unexpected surgical expense for this animal after he was purchased at auction. Nevada as a gelding with his owner Marilyn (B). He has gained another BCS, and his owner has done a good job starting him under saddle.

at each level as you ask your horse for more and more specialized riding exercises (figs. 17.5 A & B).

THE BEST GIFT

You have fully restored your horse's health and given him purpose. He will take direction from you while you are in the saddle, and he is wearing a bridle. You should be able to choose the direction (left, right, or straight) and the gait (walk, trot, or canter).

Understand that the best gift you can give your horse is great ground manners and a good training base, as a well-trained horse can have a happy and productive life and retain his home.

Working for 20 to 30 minutes several times a week will help solidify your horse's skills as you add new concepts. As you have experienced through working with your rescue horse, a smaller amount of quality training is effective. A good relationship between human and horse along with solid basic skills and understanding will go a long way.

Although we are at the end of our book, you are at the beginning of your horse's career as a healthy riding companion. Whether you keep him for yourself, or have prepared him for rehoming or adoption, you have given him a new start on life. The whole world of riding awaits. Pet him and enjoy the day, because every day you have the privilege of riding is a good day! Rescuing a horse is never a simple journey, but with experience and knowledge, the process will become easier each time. The horses are so fortunate to have you in this world to help them.

Thank you.

END NOTES

[1] https://www.dictionary.com/browse/rescue, accessed February 1, 2018.

[2] Malinda Larkin, "Dry conditions hitting horse owners, rescue groups in the wallet," *Journal of the American Veterinary Medical Association* 241, no. 8 (Oct 15, 2012) 980, 982-5, https://www.avma.org/News/JAVMANews/Pages/121015a.aspx.

[3] Roger Brambell, "Report of the Technical Committee to Enquire Into the Welfare of Animals Kept Under Intensive Livestock Husbandry Systems," (Great Britain. Parliament, 1965, and the 1979 United Kingdom Farm Animal Welfare Council): 1-84.

[4] Bruce H. Rittenhouse, "At a Crossroads: Bureau of Land Management's Wild Horse and Burro Program," *Proceedings of the American Association of Equine Practitioners* 64 (2018): 57-68.

[5] Callie Hendrickson, "Managing Healthy Wild Horses and Burros on Healthy Rangelands: Tools and the Toolbox," *Proceedings of the American Association of Equine Practitioners* 64 (2018): 69-73.

[6] Tom Lenz, "The Unwanted Horse in the U.S.," American Association of Equine Practitioners (July 29th, 2008), last accessed April 22, 2019, https://aaep.org/horsehealth/unwanted-horse-us.

[7] Wendy Williams, "Watching Wild Horses," *The Horse, The Epic History of Our Noble Companion* (New York: Scientific American/ Farrar, Straus and Giroux, 2015): 11-44.

[8] C. Jill Stowe, *Results from 2012 AHP Equine Industry Survey*, (American Horse Publications, June 15, 2012). https://www.americanhorsepubs.org/wp-content/uploads/2012/06/AHP_FinalReport_2012_final.pdf, last accessed May 18, 2019.

[9] Animal Welfare Institute, "Horse Slaughter Statistics," last accessed April 11, 2019, https://awionline.org/content/horse-slaughter-statistics.

[10] Tara A. Okuma, Rosalee S. Hellberg, "Identification of meat species in pet food using a real-time polymerase chain reaction (PCR) assay," *Food Control* 50 (April 2015): 9-17.

[11] Deloitte Consulting, LLP. 2018 "The Economic Impact of the U.S. Horse Industry," National Report for the American Horse Council Foundation: Louisville, KY, USA, 2018.

[12] The Jockey Club, "Annual North American Foal Crop," http://www.jockeyclub.com/default.asp?section=FB&area=2, last accessed April 22, 2019.

[13] Melissa Hines, email message to author regarding scientific abstract in progress, April 18, 2019. Victoria A. Hughes, Melissa Hines et al., "Retrospective analysis of clinical health markers as indicators of death in malnourished equids," University of Tennessee Institute of Agriculture.

[14] The United Horse Coalition, https://unitedhorsecoalition.org/, accessed March 12, 2018.

[15] The United Horse Coalition, https://unitedhorsecoalition.org/, accessed March 12, 2018.

[16] John W. Lee, Jr., Brand Tanner, and Alina Vale, *AAEP Care Guidelines for Rescue and Retirement Facilities* (Lexington, Kentucky: American Association of Equine Practitioners, 2019).

[17] Grant Miller, Carolyn Stull, and Gregory Ferraro, *A Guide: Minimum Standards of Horse Care in the State of California* (Davis, California: University of California, Davis, Center for Equine Health, 2014).

[18] Emily Weiss et al., "Estimating the Availability of Potential Homes for Unwanted Horses in the United States," *Animals* 7, no. 7 (July 2017): 53. https://doi.org/10.3390/ani7070053.

[19] Kathryn E. Holcomb et al., "Characteristics of Relinquishing and Adoptive Owners of Horses Associated with U.S. Nonprofit Equine Rescue Organizations," *Journal of Applied Animal Welfare Science* 15 (2012): 21-31.

[20] Jennifer Williams, "Working With Rescues to Establish Best Practices and Safety Nets for Early Problem Solving," *Proceedings of the American Association of Equine Practitioners* 62 (2016): 215-219.

[21] Carolyn L. Stull, "The journey to slaughter for North American horses," *Animal Frontiers* 2, no. 3 (July 2012): 68-71. https://doi.org/10.2527/af.2012-0052.

[22] Barbara Padalino et al., "Survey of horse transportation in Australia: issues and practices," *Australian Veterinary Journal* 94, no. 10 (October 2016): 349-357. https://doi.org/10.1111/avj.12486.

[23] Carolyn L. Stull et al. "Immunological response to long-term transport stress in mature horses and effects of adaptogenic dietary supplementation as an immunomodulator," *Equine Veterinary Journal* 36, no 7 (November 2004): 583-589.

[24] Carolyn L. Stull and AnneV. Rodiek, "Physiological responses of horses to 24 hours of transportation using a commercial van during summer conditions." *Journal of Animal Science* 78, no.6 (June 2000): 1458-1466.

[25] Barbara Padalino et al., "Risk factors in equine transport-related health problems: A survey of the Australian equine industry," *Equine Veterinary Journal* 49, no. 4 (August 2016). https://doi.org/10.1111/evj.12361.

[26] M. Allano et al., "Influence of short distance transportation on tracheal bacterial content and lower airway cytology in horses." *Veterinary Journal* 47 (August 2016): 47-49.

[27] D.J. Rackyleft et al., "Towards an understanding of equine pleuropneumonia: factors relevant for control," *Australian Veterinary Journal* 78, no. 5. (March 2008) https://doi/org/10.1111/j/1751-0813.2000.tb11788.x.

[28] Carolyn L. Stull et al., "Immunophysiological responses of horses to a 12-hour rest during 24 hours of road transport." *Veterinary Record* 162, no. 19 (May 2008): 609-614.

[29] Katherine A. Houpt and Carissa L. Wickens, "Chapter 18: Handling and transport of horses," in *Livestock Handling and Transport, 4th Edition*, ed. Temple Grandin. (Boston: CABI, 2014): 315-341.

[30] Carolyn L. Stull and Anne V. Rodiek, "Effects of cross-tying horses during 24 h of road transport." *Equine Veterinary Journal* 34, no. 6 (September 2002): 550-555.

[31] "Frequently Asked Questions" https://www.blm.gov/sites/blm.gov/files/Wildhorse_NNCC_FAQ.pdf, accessed November 7, 2019.

[32] "BLM Adoption Requirements," https://www.blm.gov/sites/blm.gov/files/wildhorse_adoption-requirements.pdf, accessed November 7, 2019.

[33] "Legal Protections for Farm Animals During Transport," https://awionline.org/sites/default/files/uploads/documents/fa-legalprotectionsduringtransport-12262013.pdf, accessed November 7, 2019.

[34] "AVMA Supports Horse Transportation Safety Act," https://www.avma.org/Advocacy/National/Congress/Documents/IB_S1459_HTSA_21April2014_Final.pdf.

[35] Temple Grandin, Kasie McGee, and Jennifer Lanier, "Survey of Trucking Practices and Injury to Slaughter Horses," Department of Animal Sciences, Colorado State University, Fort Collins, CO 80523-1171. http://www.grandin.com/references/horse.transport.html.

[36] R. Cyril Roy et al., "Injuries in horses transported to slaughter in Canada," *Canadian Journal of Animal Science* 95 (2015): 523-531. http://www.doi.org/10.4141/CJAS-2015-032.

[37] USDA Equine Identification, https://www.aphis.usda.gov/aphis/ourfocus/animalhealth/nvap/NVAP-Reference-Guide/Animal-Identification/Equine-Identification, accessed July 1, 2019.

[38] Stephanie Valberg et al., "Skeletal muscle metabolic response to exercise in horses with 'tying-up' due to polysaccharide storage myopathy." *Equine Veterinary Journal*

31, no.1 (January 1999): 43-47. https://doi.org/10.1111/j.2042-3306-1999.tb03789.x.

[39] Thomas W. McGowan et al., "Prevalence, risk factors and clinical signs predictive for equine pituitary pars intermedia dysfunction in aged horses," *Equine Veterinary Journal* 45, no. 1 (May 2012). https://doi.org/10.1111/j.2042-3306.2012.00578.x.

[40] J.L. Ireland and Cathy M. McGowan, "Epidemiology of pituitary pars intermedia dysfunction: A systematic literature review of clinical presentation, disease prevalence and risk factors," *The Veterinary Journal* 235 (May 2018): 22-33. https://doi.org/10.1016/j.tvjl.2018.3.002.

[41] Terry L. Whiting et al., "Chronically starved horses: Predicting survival, economic, and ethical considerations," *Canadian Veterinary Journal* 46, no. 4 (April 2005): 320-324.

[42] Don R. Henneke et al., "Relationship between condition score, physical measurements and body fat percentage in mares," *Equine Veterinary Journal* 15, no. 4 (October 1983): 371-372.

[43] Martin A. Crook, "The Importance of the Refeeding Syndrome," *Nutrition* 17, no 7-8 (July-August 2001): 632-637. https://doi.org/10.1016/s)899-9007(01)00542-1.

[44] Carolyn L. Stull and C.L. Whitham, "Metabolic responses of chronically starved horses to refeeding with three isoenergetic diets," *Journal of the American Veterinary Medical Association* 212, no. 9 (March 1, 1998): 691-696.

[45] Carolyn Stull, "Nutrition for Rehabilitating the Starved Horse," *UC Davis Center for Equine Health Horse Report*, July 2012, 1, 3-4.

[46] Carolyn L. Stull and Anne V. Rodiek, "Responses of blood glucose, insulin and cortisol concentrations to common equine diets." *Journal of Nutrition* 118, no. 2 (February 1988): 206-213. https://doi.org/10.1093/jn/118.2.206.

[47] Caroline McGregor Argo, "Feeding thin and starved horses," in *Equine Applied and Clinical Nutrition: Health, Welfare and Performance*, eds. Raymond J. Goer, Patricia A. Harris, and Manfred Coenen (Philadelphia: Saunders, 2013), 503-510.

[48] Sarah L. Ralston and Patricia A. Harris, "Nutritional considerations for aged horses," in *Equine Applied and Clinical Nutrition: Health, Welfare and Performance*, eds. Raymond J. Goer, Patricia A. Harris, and Manfred Coenen (Philadelphia: Saunders, 2013), 289-300.

[49] Derek Cuddeford, "Factors affecting feed intake," in *Equine Applied and Clinical Nutrition: Health, Welfare and Performance*, eds. Raymond J. Goer, Patricia A. Harris, and Manfred Coenen (Philadelphia: Saunders, 2013), 64-77.

[50] Carolyn L. Stull et al., "Fat Supplementation to Alfalfa Diets for Refeeding the Starved Horse," *The Professional Animal Scientist* 19 (2003): 47-54.

[51] Anne M. Desrochers et al., "Efficacy of *Saccharomyces boulardii* for treatment of horses with acute enterocolitis." *Journal of the American Veterinary Medical Association* 227, no.6 (September 15, 2005): 954-959. https://doi.org/10.2460/javma.2005.227.954.

[52] Claudia Sonder, "Director's Message: It Takes a Village," *UC Davis Center for Equine Health Horse Report*, July 2012, 2.

[53] David Baker and Natacha Keramidas, "The psychology of hunger," *Monitor on Psychology*, 44, no. 9 (October 2013): 66. http://www.apa.org/monitor/2013/10/hunger.aspx.

[54] John Maas and Meri Stratton Phelps "Alterations in Body Weight or Size," in *Large Animal Internal Medicine* (Maryland Heights, Missouri: Mosby, 2005): 169.

[55] Becky Hothersall and Christine J. Nicol, "Effects of diet on behavior - normal and abnormal," in *Equine Applied and Clinical Nutrition: Health, Welfare and Performance*, eds. Raymond J. Goer, Patricia A. Harris, and Manfred Coenen (Philadelphia: Saunders, 2013), 443-451.

[56] Elke Hartmann et al., "Management of horses with focus on blanketing and clipping practices reported by members of the Swedish and Norweigian equestrian community," *Journal of Animal Science* 95, no. 3 (March 2017): 1104-1117. https://doi.org/10.2527/jas.2016.1146.

[57] Jennifer Williams, *How to Start and Run a Rescue*, (Gaithersburg, Maryland: Primedia Equine Network, 2007).

[58] Gordon J. Baker and Keith J. Chandler, "Dentistry in the Geriatric Horse," in *Equine Geriatric Medicine and Surgery*, ed. Joseph Bertone (Philadelphia: Saunders, 2006), 51-58.

[59] "Incidence of Colic in U.S. Horses," United States Department of Agriculture, National Animal Health Monitoring System (Veterinary Service Info Sheet, October 2001). https://www.aphis.usda.gov/animal_health/nahms/equine/downloads/equine98/Equine98_is_Colic.pdf.

[60] Mary K. Tinker et al., "Prospective study of equine colic incidence and mortality, "*Equine Veterinary Journal* 29, no. 6 (November 1997): 448-453. https://doi.org/10.1111/j.2042-3306.1997.tb03157.x.

[61] L.M. Mesa et al., "Aquatic toxicity of ivermectin in cattle dung assessed using microcosms," *Ecotoxicology and Environmental Safety* 144 (October 2017): 422-429. https://doi.org/10.1016/j.ecoenv.2017.06.016.

[62] N. Schweitzer "Effects of ivermectin-spiked cattle dung on a water-sediment systme with the aquatic invertebrates *Daphnia magna* and *Chironomus riparius*," *Aquatic Toxicology* 97, no. 4 (May 10, 2010) 304-313.

[63] Jessica C. Gould et al., "The effects of windrow composting on the viability of Parascaris equorum eggs." *Veterinary Parasitology* 191 no. 1-2 (January 16, 2013): 73-80. https://doi.org/10.1016/j.vetpar.2012.08.017.

[64] Laurent Hébert, et al., "Viability of *Rhodocoddus equi* and *Parascaris equorum* eggs exposed to high temperatures," *Current Microbiology* 60, no. 1 (January 2010): 38-41. https://doi.org/10.1007/s00284-009-9497-5.

[65] Lindsay Keller, "Count Your Eggs Before They Hatch," *America's Horse*, May 2017, 16-20.

[66] Jennie A.H. Crawley, "Testing storage methods of faecal samples for subsequent measurement of helminth egg numbers in the domestic horse," *Veterinary Parasitology* 221 (May 15, 2016): 130-133. https://doi.org/10.1016/j.vetpar.2016.03.012.

[67] Kurt Pfister, "New Perspectives in Equine Intestinal Parasitic Disease: Insights in Monitoring Helminth Infections," *Veterinary Clinics of North America, Equine Practice* 34 (2018): 141-153. https://doi.org/10.1016/j/cveq/2017.11.009.

[68] Lindsay Keller, "Deworming Without Dust," *America's Horse*, May 2017, 10-13.

[69] Amanda A. Adams, "Immunosenescence and How it Affects Care of the Older Horse," *Proceedings of the American Association of Equine Practitioners* 62 (2016): 481-490.

[70] Nancy S. Loving, "Equine Immunity From Birth to Old Age," *The Horse*, April 2018, 23-28.

[71] Alison M. Harvey, "Duration of serum antibody response to rabies vaccination in horses," *Journal of the American Veterinary Medical Association* 249, no. 4 (August 15, 2016): 411-418.

[72] Nancy Rich-Gutierrez. "You Are Not A Bad Horse Owner, 8 reasons why your horse might need shoes." https://horsenetwork.com/2017/02/you-are-not-bad-horse-owner/

[73] Andrea A. Floyd and Richard A. Mansmann. *Equine Podiatry*. Saunders; 1 edition (May 30, 2007)

[74] Kevin G. Keegan et al., "Effectiveness of administration of phenylbutazone alone or concurrent administration of phenylbutazone and flunixin meglumine to alleviate lameness in horses," *American Journal of Veterinary Research* 69. No. 2 (February 2008): 167-173. https://doi.org/10.2460/ajvr.69.2.167.

[75] C.G. MacAllister, et al, "Comparison of adverse effects of phenylbutazone, flunixin meglumine, and ketoprofen in horses." *Journal of the American Veterinary Medical Association*, 202, no. 1 (January 1, 1993): 71-77.

[76] Ali Asghar Mozaffari et al., "A comparative study on the adverse effects of flunixin, ketoprofen and phenylbutazone in miniature donkeys: Haematological, biochemical and pathological findings." *New Zealand Veterinary Journal*, 58,

no. 5 (October 2010): 224-228. https://doi.org/10.1080/00480169.2010.69295.

[77] Pierre-Louis Toutain et al., "Plasma concentrations and therapeutic efficacy of phenylbutazone and flunixin meglumine in the horse: pharmacokinetic/pharmacodynamic modelling." *Journal of Veterinary Pharmacology and Therapeutics* 17, no. 6 (December 1994): 459-469. https://doi.org/10.1111/j.1365-2885.1994.tb00278.x.

[78] Michèle Y. Doucet et al., "Comparison of efficacy and safety of paste formulations of firocoxib and phenylbutazone in horses with naturally occurring osteoarthritis." *Journal of the American Veterinary Medical Association* 232, no. 1 (January 1, 2008): 91-97. https://doi.org/10.2460/javma.232.1.91.

[79] Caroline G. Gillespie et al. "Methods and Variables Associated with the Risk of Septic Arthritis Following Intra-Articular Injections in Horses: A Survey of Veterinarians." *Veterinary Surgery* 45, no.8 (September 2016). https://doi.org/10.1111/vsu.12563.

[80] Catherine M. Steel et al., "Risk of septic arthritis after intra-articular medication: a study of 16,624 injections in Thoroughbred racehorses." *Australian Veterinary Journal* 91, no. 7 (July 2013): 268-273. https://doi.org/10.1111/avj.12073.

[81] S.M. Rosanowski et al., "Open standing castration in Thoroughbred racehorses in Hong Kong: Prevalence and severity of complications 30 days post-castration," *Equine Veterinary Journal* 50, no. 3 (February 2018). https://doi.org/10.1111/evj.12758.

[82] P. Busk et al., "Administration of perioperative penicillin reduces postoperative serum amyloid A response in horses being castrated standing," *Veterinary Surgery* 39, no. 5 (July 2010): 638-643. https://doi.org/10.1111/j.1532-950X.2010.00704.x.

[83] S.W. Line et al., "Effect of prepubertal versus postpubertal castration on sexual and aggressive behavior in male horses," *Journal of the Americal Veterinary Medical Association* 186, no. 3 (February 1, 1985): 249-251.

[84] Lori A. Bidwell, "How to Anesthetize Donkeys for Surgical Procedures in the Field," *Proceedings of the American Association of Equine Practitioners* 56 (2010): 38-40.

[85] Susanne Eriksson, "Prevalence and genetic parameters for cryptorchidism in Swedish-born Icelandic horses," *Livestock Science* 180 (October 2015): 1-5. https://doi.org/10.1016/j/livsci/2015/06/022.

[86] H.M. Hayes, "Epidemiological features of 5009 cases of equine cryptorchism," *Equine Veterinary Journal* 18, no. 6 (November 1986). https://doi.org/10/1111/j.2042-3306.1986.tb03692.x.

[87] Mathieu Diribarne, "Polymorphism Analysis of Microsatellites Associated with Seven Candidate Genes for Equine Cryptorchidism," *Journal of Equine Veterinary Science* 29, no. 1 (January 2009): 37-41. https://doi.org/10.1016/j/jevs.2008.11.003.

[88] Suzanne M. Pratt et al., "Malignant Sertoli cell tumor in the retained abdominal testis of a unilaterally cryptorchid horse," *Journal of the American Veterinary Medical Association* 222, no. 4 (February 15, 2003): 486-90.

[89] Natalie Voss, "Something's Missing Here: Explaining Ridgelings," published December 6, 2013. https://www.paulickreport.com/news/ray-s-paddock/somethings-missing-here-explaining-ridglings/. Accessed November 30, 2018.

[90] Patrick M. McCue, "The Proud-Cut Gelding," Colorado State University Equine Reproduction Laboratory. http://csu-cvmbs.colostate.edu/Documents/Learnstall9-proudcut-apr09.pdf.

[91] Patrick M. McCue, "Ovarian Tumors," Colorado State University Equine Reproduction Laboratory. http://csu-cvmbs.colostate.edu/Documents/Learnmares47-reprodprob-ovtum-apr09.pdf

[92] James R. Crabtree, "Can ovariectomy be justified on grounds of behaviour?" *Equine Veterinary Education* (January 2016): 58-60.

[93] Foal Watch by Chemetrics. https://www.foalingwatch.com/ or 1-800-356-3072.

[94] Predict-a-foal by Animal Reproductive Services https://www.arssales.com/epfo-predictafoal.html or 1-800-300-5143.

[95] Kenji Korosue et al., "Comparison of pH and refractometery index with calcium concentrations in preparturient mammary gland secretions of mares," *Journal of the American Veterinary Medical Association* 242, no. 2 (January 15, 2013): 242-248.

[96] Cristina Rosales, et al., "Periparturient characteristics of mares and their foals on a New Zealand Thoroughbred stud farm," *New Zealand Veterinary Journal* 65, no. 1(January 2017): 24-29. https://doi.org/10.1080.00480169.2016.1244021.

[97] Patrick M. McCue, "Meconium Impaction," Colorado State University Equine Reproduction Laboratory. http://csu-cvmbs.colostate.edu/Documents/Learnfoals9-meconiumimpact-apr09.pdf.

[98] Nicola Pusterla et al., "Evaluation of the SNAP foal IgG test for the semiquantitative measurement of immunoglobulin G in foals," *Veterinary Record* 151, no. 9 (August 31, 2002): 258-260. https://doi.org/10.1136/vr.151.9.258

[99] Brett Tennent-Brown, "Plasma therapy in foals and adult horses." *Compendium of Continuing Education, Veterinary* 33, no. 10 (October 2011).

[100] Elisa Rampacci et al., "Umbilical infections in foals: microbiological investigation and management," *The Veterinary Record* 180, no. 22 (June 3, 2017): 543. https://doi.org/10.1136/vr.103999.

[101] Robert H. Mealey and Maureen T. Long, "Mechanisms of Disease and Immunity," in *Equine Internal Medicine (Fourth Edition)*, eds. Stephen M. Reed, Warwick M. Bayly, and Debra C. Sellon, 3-78.

[102] Sarah J. Stoneham, "Feeding orphan and sick foals," in *Equine Applied and Clinical Nutrition: Health, Welfare and Performance*, eds. Raymond J. Goer, Patricia A. Harris, and Manfred Coenen (Philadelphia: Saunders, 2013), 618-627.

[103] Virginia Ann Buechner-Maxwell and Craig D. Thatcher, "Neonatal Nutrition," in *Equine Neonatal Medicine*, (Philadelphia: Saunders, 2006), 51-74.

[104] Mary Rose Paradis, "Feeding the Orphan Foal," *Proceedings of the American Association of Equine Practitioners* 58 (2012): 402-406.

[105] Mare's Match® is available from Purina Animal Nutrition. https://www.purinamills.com/horse-feed/products/detail/mare-s-match-foal-milk-replacer, 1-800-227-8941, P.O. Box 66812, St. Louis, MO 63166-6812.

[106] "Foal Growth, Special Care and Nutrition," The American Association of Equine Practitioners. https://aaep.org/horsehealth/foal-growth-special-care-and-nutrition.

[107] Foal-Lac® pellets are available from Pet-Ag®. https://www.petag.com/products/milk-replacers/equine-milk-replacers/foal-lac-pellets, 1-800-323-6878, 225 Keyes Avenue, Hampshire, IL 60140.

[108] Z. A. Jelan, et al., "Growth rates in Thoroughbred foals," *Pferdeheilkunde* 12, no. 3 (May 1996): 291-295. https://doi.org/10.21836/PEM19960326.

[109] Carleigh Fedorka, "Nurse mares, why we need them, and how to stop the production of nurse mare foals: A rebuttal to Last Chance Corral," *A Yankee in Paris* blog. https://ayankeeinparis.com/2016/10/10/nursemares-why-we-need-them-and-how-to-stop-the-production-of-nursemare-foals-a-rebuttal-to-last-chance-corral/. Last accessed April 3, 2018.

[110] Ryan Bell, "Nurse Foals: The Throwaway Horses," *Western Horseman*, January 2017.

[111] Katherine A. Houpt and Carissa L. Wickens, "Chapter 18: Handling and transport of horses," in *Livestock Handling and Transport, 4th Edition*, ed. Temple Grandin. (Boston: CABI, 2014): 315-341.

[112] Rebecca Watson, "Let sleeping horses lie?" *Equine Health* 2017 no. 37 (September 2017). https://doi.org/10.12968/eqhe.2017.37.33.

[113] D.C. Williams, et. al., "Qualitative and Quantitative Characteristics of the Electroencephalogram in Normal Horses during Spontaneous Drowsiness and Sleep," *Journal of Veterinary Internal Medicine* 22, no. 3 (July 2008). https://doi/abs/10.1111/j.1939-1676.2008.0096.x.

[114] Robert E. Holland, Jr., "Conditions, Diseases, and Injuries of the Older Horses for Horse Owners," in *Equine Geriatric Medicine and Surgery*, ed. Joseph Bertone (Philadelphia: Saunders, 2006), 245-251.

[115] Hussni O. Mohammed et al., "Vitamin E deficiency and risk of equine motor neuron disease," *Acta Veterinaria Scandinavia* 49, no. 17 (July 2007). https://doi.10.1186/1751-0147-49-17.

[116] Rebecca Gimenez, Tomas Gimenez, and Kimberley A. May, *Technical Large Animal Emergency Rescue* (New Jersey: Wiley-Blackwell, 2008).

[117] Rebecca Gimenez, "How to Manipulate a Recumbent Horse (Entrapment, Clinical, or Technical Emergency Rescue Situations)," *Proceedings of the American Association of Equine Practitioners* 63 (2017): 403-412.

[118] "Maintenance of Horses in Slings," in *Current Therapy in Equine Medicine, 6th Edition,* eds. N. Edward Robinson and Kim A. Sprayberry (Philadelphia: Saunders, 2008): 921.

[119] "Community Emergency Response Team," Official Website of the Department of Homeland Security. ready.gov/community-emergency-response-team, accessed September 21, 2018.

[120] Peter Hoeppe, "Trends in weather related disasters – Consequences for insurers and society," *Weather and Climate Extremes* 11 (March 2016): 70-79. https://doi.org/10.1016/j.wace.2015.10.002.

[121] Federal Emergency Management Agency (FEMA) 2017 survey, fewer than 40% of people have an emergency plan. https://community.fema.gov/resource/1549551304000/ICPD_AP_Story_Survey_PDF, and

[122] Rebecca Husted et al., "How to Develop and Equine Veterinary Facility All-Hazards Sheltering and Evacuation Plan," *Proceedings of the American Association of Equine Practitioners* 64 (2018): 74-86.

[123] Ann Harris, "Ralph's Responders," *America's Horse,* May, 2017, 50-51. lsart.org/ralphs-responders.pml.

[124] Ky Evan Mortensen, *Horses of the Storm* (Lexington, Kentucky: Eclipse Press, 2008).

[125] Ky Evan Mortensen, *Horses of the Storm* (Lexington, Kentucky: Eclipse Press, 2008).

[126] FEMA Resources https://www.fema.gov/incident-command-system-resources.

[127] Rebecca Husted (Gimenez), http://www.TLAER.org, accessed September 9, 2018.

[128] Tomas Gimenez et al., "How to Effectively Perform Emergency Rescue of Equines," *Proceedings of the American Association of Equine Practitioners* 48 (2002): 276-281.

[129] Kenneth Marcella, "Equine rescue 101: Aiding a downed horse, Practitioners must protect rescuers as well as rescuees," *DVM 360*, Jan 2006. http://veterinarynews.dvm360.com/equine-rescue-101-aiding-downed-horse.

[130] Heather Smith Thomas, "Navigating Natural Disasters with Horses," *The Horse* March 2, 2015.

[131] Pat Raia, "Narrow Escape," *The Horse*, February 2017, 26-30.

[132] Elizabeth W. Herbert, "Findings and strategies for treating horses injured in open range fires," *Equine Veterinary Education* 30, no. 4 (April 2018): 177-186. https://doi.org/10/1111/eve.12806.

[133] Derek C. Knottenbelt, "Management of Burn Injuries," in *Current Therapy in Equine Medicine, 6th Edition,* eds. N. Edward Robinson and Kim A. Sprayberry (Philadelphia: Aaunders, 2008): 220-225

[134] Susan C. Kahler, "When Fire Strikes Home: Tending to the needs of pets affected by residential fires," *Journal of the American Veterinary Medical Association* 252, no. 4 (February 15, 2018): 376-383.

[135] Oliver Knes et al., "Veterinarians and Humane Endings: When Is It the Right Time to Euthanize a Companion Animal?" *Frontiers in Veterinary Science* 4 no. 45 (April 2017). https://doi.org/10.3389/fvets.2017.00045.

[136] Thomas W. McGowan et al., "Euthanasia in Aged Horses: Relationship between the Owner's Personality and Their Opinions on, and Experience of, Euthanasia of Horses," *Journal Anthrozoös: A multidisciplinary journal of the interactions of people and animals* 25 no. 3 (2012): 261-275. https://doi.org/10.2752/175303712X13403555186091.

[137] Carolyn Butler and Laurel Lagoni, "Euthanasia and Grief Support in an Equine Bond-Centered Practice," in *Equine Geriatric Medicine and Surgery*, ed. Joseph Bertone (Philadelphia: Saunders, 2006), 231-243.

[138] "Euthanasia Guidelines," revised 2016. https://aaep.org/euthanasia-guidelines, accessed August 5, 2018.

[139] Emanuela Dalla Costa et al., "Development of the Horse Grimace Scale (HGS) as a pain assessment tool in horses undergoing routine castration." *PLoS One* 9 no. 3 (March 19, 2014): e92281. https://doi.org/10.1371/journal.pone.0092281.

[140] "Equine 2015 Baseline Reference of Equine Health and Management in the United States," United States Department of Agricultures, National Animal Health Monitoring System (December 2016).

[141] Adriana G. Silva and Martin O. Furr, "Diagnoses, clinical pathology findings, and treatment outcome of geriatric horses: 345 cases (2006–2010)," *Journal of The American Veterinary Medical Association* 243, no. 12 (December 15, 2010): 1762-1768.

[142] J.K. Shearer and P. Nicoletti. "Humane euthanasia of sick, injured and/or debilitated livestock," University of Florida IFAS Extension. http://neacha.org/resources/Humane.livestock.Euthanasia.pdf.

[143] Amanda Abnee, "Dead Animal Disposal," University of Kentucky Cooperative Extension Service. https://kyhorsevet.com/wp-content/uploads/Dead_Animal_Disposal_UK.pdf, accessed June 15, 2019

[144] Claudia Hartley and Rachael A. Grundon, "Chapter 5: Diseases and surgery of the globe and orbit," in *Equine Ophthalmology* (3rd Edition), ed. Brian C. Gilger (New Jersey: Wiley-Blackwell, 2016), 151.

[145] Erica Larson, "Understanding Equine Vision," *The Horse*, Oct 7, 2012. https://thehorse.com/118318/understanding-equine-vision/.

[146] Hilary M. Clayton, Peter F. Flood, Diana S. Rosenstein, *Clinical Anatomy of the Horse*, (Maryland Heights, Missouri: Mosby, 2005): 12, 18.

[147] Lee Benson, "The Anatomy of the Ear," *The Horse*, May 1, 1999. https://thehorse.com/14457/the-anatomy-of-the-ear/.

[148] Alexandra Kupke et al., "Intranasal Location and Immunohistochemical Characterization of the Equine Olfactory Epithelium," *Frontiers in Neuroanatomy* 10, no. 97 (October 13, 2016). https://doiorg/10/3389/fnana.2016.00097.

[149] Jennifer L. Williams et al., "The efficacy of a secondary reinforcer (clicker) during acquisition and extinction of an operant task in horses" *Applied Animal Behaviour Science* 88, no. 3–4 (October 2004): 331-341. https://doi.org/10.1016/j.applanim.2004.03.008.

[150] P. Ivan Pavlov, "Conditioned reflexes: An investigation of the physiological activity of the cerebral cortex," 1927 lecture, printed in *Annals of Neurosciences* 17, no. 3 (July 2010): 136–141. https://doi.org/10.5214/ans.0972-7531.1017309.

[151] Sue McDonnell personal communication at the American Veterinary Medical Association Conference (July 2018). Magnetic Resonance Imaging (MRI) of a horse's brain post-starvation showed decreased to absent neural tissue.

[152] Christa Lesté-Lasserre, "Fear In Horses," *thehorse.com* Factsheet (2014), sponsored by Ceva Pharmaceuticals.

[153] Sue McDonnell "What Does 'Licking and Chewing' in Horses Mean?" *The Horse*, Feb 28, 2019. https://thehorse.com/18825/what-does-licking-and-chewing-in-horses-mean/.

[154] Temple Grandin. "Safe Handling of Large Animals," *Occupational medicine: State of the Art Reviews*, 14, no. 2 (April-June 1999): 195.

[155] Benjamin Flakoll et al., "Twitching in veterinary procedures: How does this technique subdue horses?" *Journal of Veterinary Behavior* 18 (March–April 2017): 23-28. https://doi.org/10.1016/j.jveb.2016.12.004.

156 E. Lagerweij et al., "The twitch in horses: a variant of acupuncture," *Science* 225, no. 4667 (September 14, 1984): 1172-1174. https://doi.org/10.1126/science.6089344.

157 Ahmed B. Ali, et al, "Assessing the influence of upper lip twitching in naive horses during an aversive husbandry procedure (ear clipping)," *Journal of Veterinary Behavior* 21 (September-October 2017): 20-25. https://doi.org/10.1016/j.veb.2017.07.001.

158 Jeannine M. Berger et al., "Behavior and physiological responses of weaned foals treated with equine appeasing pheromone: A double-blinded, placebo-controlled, randomized trial," *Journal of Veterinary Behavior* 8, no. 4 (July-August 2013): 265-277. https://doi.org/10.1016/j.veb.2012.09.003.

159 Elke D. Eckert et al., "A 57-year follow-up investigation and review of the Minnesota study on human starvation and its relevance to eating disorders," *Archives of Psychology* 2, no. 3 (March 2018). https://archivesofpsychology.org/index.php/aop/article/view/50.

160 Jennifer Williams, "Starting the Older Horse," *Equus*, April 2013. https://equusmagazine.com/horse-care/on-behavior-starting-the-older-horse-8602.

161 Jess Holloway, Holloway's Pretty Good Horse Barn and Training. Personal communication. https://www.hollowaysprettygoodhorsebarn.com/.

162 "BLM Adoption Requirements," Bureau of Land Management, last accessed July 1, 2019. https://www.blm.gov/sites/blm.gov/files/wildhorse_adoptionrequirements.pdf.

163 Janice Cartwright, Montana Horse Sense. Personal communication. https://www.montanahorsesense.com/.

164 Elyssa M. Payne et al., "Evidence of horsemanship and dogmanship and their application in veterinary contexts," *The Veterinary Journal* 204, no. 3 (June 2015): 247-254. https://doi.org/10.1016/j.tvjl.2015.04.004.

165 Elke Hartmann et al., "Training young horses to social separation: Effect of a companion horse on training efficiency," *Equine Veterinary Journal* 43, no. 5 (September 2011): 580-584. https://doi.org/10.1111/j.2042-3306.2010.00326.x.

166 Sue McDonnell, "How to Rehabilitate Horses with Injection Shyness (Or Any Procedure Non-Compliance)," *Proceedings of the American Association of Equine Practitioners* 46 (2000): 168-172.

167 Katherine Reid et al., "Anxiety and pain in horses measured by heart rate variability and behavior," *Journal of Veterinary Behavior* 22 (November-December 2017): 1-6. https://doi.org/10.1016/j.jveb.2017.09.002.

168 Kathrine J. Wågø et al., "The importance of needle gauge for pain during injection of lidocaine," *Journal of Plastic Surgery and Hand Surgery* 50, no. 2 (2016): 115-118, https://doi.org/10.3109/2000656X.2015.1111223.

169 Stephanie Barnette, Skogen-Barnette Horses. Personal communication. https://www.skogenbarnettehorses.com/.

170 Dan James and Dan Steers, *Long Reining with Double Dan: Safe, Controlled Ground Techniques for Building Partnership, Achieving Softness, and Overcoming Training and Behavioral Issues.* (Vermont: Trafalgar Square Books, 2016).

Acknowledgments

This book would not be possible without support and contributions from family, friends, and equine professionals.

Thank you first and foremost to my husband, Sid. He is the only reason this work is possible; he made sure that our herd and I managed to eat during the really long days.

Of course, my parents, Ron and Amie Green, who somehow managed to give me enough drive to complete this daunting effort deserve my thanks.

Karen Lehmann (of Phrases Incorporated) was so very helpful in breaking outside of her box and making sure I was on track with this work.

The people who have spent the most time reading this are a group of non-horsey friends in the Bozeman Writers' Group. Most knew nothing about horses when I started. Their ability to make sure this book is readable to the "average" person has been critical in moving it forward. Thank you to Jennifer Courtemanche, Jessica Darling, Seth Hartman, Amy San Nicolas, Ed Merritt, Sarah Simser, Steve Powell, Laura Idzerda, Theresa Nichols Schuster, Rebecca Watters, and others who have been kind enough to put up with my "boring non-fiction" as they work on their sci-fi, fantasy, and fascinating storytelling. I appreciate you all more than you could know and value everything you bring to the table.

My work family at Hardaway Veterinary Hospital has been amazing. Crystal, thank you for the incessant photo sessions, and Rachael, for your artistic talent. Many people posed for photos, read chapters, and just generally put up with me as I worked.

I have abundant gratitude for Rebecca Didier, Martha Cook, and Caroline Robbins at Trafalgar Square Books. They have taken the time to help me clarify what I needed to say about rescuing horses and provided support and encouragement along the way.

Jake Mosher was extraordinarily generous to provide me with a cover photo of rescued horses. Jennifer Williams with Bluebonnet Equine Humane Society has been amazing with encouragement, photos, and horse histories. Melissa Hines at the University of Tennessee is very knowledgeable and caring! Rebecca Husted (Gimenez) is always a pleasure to work with, and so dedicated and passionate. Janice Cartwright helped me with titles, photos, brainstorming, and horses. Brianna Rigdon and Rachael Roberts also lent me their artistic talent. Thank you all.

Patty Wilbur and Miriam Kan are two dear friends with their own writing and life aspirations who still found the time to read and critique. Steve Price helped me navigate the whole process. Robin Williams read an excessively long draft in just a couple of days, helping me reduce it to something usable. Eva Wendell was there from start to finish. Many professionals advised and supported me: Jess Holloway, Renae Jones, Ed Bullock, Stephanie Barnette, David Arnold, Cheryl Nigg, Naomi Saiz, Emily Hutton, and Am Kuglin.

Veterinarians and horse people who have mentored me over the years have made me into the person I am today. Thank you Danny and Ann Allen, Terry Berg, Sean Bowman, Joe Davis, Alexis Theiss, Linda Dahlgren, Michael Schramme, Liara Gonzalez, and Lisa Fortier. Many people over the years and distance have contributed to my personal development and thus, this book.

The Rescue groups that have inspired me should be named here: Horse Haven (Lenoir City, Tennessee), Hearts of Horse Haven (Knoxville, Tennessee), Walkin 'N Circles (Stanley, New Mexico), 3H Horses, Humans and Herds (Tijeras, New Mexico), EquiSave Foundation (Livingston, Montana), Bluebonnet Equine Humane Society (College Station, Texas), and Big Horn Ranch and Rescue (Busby, Montana).

Every week I hear, "Well, Doc, he's a rescue," so I must also reach out and tell every individual who has rescued a horse how much I appreciate you, your hard work, and your dedication to horses.

INDEX

Page numbers in *italics* indicate illustrations.

Abdominal cavity, compromise of, 83, 84, 90, 141
Abortion, 96, 99
Abscesses
  caused by strangles, 59, *59*
  in hooves, 65, 72, *72*, 74–75, *75*
  muscular, 77, *78*
Abuse, 162, 175
Accidents, 144, 159. *See also* Emergencies
Adequan, 78, 79
Adrenaline, 166
Aggression, 38, 173
Agonal breaths, 149
Alfalfa
  kidney disease caution, 43
  nutritional aspects, 33, 36
  for pregnant mares, 96
  in refeeding starved horses, 27, 30–31
American Association of Equine Practitioners guidelines, 56, 145–47
American Horse Council economic impact report, 6, 7
American Paint Horse Association, 6
American Quarter Horse Association, 6, 17
Anderson sling, *131*, 133
Anemia, 23–24, 25, 32, 110
Anesthesia
  in castration, 85–87, 91
  of debilitated horses, 85
  of donkeys and mules, 90
  of foals, 109
Anestrus, 93
Angle code freeze brand system, 17, *17*
Angular limb deformities, 106–8, *107*
Animal shelters and animal control teams, 135
Antibiotics, 75, 83, 105

Antibodies, passive transfer of, 96, 102, 110, 112
Anti-cruelty legislation, 15
Antiseptics, 81, 83
Anxiety, 173, 177–180, 204, 218
Approach-and-retreat techniques
  overview, 195–96
  uses of, 161, 204, 207, 217, 229
Arabian Horse Association, 6, 17
"Arm extensions." *See* Whips
Arthritis
  down horses and, 125, 126, 128
  foot handling considerations, 182
  lameness from, 76–77
  in overweight horses, 154
  treatment of, 76–79
Ascarids, 51, 52
Asking for help
  case histories, 120, 216
  with training, 152, 168, 181, 184, 210, 221
Aspiration pneumonia, 113
Assistance, for owners, 7–8
Avoidance behaviors, 173

Backing up, 200, 223
Bacterial infections. *See* Infections
Balance point, of flight zone, 185–86, *186*, *188*
Balking, 197, 198
Banamine, 45, 47, 77, 78, 79
Bandages and bandaging
  for contracted tendons, 105
  cost considerations, 80
  in emergencies, 140
  for wound care, 82–83, *82*
Barbiturate injections, 147, 148
Barefoot hoof care, 69–70, 72
Barn fires, 142
BCS. *See* Body Condition Score
Becker sling, *130*
Bed sores, 132, *132*
Bedding, in trailers, 13
Beet pulp, 42
Befriending technique, for untouchable horses, 186–87

Behavior
  castration and, 88–89, 91–92
  correction of, 172
  in debilitated horses, 38, 171, 185
  in foals, 115–16, 121
  retraining to correct, 221
  spaying and, 97
Bell boots, 132
Bile, 35
Bills of sale, 20
Biosecurity measures, 21, *21*
Biotin, 64
Birth control. *See also* Pregnancy
  castration, 85–93
  spaying, 97
Biting, 162
Bits, 224
Blankets and blanketing, 14, 38
Bleeding, following castration, 89–90. *See also* Wounds
Blind spots, 155
Blindness, 157
Blizzards, 142–43
Blocker Tie Ring, 193, *193*
Blood flow, in prone horses, 86
Blood pressure, 86
Blood tests
  for down horses, 125–26
  in evaluating rescue horses, 24–25, 43
  IgG test, 108
Body Condition Score (BCS)
  overview, 26–28, *27–29*
  examples of, *8*
  monitoring/documentation of, 22, 37
  training considerations, 152–54, 171–72, 200, 209, 211, 223
Body disposal, 150
Body language
  of handler, 214
  of horse, 173, 184–85, 187, 228
Body temperature
  in foals, 104
  maintaining, in emaciated horses, 38
  monitoring, 21, 60, 80, 104

overheating, 15
   thermometer desensitization, 203
Bolting, of food, 178–180
Bonding, with rescued/neglected horses, 22, 25, 170–72, 186–87, 194
Bone injuries, 83, 84, 140, 146
Boots, protective, 14
Borium, 72–73, *73*
Bot flies, 52, *52*
Bottle feeding, 113, 116
Braiding in, of identification tags, 20
Brand inspections, 20
Brands, 16–17, *17*
Breakaway equipment, 14, 20, 118, 188
Breaks, during travel, 13
Breed registry statistics, 6
Bribes, 159–161, 187
Bridles
   fit of, 224–26
   identification tags for, 19–20
   introducing, 222–24
Bucket feeding, 113, *114*, 116
Bucking, 219
Bureau of Land Management Mustang adoption guidelines, 15, 186–87
Burial, 150
Burns, 142, *143*
Bute, 79
Butt ropes, 119, *119*

Calcium, 45, 64
Calories, 33, 36
Canada, export of horses to, 6
Cancer, 43–44
Canter, 215, 217, 229
Captive bolt tools, 147–48, *148*
Carbohydrates, 27, 32–33
Carotid artery, 205–6
Carpal valgus abnormalities, 107
Carrot sticks (whip type), 173, *173*, 181
Cartwright, Janice, 189
Case histories
   asking for help, 120, 228
   blind horses, 157
   colic, 9
   emergency evacuations, 137
   euthanasia, 149
   fescue toxicosis, 95
   foaling, 99
   injuries, 70

joint infections, 70
lost horses, 192
negative reinforcement, 161
neglected horses, 4–5
obese horses, 178
orphan foal behavior, 116
pain-related behavior, 62
positive memories, 198
pregnancy/pregnant mares, 32, 95, 99
proud-cut horses, 92
rescuer devotion, 46, 226
"rideable" horses, 228
trailer loading, 12, 167
training, 120
trust, 167
unwanted horses, 216
Cast horses, 124, 128, *128*
Castration
   behavioral effects, 87, 88–89
   case histories, 229
   complications, 89–90
   of cryptorchids, 90–93, *91*
   procedures for, 85–88, *87–88*
   proud-cut horses, 91–92
Catch ropes, 118, 181
Catching horses, 121, 152, 181
Cathartics, 47
Cavalletti, 171, 223
Chain of Custody forms, 20
"Chasing," to trailer load, 13, 186
Chestnut patterns, 16
Chewing
   dental health and, 39
   by foals, 121
   of food, 179–180
   as sign of relaxation, 167
Choke, 34, 146, 178–180
Cleft palate, 109
Clicker training, 160
Clostridium tetani infections, 57
Club feet, 68–69, *68*
Coffin bones, 68–69
Coggins, Leroy, 23
Coggins tests, 20, 23–24, 137
Colic
   overview, 44, 45, 180
   case histories, 9
   in older horses, 146
   prevention, 47
   resemblance of labor to, 100
   risk factors, 15, 23, 45, 54, 97, 142
   severity of, 133
   signs of, 44–45, 124, 126
   treatment of, 47–48, 130

Color perception, 156
Colostrum
   alternatives to, 111–12
   antibody transfer through, 96, 102, 108, 110
Colts, castration of, 85–93. *See also* Foals
Communication, in emergency response, 138–39
Community emergency response teams, 134
Companion horses
   benefits of, 14, 22, 47, 193, 204
   for orphan foals, 116
   soundness of, 66
Complete Blood Count, 24–25
Complete feeds, 33, 34, 35
Composting, of manure, 51
Confidence, building, 171, 172, 196, 201, 212
Confidence EQ, 176–77
Confined spaces
   down horses in, 124
   training for manners in, 153, *153*, 196–97, 199–200, 202
Confinement, extended, 146
Confiscation, 7–8, 20, 36
Congenital problems, evaluation for, 104
Consistency, in training, 172, 182, 183, 214
Constipation, 115. *See also* Impaction
Coordination, 171, 201
Corneal reflex, 149–150
Coronary bands, 62, *63*, 73, 75
Corrections, 172. *See also* Punishment
Cortisol, 25
Costs. *See* Economic factors
Coughing, 13
Cracks, in hooves, 74–75, *74–75*
Cradling, of foals, 117–18, *118*
Cremation, 150
Crooked ankle/crooked knee, 107
Cross-cantering, 217
Cryptorchidism, 90–93, 229
Cubed feeds, 34
Curiosity, 171, 173, 185
Cushing's disease, 25

Dangerous horses, 175, 193
Darkness, visual adaptation to, 156, 158, 197, 199
Dart guns, 194
Deafness, 158

Death, confirmation of, 149. *See also* Euthanasia
Debilitated horses
   behavior in, 171, 185
   care considerations, 38, 54, 55
   down, 125
   exercise guidelines, 152–54, 171–72, 187
   hoof handling considerations, 67, 182
   paraphimosis in, 93
   pregnancy in, 93, 94
   refeeding of, 27, 30–31, 48
Decubital ulcers, 132
Deer flies, 54
Defecation, as sign of stress, 165
Dehydration, 15, 45, 126
Delayed patellar release, 223
Dental care
   floating teeth, 40–42, 40–42
   for older horses, 38–39
Depth perception, 155
Dermatophilus congolensis infections, 55
Desensitization
   approach-and-retreat in, 161, 195–96
   to handling of feet/legs, 181–83
   to injections, 205–8, *206*
   to mounting, 227
   opportunities for, 172
   to scary objects, 174–75
   to tack, 217–19, 224–25
Deworming, 23, 49–51, 52, 54, 97, 205
Diarrhea, 21, 35, 113
Dictyocaulus arnfieldi parasites, 53
Digestive health. *See also* Colic
   dentistry and, 38–42
   NSAID effects on, 77
   nutritional aspects, 26, 38, 39
   probiotics for, 35
   weight loss and, 37–38, 43
Disaster preparedness, 134–38
Disease modifying osteoarthritis drugs, 78
Diseases
   control procedures, 21–22
   freedom from, 3
   infectious, overview of, 57
   parasite vectors of, 54
Disrespectful behavior, 116, 118. *See also* Respect, training for
Distinguishing marks, 16, 20–21

Distraction techniques, 160, 175–76, 206–7
Distress, freedom from, 3
Documentation
   in emergency preparedness, 136–37, 139
   monitoring weight, 37, 44
   of ownership status, 20–21, 137
   in proving neglect, 22, 37, 49
Dog-sitting position, 125
Dominance, 169
Donkeys
   castration of, 90
   gestation period, 98
   hoof care, 64, *64*
   parasites in, 53
   stand and wait response, 166, 218
Dormosedan Gel, 177
Down horses
   overview, 122
   assessment of, 124–26
   in emergency response, 139–140
   euthanasia considerations, 146
   handler safety, 122–23, *123*
   health risks for, 124–25
   long-term maintenance of, 130–33
   repositioning, 127–29
   standing assistance techniques, 126–130
Drainage, of infections, 75, 90

Ears
   in fear response, 165
   handling of, 223–24
   movement of, 158–59
   twitch technique, 175–76
Eastern equine encephalitis, 56, 58
Economic factors
   as factor in neglect, 4–8
   in horse care, 9, 42, 80, 150
"The Economic Impact of the U.S. Horse Industry" (American Horse Council), 6, 7
Ectoparasites, 54–55
Edema, 23
Electrolytes, 45, 47, 126
Emaciated horses. *See* Debilitated horses
Emergencies. *See also* Colic; Down horses; Wounds
   natural disasters, 137, 141–44

   preparedness measures, 134–38, 201
   rescue techniques, 138, 139–140
   response teams, 138–39, 140
Emergency contact information, 136, 137
Encephalitis, 56, 57, 58
Enclosed spaces
   trailers as, 12–14, 202
   training for, 196
   visual considerations, 156, 158, 197, 199
Enclosures, guidelines for, 186
Endorphin release, 176
Enemas, 103–4
Environmental considerations, 50–51, 65. *See also* Natural disasters
Epidiymis, 91, 92
Eponychium, 101
Equine appeasing pheromone, 176–77
Equine Emergency Response Units, 139
Equine Herpes Virus, 21, 57, 59, 96
Equine Infectious Anemia, 23–24
Equine metabolic syndrome, 76–77
Equine Podiatry (Floyd and Mansmann), 70
The Equine Protection Fund of New Mexico, 229
Equioxx, 77, 79
EquiSave Foundation, *86*
Escaped horses, 142, 192
Estrogens, 97
Euthanasia
   overview, 150
   advance planning for, 145
   compassionate guidelines, 145–47
   consent documents, 147, *147*
   cost of, 150
   due to injury, 83–84
   indications, 25, 42, 70, 115–16, 125, 130, 131, 140
   procedures, 147–150
Evacuation planning, 134–38
Evisceration, 90
Exercise
   BCS considerations, 152–54, 171–72, 187
   changes in, 45
   groundwork as, 211
   to reduce castration swelling, 89, 90

for strengthening horses, 211, 217, 220–21, 223
at trot, 213
Expectations, setting, 172
Eyes
adjustment to dark, 156, 158, 197, 199
anatomy of, 156
covering of, 126
darting motion in, 125
injuries to, 140–41
signs of tension/fear in, 164, 165

Facial crest, 190, 191
Fairness
as euthanasia consideration, 25, 115–16
in training, 145–46, 168, 172
Falls, 124
Farriers, 63–64, 121, 182–83
Fats. *See* Oils and fats
Fear
vs. curiosity, 173
freedom from, 3
medically addressing, 175
physiology of, 166–67
recognizing, 165
signs of, 164–66
of trailer loading, 200
training to overcome, 162–64, 168, 184–85, 200, 221
unintentional reward of, 198
of whips, 173–75
Fecal egg counts, 49, 52–53, 52
Fecal evaluations, 23
Fecal output, monitoring, 45
Fedorka, Carleigh, 117
Feeder designs, 177–79, 177–79
Feeding
changes in, 45, 47, 115
of orphan foals, 111–16, 113–14
re-feeding considerations, 5, 27, 30–31, 36–38
in trailers, for desensitization, 200
during travel, 13
unwanted behaviors around, 38, 177–180
in winter conditions, 143
Feet. *See also* Hoof care
abscesses in, 72
anatomy of, 61–63, 63, 71, 71
chronic lameness and, 76
conformation of, 67–69, 67–69
of foals, 101

growth rate of, 71
handling of, 120–21, 152, 180–83
hoof growth and structure, 64–65
movement of, in fear response, 161, 165, 175
Fences and fencing, 142, 186
Fescue toxicosis, 94, 96, 102
Fetlock bands, 19
Fetlocks
abnormalities of, in foals, 107
protection of, 132
Fever, 21, 60, 104, 108. *See also* Infections
Fiber, indigestible, 33
Fidgeting, 187
Field anesthesia, 85–86, 86
Field of view, 155–56, 156
Fires, 142
Firmness, in training, 120
Firocoxib, 77, 79
First aid
basic techniques, 81–84, 140–41
for down horses, 126
kits for, 81, 136
Five Freedoms, 3
Flat halters, 181, 188
Flax seed, 47
Flehmen response, 88, 89
Flexion tests, 222, 222
Flight response, 165, 173, 181, 185, 194, 226
Flight zone, 185–86, 186
Floating
of damaged hooves, 73–74, 74
of teeth, 40–42, 40–41
Flooding, 138
Floyd, Andrea, 70
Flunixin meglumine. *See* Banamine
Fly spray, 54
Foaling
birthing process, 98–102, 100–102
complications of, 99, 101–2
signs of, 92, 95, 98–100, 98
Foal-Lac, 115
Foals
abnormalities in, 106–8, 107
adoption of, 117
behavior of, 110, 115–16
early handling of, 116–17
health evaluations for, 104–9
immature, 107

milestone timeline, 115
monitoring growth of, 115
orphan, 110–16, 113–14, 117
positioning of, during birth, 101, 101
training of, 116–121
Footing
euthanasia considerations, 148–49
for helping down horses, 127
hoof growth and, 65
horse's examination of, 156, 197, 199
in trailers, 12, 13
Forage
calorie estimates, 36
foals' consumption of, 115
in refeeding starved horses, 30–31
selection of, 32–34
Forelegs, handling of, 182
Forward assist repositioning, 129, 129, 144
Fractures, 84, 140, 146
Freeze brands, 16–17, 17
Fungal infections, 55, 65

Gaited horses, 215
Gallbladder, lack of, 35
Gas colic, 45, 47
Gastroguard, 44
Gastrointestinal tract. *See* Digestive health
Gastroscopy, 44
Geldings, 22, 88–89, 169, 212. *See also* Castration
Genetics
health factors, 65, 90
identification systems using, 18
Girth area, 218
Glucosamine, 78, 79
Go Bucket, recommendations for, 136
Goats, as companions, 22
Grain
overview, 34–35
calorie estimates, 36
carbohydrates in, 32–33
as distraction, 206–7
eliminating, 47
in refeeding syndrome, 30
Grass hay, 30–31, 33, 33, 36
Grasses and grazing, 47, 94, 96, 102
Gravel, ingestion of, 177, 177
Grazing. *See* Grasses and grazing

Grinding teeth, 39, 39
Grooming
   in bonding/training, 172, 204
   desensitization to, 121, 161, 181
   health considerations, 55
   mutual, 187, 188
Ground poles, 153, 171, 223
Ground-driving, 154, 224–25, 225
Groundwork
   BCS considerations, 153
   longeing, 212–15, 213, 217
   purpose of, 209
   safety considerations for, 209–10
Gums, evaluating, 81, 203
Gut bacteria, 35, 110
Gut motility, 45, 48
Guttural pouches, infection of, 59, 59

Habronema parasites, 52, 53
Hair coat
   dirty, 55
   external parasites and, 22–23, 54
   slow-shedding, 25
   thick, body evaluation and, 26, 38
Halter training. *See also* Handling
   for adult horses, 184, 190–93
   building horse's confidence with, 171
   for foals, 116–120, 118–19
   health care considerations, 47
   importance of, 152, 194, 200
Halters
   embedded, 53
   fit of, 190
   identification tags for, 19–20, 19
   types of, 188–190
Halting, on longe, 214–15
Handlers and rescuers. *See also* Safety considerations
   devotion of, 46, 226
   emotional health of, 150, 172
Handling
   from both sides, 207, 213–14, 217, 226
   training for, 47, 152, 161, 199
Handwashing, 21
Hard keepers, 35, 38
Hay
   feeders and nets for, 14, 31, 177–79, 177–79
   for pregnant mares, 94, 96
   in refeeding starved horses, 30–31
   selection of, 32–34, 33
Head
   control of, 214
   injuries to, 83
Head bob, in evaluating lameness, 69
Head bumpers, 14
Healing, delayed, 80
Health evaluations, prior to training, 210–11. *See also* Veterinary examinations
Hearing, 158–59
Heart murmurs, 104. *See also* Pulse rate
Heat waves, 142
Hemorrhages, 89–90
Henneke, Don, 26. *See also* Body Condition Score
Herd dynamics
   around feeding, 177–180
   new horse socialization, 169–170
   orphan foals and, 115–16
   punishment in, 162
   rescue horses and, 22
Herd-bound horses, 204
Hernia, umbilical, 109
Herpes. *See* Equine Herpes Virus
High flankers, 90
High-shedders, 51, 52
Hind legs, handling of, 182
Hoof boots, 71
Hoof care. *See also* Feet
   for foals, 107, 121
   foot angle in, 72
   in managing lameness, 66–73
   neglect of, 3, 67–69, 67–69, 185
   routine trimming, 63–64
   shoeing, 69–73, 71–74
   training for, 120–21, 152, 181–83
Hoof testers, 222
Hormones, 93, 97, 99
Horse flies, 54
Horse Transportation Safety Act, 15
Horse/human relationships, 159, 178
Horses, population estimates, 4, 6–7. *See also* Debilitated horses; Rescue horses; Unwanted horses

Horses of the Storm (Mortenson), 138–39
Hospital environments, training for, 198, 202
Hot brands, 16–17, 17
Hunger, freedom from, 3. *See also* Feeding
Hurricanes, 136–37, 138, 142
Husted, Rebecca Gimenez 139
Hyaluronic acid, 78, 79
Hydration. *See* Water
Hyperadrenocorticism, 25
Hypothermia, 126, 144
Hypsodont teeth, 39, 39

Identification
   in emergency preparedness, 136–37, 138, 139
   permanent, 16–19, 17
   temporary, 19–20, 19
   for travel, 13
Immune system, 22, 53, 59, 102, 108
Immunoglobulin class G (IgG) test, 108, 108, 112
Impaction
   colic, 45, 180
   of meconium, 103–4
Impoundment, 36
Incident command, 138–39
Infections
   from castration, 88, 90
   in hooves, 65, 75
   infectious disease overview, 57
   in joints, 80, 83, 106
   skin conditions, 55
   treatment of, 84
   of umbilicus, 109
   weight loss from, 43
Influenza, 21, 57, 59
In-hand work, 224. *See also* Ground-driving; Longeing
Injections, training for, 205–8, 206. *See also* Sedation; Vaccines
Injuries
   from abuse, 162
   to bones, 83, 84, 140, 146
   freedom from, 3
   to hooves, 73–74
   preventing, 169–170
   during travel, 14
Insects, beneficial, 50–51. *See also* Parasites
Insulin response, 27, 30, 32
Internal organs, injuries to, 83, 133

Internet resources, 7
Intranasal treatments, 208
Intravenous fluids, 30
Intrinsic rewards, 159–161
Iris patterns, 16
Ivermectin, 49

JNP Horses, 117
Jockey Club of North America, 6, 19
Joint infections, 80, 83, 106
Joint injections, 78–79, 84
Jugular vein, 205–6

Keratin, 62, 64
Keys, Ancel, 38
Kicking, 180, 181, 183, 219
Kidneys, 43, 144
Knees, 125

Labor. *See* Foaling
Laboratory testing, 23–25, 43, 108, 125–26. *See also* Veterinary examinations
Lameness
　overview, 84
　causes of, 73–77, 80
　chronic, 76
　evaluating for, 67–69, 154, 217
　hoof care in management of, 66–73
Laminae, 63, 63
Laminitis, 25, 69, 69, 75–76, 76, 154
Landfill disposal, 150
Last Chance Corral, 117
Lateral movements, 171
Law enforcement
　euthanasia authority, 148
　rescue partnerships with, 7
Leading, in new situations, 196–97. *See also* Halter training
Leads, in canter, 215
Learning
　by horses, 166–67, 173
　by humans, 168 (*see also* Asking for help)
Leg bands, for identification, 19, 20
Leg wraps, for shipping, 14
Legal considerations
　around re-feeding, 36–38
　Coggins tests, 23–24
　proof of ownership, 20–21, 137
　proving neglect, 22, 37, 49
　transportation regulations, 15

Legs
　abnormalities of, in foals, 105–7, 106–7
　handling of, 120–21, 180–81
　wound care, 82–83, 82, 140, 141
Legumes, 33
Levamisole, 49
Lice, 54
Licking, 167, 197
Lifespan, of horses, 6
Ligaments, in upward fixation of patella, 223
Light perception, 156
Lip tattoos, 17
Liver function, 35, 43
Lockjaw, 57–58
Long reins, 224–25
Longeing
　basic training for, 212–15, 213
　BCS considerations, 153–54
　equipment for, 209, 224
　halts, 214–15
　trot/canter in, 215, 217
　working mindset for, 219
Loose horses, 142
Lost horses, 192
Lungworms, 53

Maggot infestations, 53, 53
Malabsorption issues, 38
Malnourishment, 2–3, 25. *See also* Starvation
Mane, identification braided into, 20
Manners. *See* Halter training; Respect, training for
Mansmann, Richard, 70
Manure
　eating of, by foals, 110
　management of, 50, 51–52
　monitoring, 23, 45
Mares, 22, 169. *See also* Pregnancy
Mastitis, 110
McGonigle, Tracy, 2–3
McMaster's fecal evaluation, 52
Meconium, passage of, 103–4
Medical conditions, in euthanasia considerations, 146
Medical procedures, training for, 175, 194, 202–8. *See also* Veterinary examinations
Medical records, 22
Melanocytes, deafness link, 158
Memories, negative, 162, 163, 166, 221

Mental status, training and, 211–12
Metabolic issues
　case histories, 5
　insulin resistance, 32
　as reason for down horses, 124
　refeeding syndrome, 27, 31
　from starvation, 37–38, 131
Mexico, export of horses to, 6
Microchipping, 18–19, 18, 136–37
Milk
　production of, 95, 110
　replacer products, 112–13, 113, 115
　testing of, 99, 99
Molasses, cautions regarding, 205
Monocular vision, 155
Montana Horse Sense, 189
Mortenson, Ky Evan, 138
Mosquitoes/mosquito-borne viruses, 54, 58
Mounting, 226–27
Mouth, handling of, 204–5, 205
Mouthing, by foals, 121
Movement. *See also* Exercise
　monitoring, 69
　training for, 185–86
　visual sensitivity to, 158
Mucous membranes, 81
Mud fever, 55, 55
Mules
　bridling, 223–24
　castration of, 90
　gestation period, 98
　hoof care, 64
　immune disease risk, 110
　stand and wait response, 166, 218
Muscles
　damage to, 27, 86, 128
　development of, 153, 171–72, 201, 210, 215, 220–21
Mustangs
　adoption guidelines, 15, 186–87
　characteristics of, 65
　training considerations, 181, 199, 211

Name tags, 19–20, 19
Nasal discharge, 42
Nasoincisive notch, 190, 191
National Animal Identification System, 18
Natural disasters
　health consequences of,

141–44
  preparedness measures, 134–38, 201
  response teams, 138–39
Neck collars, 19, 20
Neck twitch, 176
Necropsy, 150
Needle-shy horses, 207
Negative reinforcement, 161
Neglect
  as cause of starvation, 26
  documentation of, 22, 37, 49
  economic factors in, 3–7
  of hooves, 67–69, 67–69, 185
  temporary vs. permanent, 7–8
Neonatal Isoerythrolysis, 110
Neosporin, 83
Nervous horses, 173, 177–180, 204, 218
Nervous system diseases, 57
Netposse.com, 7
Neurologic conditions, 57, 124, 131, *131*
Neurologic status, of down horses, 125
Non-steroidal anti-inflammatory drugs (NSAIDs), 75, 77–78, 79
Non-structural carbohydrates, 32–33
Nose/nostrils, handling of, 208
Novelty, desensitizing horses to, 173
NSAIDs. *See* Non-steroidal anti-inflammatory drugs
Nurse mares, 116, 117
Nursing, 96–97
Nutrient absorption, 180
Nutrient analysis, 32–34
Nutrition. *See also* Feeding
  hoof growth and, 64–65
  for orphan foals, 111–16, *113–14*
  for pregnant mares, 94–96
Nystagmus, 125

Obesity, 154, 177–78
Obstacles, training with, 171
Oils and fats
  in colic prevention, 47
  digestion of, 35
  hoof growth effects, 64
  for weight gain, 33, 36, 42
Ointments, topical, 83, 132
Older horses
  behavior, 185
  case histories, 18
  dental care, 38–39, 40, 41, 42

down, 130
euthanasia considerations, 146
health considerations, 53, 59, 77–79
in herd dynamics, 169
hoof care, 67
Omeprazole, 44
Oral medications, 204–5, *205*
Orchid, 42, 43
Organ failure, 44
Orphan foals, 110–16, *117*
Ovarian tumors, 97
Overeating, in response to starvation, 177–78
Overheating, 15
Overweight horses, 154, 177–78
Ownership
  in neglect cases, 22
  proof/documentation of, 20–21, 137
  transfers of, 6–7, 20

Pads, in shoeing, 72, *72*
Pain
  behavior related to, 62
  from colic, 44–45
  control of, 47
  as euthanasia consideration, 146
  freedom from, 3
  medications for, 75, 77–79
  as reason for down horses, 124, 126
  shoeing for relief of, 71–72
  signs of, 146
Palate, cleft, 109
Palpation, for pregnancy, 93
Pan feeding, 113, *114*
Paraphimosis, 93
Parasites
  external, 54–55
  internal, 49–54
  monitoring for, 21, 23
  passed to nursing foals, 96–97
  weight loss from, 43
Passive transfer, of immunity, 102, 108, 112
Pasture management, 50. *See also* Grasses and grazing
Patella, upward fixation of, 223
Patent urachus, 109
Patience, 197. *See also* Stop, wait, and read technique
Pavlov feeding experiments, 160
Pawing
  as sign of colic, 44

as sign of labor, 100
as sign of thinking, 167, 197, *197*, 202
unwanted behavior, 177
Pelleted feeds, 34, 42, 115
Penetrating captive bolt, 147–48, *148*
Penis, 90, 93
Peritonitis, 43
Permethrin sprays, 54–55
Personal space, 185
Phenylbutazone, 77, 79
Pheromones, 88, 176–77
Phosphorus, 64
Physical examinations. *See* Veterinary examinations
Physiology
  of fear, 166–67
  of senses, 155–59
Pinworms, 52, *52*
Pituitary Pars Intermedia Dysfunction (PPID), 24, *24*, 25, 53
Placenta, passing of, 101–2, *102*
Plasma transfusions, for immunity transfer, 108, 110, 112
Platelets, 25
Pleuropneumonia, 60
Pneumonia, 86, 104–5, 109, 113
Polysulfated glycosaminoglycan, 78
Population
  control of, 85
  estimates of, 6–7
Positive reinforcement
  overview, 159
  primary vs. secondary, 160
  uses of, 182, 187, 200
Post-mortem examinations, 150
Potassium, 45
Potassium chloride, 147, 148
PPID. *See* Pituitary Pars Intermedia Dysfunction
Pre-drive checklist, 11
Pregnancy
  accidental/unexpected, 89, 92, 95
  case histories, 32, 92
  in emaciated horses, 93, 94
  evaluation for, 93–94
  nutritional considerations, 94–96
  prevention of, 97
  vaccine recommendations, 59
Pressure sores, 132, *132*, 133
Pressure-and-release
  in halter training, 120, 192–93

timing in, 175
Preventive care, 49–60
Previcox, 77, 79
Probiotics, 35
Progesterone, 97
Proof of ownership, 20–21, 137
Protective equipment
    for skin abrasions, 132, 132
    for travel, 14
Protein, 30–31, 64
Proud-cut horses, 91–93
Psyllium husk, 23
"Pulling" horse in, on longe, 214
Pulse rate, 80–81, 104
Punishment, 161–62, 171, 172
Purpura hemorrhagica, 60
Pushy horses, 118, 160–61, 170–71. *See also* Respect, training for
Pyrethrin sprays, 54–55

Quality of life, 130, 131
Quarantine
    enclosures for, 186
    procedures, 21–22, 96, 169–170, 172
Quarter cracks, 74
Quarter Horses, 117
Quid, 42, 42

Rabbits, horses compared to, 165
Rabies, 56, 57, 58
Rain rot, 55
Rectal exams, 47–48, 203–4
Red bag, 101–2
Red blood cells, 23, 25
Re-feeding
    legal considerations, 36–38
    syndrome associated with, 5, 27, 30–31
Registration
    of brands, 16–17
    breed registries, 6
    in documentation of ownership, 20
    identification techniques, 16–18
Reinforcement withdrawal, 161
Reins, desensitization to, 224–25
Rejection, of foals, 110
Relaxation, signs of, 163, 167, 168
Relaxin, 99
Remus Memorial Horse Sanctuary, 42
Repetition, in training, 163
Rescue
    disaster-related, 134, 138–140, 138
    facilities, statistics regarding, 6
    need for, 6
    volunteer opportunities, 7, 168
Rescue horses. *See also* Debilitated horses; Unwanted horses
    overview, 2
    bonding with, 22
    case histories, 2, 4–5
    euthanasia of, 145
    transportation of, 16
    unknown training status, 163, 221, 228
Resistance, in parasites, 49–50
Respect, training for, 116, 160, 170–71, 196–208, 216, 230
Respiration rate, 81, 104–5, 149
Respiratory illnesses
    overview, 57
    causes of, 53, 59–60
    control of, 21–22
    diagnosis, 60
    risk factors, 60
    travel-related, 13, 22
    treatment of, 60
    vaccine prevention, 56
Restarting, training rescued horses as, 221
Rewards. *See also* Positive reinforcement
    intrinsic, 159–160
    treats as, 160, 205, 206–7
    types of, 161
    uses of, 193, 199, 202–3, 207
Rhinopneumonitis. *See* Equine Herpes Virus
Ribs, damaged during foaling, 109
"Ridable" horses, 228
Riding
    evaluating for, 154
    hoof wear and, 71
    mounting, 226–27
    preparation for, 209, 220–22
    progressive work, 227, 229
    tacking up, 217–19, 222–24
Rim shoes, 72–73, 73
Ringworm, 55
Rolling, of down horses, 128, 128
Rope halters, 14, 189–190, 189, 191
Ropes, lifting feet with, 183
Roping, of horses, 194
Rotational deworming, 50, 54

Round pens, 118, 187
Roundworms, 50
Routines, 170–71
Rubbing, as positive reinforcement, 187

Saccharomyces boulardii, 35
Saddle pads, 217–18
Saddles and saddling, 218–19
Safety considerations
    down horses, 122–23, 123
    in emergency response, 139–140, 144
    during euthanasia, 148–49
    foot handling, 181
    for groundwork, 209–10
    for riders, 220–22
    trailering and transportation, 10–13
    tying, 193–94
Salmonella infections, 21
Salt blocks, 30–31, 47
Sand, ingestion of, 177
Sand colic, 9, 23, 23
Scary objects, 174–75, 196–97, 197, 217
Scratching, as positive reinforcement, 187
Screening, for respiratory illnesses, 60
Sedation
    alternatives to, 176
    of fearful horses, 177, 194, 202
    of needle-shy horses, 207–8
    standing, 86–87, 87
Senior feeds, 33, 34, 35, 42
Sensory physiology, 155–59
Sepsis, 106
Serum biochemistry panel, 25
Shavings, 13
Shayne, 42
Sheath, swelling in, 89
Sheet bend knot, for tail ropes, 126, 127
Shelter in place, 135
Shipping. *See* Transportation
Shipping fever, 60
Shivers, 180
Shoeing, 69–73, 71–74
Shy horses, 171
Sideways drag repositioning, 129, 129
Silver sulfadiazine (SSD), 83, 132
Sinus infections, 42
Skin conditions
    injuries, 142, 143

pressure sores, 132, *132*
Slaughter/slaughter facilities, 5–6, 15
Sleeping patterns, 123–24
Sleeping sickness, 57, 58
Sliding, of down horses, 129, *129*
Slings, 130–31, *130–31*, 133
Slow-feeders, for hay, 180–81, *180*
Small animal population control, 85
Smell, sense of, 159
Smooth-mouthed horses, 41, *42*
Snaffle bits, 224
Snow events, 142–43
Social media, as resource, 7
Socialization. *See also* Respect, training for
 of new horses, 169–170, 216
 of orphan foals, 115–16
Sole abscesses, 72, *72*
Splint bones, fracture of, 84
Splints (supportive bandages), 105, 140
Spook response, 166
SSD (silver sulfadiazine), 83, 132
Stable flies, 54
Stallions
 adoptability, 212
 behaviors in, 88–89
 castration of, 85–93
 cryptorchidism in, 90–93, 229
 socialization of, 216
Standardbred horses, 6, 17
Standing
 assistance, for down horses, 129–130
 in desensitization training, 207
 in halter training, 192
 while tied, 184, 193–94
"Standing and waiting" response, 166
Standing sedation, 86–87, *87*
Staphylococcus infections, 55
Startle response, 166, 180
Starvation, 26, 37–38, 80, 177–180. *See also* Body Condition Score; Debilitated horses
Steroid injections, 78–79
Stifle joint, 223
Stitches, 81
Stocks, 196, *196*, 202, 207
Stomach tubes, 47
Stomach worms, 53
Stop, wait, and read technique, 155, 167

Strangles, 21, 57, 59
Strengthening exercises, 211, 217, 220–21, 223
Streptococcus infections. *See* Strangles
Stress
 effects of, 22, 35, 77
 mental, 38
 post-disaster, 142
 signs of, 165
 of training, 192
 travel-related, 13–15
Strongyles, small, 50, 52, *52*
Structure fires, 142
Stubbornness, 166
Studs (traction device), 72, *73*
Suckling, 102–3, *103*
Summer sores, 53
Sutures, 81
Swamp fever, 23–24
Sweating, 15, 25, 44, 47
Sweet feeds, 32–33
Sweeteners, for oral medications, 204–5
Swelling, 87–88, 89
Syringes, desensitization to, 204–8, *205*, *206*

Tacking up, 217–19
Tail
 flagging of, *111*
 handling of, 203, 204
 identification braided into, 20
 swishing of, 165
Tail ropes, 126, *127*, 129–130
Tapetum lucidum, 156, 158
Tapeworms, 52–53
Tarps, desensitization to, 195–96
Technical Large Animal Emergency Rescue, 138–39, *139*
Teeth
 in determining age, 18
 maintenance of, 38–42, *40–41*
Temperature. *See* Body temperature; Weather
Tendons
 deep digital flexor, 63
 in foals, 105–6, *105–6*
Tennessee Walking Horse Breeders and Exhibitors' Association, 6
Tension, signs of, 163
Testes, retention of, 90–93
Testosterone, 88, 97
Tetanus/tetanus vaccines, 56, 57–58, 87

Therapy horses, 221
Thermometer desensitization, 203–4
Thin horses. *See* Body Condition Score; Emaciated horses
Thinking, signs of, 167, 185, 197, *197*, 202
Thirst, freedom from, 3. *See also* Water
Thoroughbred horses
 hoof characteristics, 65
 lip tattoos, 17–18, *17*
 registration statistics, 6
Thrush, 65, *65*
Ticks, 54, *54*
Timid horses, 171
Timing
 in pressure and release, 175
 of punishment, 162
Toe cracks, 75
Tornadoes, 142
Touch, desensitization to, 181, 184, 187–88, 203. *See also* Handling, training for
Toxicity
 of dewormers, 50–51
 fescue toxicosis, 94, 96, 102
Traceability, 20
Traction, devices for, 72–73, *73*. *See also* Footing
Trailers and trailering
 in emergency preparedness, 135
 horse's position in, 202
 inspection checklist, 11
 loading, 135–36, *141*, 166, 199–202
 maintenance of, 10–11
 regulations regarding, 15
 safety considerations, 12–13, 15, *141*, 166
 unloading, 200–201
Training
 overview, 152, 168, 219
 asking for help, 152, 168, 181, 184, 210, 216, 221
 BCS considerations, 152, 200, 209, 211, 220, 223
 vs. bribery, 160
 consistency in, 172, 182, 183, 214
 enclosures for, 186
 of fearful horses, 162–64
 firmness in, 120
 health evaluations for, 210–11
 horse's mental status and, 211–12

key principles in, 159–162
lack of, as factor for
  unwanted horses, 152, 230
for medical procedures, 202–8
of Mustangs, 186–87
observation in, 167
repetition in, 163
session duration, 116, 118
stress of, 172–75, 192
unknown extent of, in rescue
  horses, 163, 221, 228
for versatility, 214–15
Transportation
  driver safety, 11–12
  in emergency evacuations,
    135–36
  federal regulations, 15
  practice hauling, 201–2
  pre-drive checklist, 11
  stress of, 13–15
  trailer safety, 10–13
  of untrained horses, 15
  water consumption during,
    45, 47
Travel. *See* Transportation
Treats, 160, 205, 206–7
Triple antibiotic ointment, 132
Trot
  defined, 215
  in lameness evaluation, 69
  on longe, 215
  under saddle, 229
  in strengthening, 213
Truck maintenance, 10–11, 135
Trust
  approach-and-retreat in, 217
  developing, 155, 163–64, 212
  training foundations for,
    170–72
  tying and, 193–94
Tubing, 47
Tumors, 43, 97
Twitches, 175–76, 207
Tying
  of rope halters, 189–190, 189
  safety considerations, 181, 218
  training for, 193–94
  during travel, 14

Udder
  development of, 95, 98, 98
  infection of, 110
Ulcerguard, 44
Ulcers

decubital, 132
gastric, 14, 44, 77
Ultrasound evaluations, for
  pregnancy, 93–94
Umbilicus, 109, 109
United Horse Coalition, 7
Unloading, 200–201
Unwanted behavior
  around feeding, 177–180
  eliminating, 162
  unintentionally taught, 163
Unwanted horses
  overview, 3–7
  behavior/rideability of, 4, 152,
    163, 221, 228, 230
  case histories, 216
  cryptorchidism and, 91
  euthanasia of, 148
  lameness and, 61
  population estimates, 4
Urgent rescue situations, 138–144
Urine, 13
U.S. Department of Agriculture
  slaughter facility oversight, 5–6
U.S. Hunter Jumper Association,
  19
U.S. Trotting Association, 6
Uterine-placental barrier, 96

Vaccines
  overview, 60
  for pregnant mares, 96–97
  quarantine and, 21–22
  recommendations regarding,
    55–60
  training for, 205–8, 206
Venezuelan encephalitis, 58
Versatility, training for, 214–15
Veterinary examinations
  overview, 22–25
  prior to riding, 220
  training for, 203–4
Vetricyn, 83
Vision, 155–56, 158, 197
Vital signs, monitoring, 125, 140
Volunteers, in disasters, 138–39.
  See also Handlers and rescuers

Waiting. *See* Stop, wait, and read
  technique
Walk, on longe, 214
Water
  access to, 113, 142–43, 144
  consumption of, 13, 30–31,
    45, 47
  dehydration, 15, 45, 126
Water rescues, 138, 144
Waxing, of udder, 98–99, 98
Weakened horses. *See*
  Debilitated horses
Weaning, 110
Weather
  behavior and, 159
  disasters related to, 141–44
Wedge shoes, 72
Weight. *See also* Body Condition
  Score; Re-feeding
  gain, 35, 36, 38
  loss, 13, 27, 39, 43–44, 146
  monitoring, 30, 37, 44
  shifting of, 181
Weight tapes, 36, 37
Well-being, of horses, 22
West Nile Virus, 56, 57, 58–59
Western equine encephalitis,
  56, 58
Westfall, Stacy, 117
Whips, 173–75, 173
White blood cells, 25
White line disease, 65
White-associated deafness, 158
Wildfires, 142
Will to live, 131
Wind events, 142
Winter conditions, 38, 142–43
Withers, touching, 187–88
Wounds
  care of, 53, 82–83, 83
  chronic, 79–80
  cleaning of, 81
  complicated, 83–84
  emergency first aid, 140–41
  evaluating, 80–81
  neglect as factor in, 79–80
  treatment of, 81–84

"A Yankee in Paris" (blog), 117
Young horses
  dental care, 40
  euthanasia considerations,
    146–47
  in herd dynamics, 169
  hoof care, 63
  internal parasites, 53
  respiratory illnesses in, 59